IDRC–042e

Low–Cost Rural Health Care and Health Manpower Training

An annotated bibliography with special emphasis on developing countries

Volume 1

Shahid Akhtar

(This is the first volume in a series of annotated bibliographies on low-cost rural health care and health manpower training. These volumes will be published irregularly.)

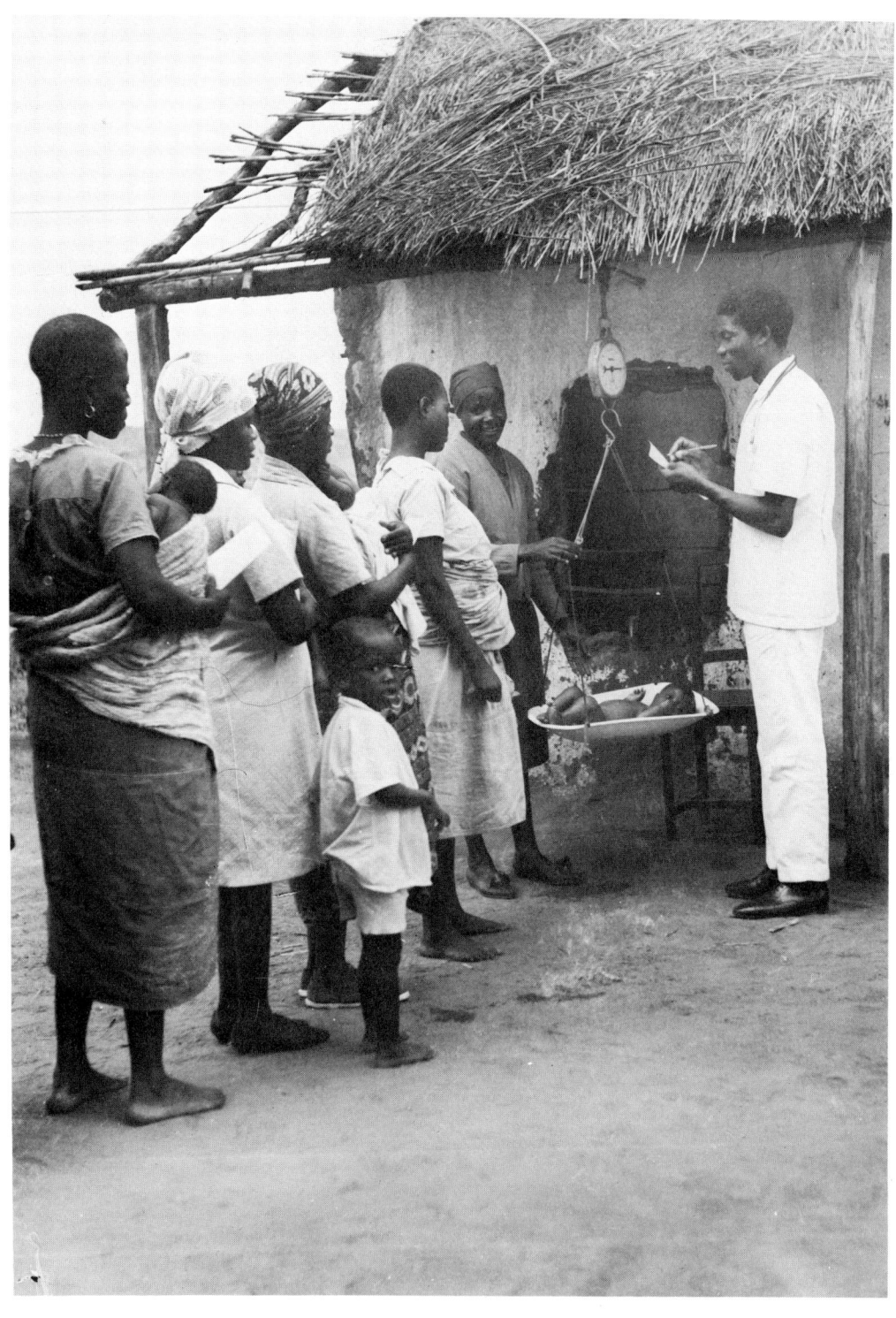

A medical assistant in Malawi registers the weight of a baby at a mobile clinic in a small village and advises the mother.

Abstract This bibliography is an attempt to coordinate information on nontraditional health care delivery systems in remote regions of the world, especially in developing countries. The literature abstracted focusses primarily on new models of health care delivery, and on the training and utilization of auxiliary health workers. It is intended to be of use to: (*a*) persons who are involved in planning, operating, and evaluating systems to provide rural health services; (*b*) persons concerned with the training of auxiliary health workers to staff such systems; and (*c*) organizations that are supporting research into the problems of organizing and staffing health care delivery systems.

Résumé Cette bibliographie tente de coordonner une information sur les différentes méthodes de distribuer des soins aux populations rurales à travers le monde, et surtout dans les pays en voie de développement. La documentation existante a trait surtout à la formation du personnel auxiliare de santé. C'est notre intention de la mettre à la portée des animateurs de programmes visant à fournir des soins médicaux, du personnel enseignant, et des organisations qui offrent un appui financier pour des recherches dans ce domaine.

Resumene Esta bibliografía representa un esfuerzo por coordinar la información existente sobre nuevos tipos de sistemas de prestación de servicios de salud que están siendo experimentados en varias regiones remotas o aisladas del mundo y en particular en aquéllas de los países en vías de desarrollo. La literatura aquí resumida abarca principalmente los nuevos modelos de prestación de servicios de salud, así como los aspectos de capacitación y utilización de personal auxiliar de salud. Esta bibliografía constituye un instrumento de trabajo especialmente útil para: (*a*) las personas que participan en las etapas de planificación, implantación y evaluación de servicios salud para las zonas rurales; (*b*) las personas dedicadas a la capacitación del personal auxiliar destinado a trabajar en los servicios mencionados; (*c*) las organizaciones que están apoyando y promoviendo la búsqueda de soluciones a los problemas de organización y de dotación de personal de los sistemas de prestación de servicios de salud.

ISBN: 0-88936-051-0
UDC: 016:613
©1975 International Development Research Centre
Postal Address: Box 8500, Ottawa, Canada K1G 3H9
Head Office: 60 Queen Street, Ottawa
Microfiche Edition $1

Contents

Preface   7

Introduction — Rural Health Care: Issues
                and Alternatives   11

I   Reference Works   17

II   Organization and Planning   21
      1   Health manpower   21
      2   Organization and administration   26
      3   Planning   38
      4   Geographic distribution of health services   52
      5   Financial aspects   55
      6   Cultural aspects   57
      7   Epidemiological, family planning,
         MCH, and nutritional studies   57

III Primary Health Care — Implementation   67
      1   Rural inpatient care   67
      2   Rural outpatient care   68
      3   Mobile units and services   75
      4   Community health education   78

IV   Primary Health Manpower — Training and Utilization   83
      1   Primary medical care   83
         1   Professional   83
         2   Lower- and middle-level health workers   91
      2   Primary nursing care   104
         1   Professional   104
         2   Nonprofessional   105
      3   Primary family planning and midwifery care   107
         1   Professional   107
         2   Nonprofessional   110
      4   Primary dental care   111
         1   Professional   111
         2   Nonprofessional   112
      5   Primary laboratory care   112
      6   Primary environmental health   113
      7   Teaching aids   114
         1   Rural health care   114
         2   Family planning and midwifery   119

Contents *(concluded)*

V   Formal Evaluative Studies   123
         1   Health manpower   123
         2   Organization and administration   125
         3   Planning   133
         4   Geographic distribution of health services   134
         5   Financial aspects   136
         6   Cultural aspects   136
         7   Epidemiological, family planning,
            MCH, and nutritional studies   136

Appendix 1.   Abbreviations and Acronyms   143

Author Index   145

Geographical Index   152

Subject Index   155

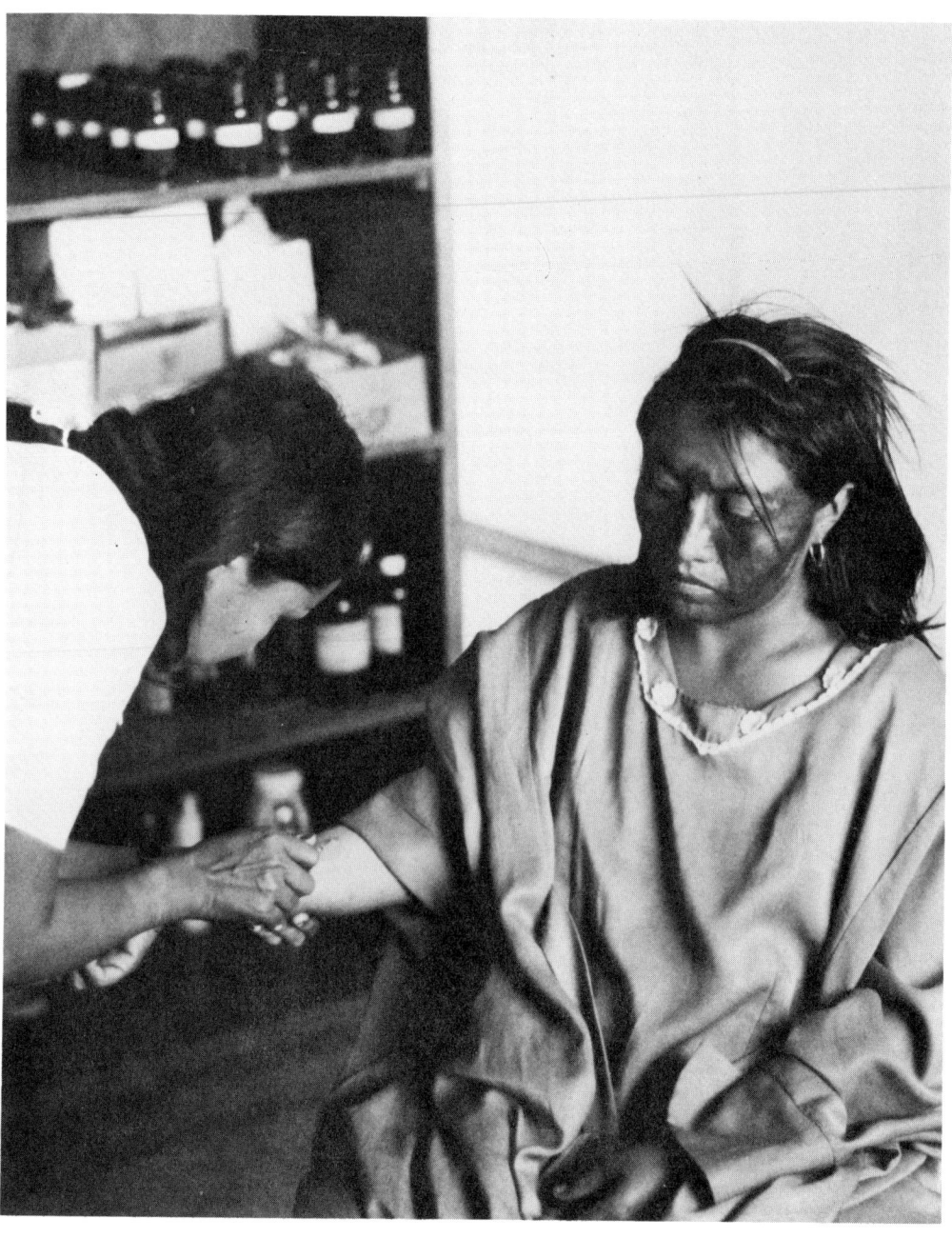

Medical auxiliary in Venezuela (CIMDER Project). Patient is a Guayira Indian.

Preface

There is little coordinated information currently available to guide persons responsible for planning and operating nontraditional systems of health care in remote regions of the world. Often the successes and failures of experimental systems are recorded only in mimeographed documents that do not find their way into international information systems. Although information does exist on the barefoot doctors of China, the feldshers of the USSR, and the traditional midwives of various cultures, it is usually "fugitive," i.e., widely scattered and difficult to come by. A system is needed to pull together such information in order to extract the knowledge that might be derived from various experiences.

In an effort to fill the information gap on rural health care in developing countries, the International Development Research Centre (IDRC) is establishing a computerized data base on alternative ways of delivering primary health care to remote regions, particularly in developing countries.

The material being collected focusses primarily on new models of health care delivery, and the training and utilization of auxiliary health workers. It is selected on the premise that its users would include: (a) those persons in developing countries who are planning, operating, or evaluating systems to provide health services and those persons concerned with the training of auxiliary health workers to staff such systems; and (b) organizations, such as IDRC, that are supporting research into the problems of organizing and staffing systems for health care services in remote regions. Thus, the boundaries of interest of this service have been set to include information useful to persons working in programmes in developing countries or regions.

Material for this collection was gathered in several ways. In a special effort to retrieve the unpublished "fugitive" literature, such as theses, essays, papers, and reports produced for limited distribution, personal approaches were made to over 1200 individuals and institutes throughout the world. Manual searches of numerous abstracting/indexing journals, bibliographies, professional journals, etc., were supplemented by special computer searches commissioned from a number of sources. Approximately 4000 documents in various languages have been received so far. These include articles, reports, and studies on alternative or unique models of health care delivery, bibliographies, course and job descriptions, teaching aids and manuals, syllabuses, etc. As additional literature becomes available, it too is added to the data base.

From time to time, annotated bibliographies will be published from this data base. The first such bibliography to appear was on health care in the People's Republic of China.[1] It presents information on the approaches taken by China in delivering primary health care to its population.

The present bibliography is the first volume of a multivolume bibliography we intend to publish on approaches taken throughout the world. Each volume in this series will contain at least 700 entries with abstracts. However, although we are continuing to record the new literature still coming in as a result of the mechanisms we have already established, we have slowed down the active pursuit of additional material until we have some feedback from the various people and organizations for whose benefit this service was set up. *We therefore urge you* to write and tell us whether or not you have found these bibliographies useful, and to continue sending us any documents you feel should be included in subsequent volumes. Your efforts will not only help us to evaluate the service, but also guide us in assembling later volumes. The decision as to whether or not IDRC should continue to provide this service will be largely based upon this feedback. The service therefore depends entirely upon you for its existence.

---

[1] Akhtar, Shahid. *Health Care in the People's Republic of China: A Bibliography with Abstracts.* Ottawa, International Development Research Centre (IDRC-038e), 1975. 182p.

The scope of this bibliography, and that of the forthcoming issues, includes material on the following subjects:

1) planning, financing, organization, utilization, and evaluation of systems designed to provide overall health care to people who lack access to conventional hospital and physician services, with special emphasis on rural areas and on metropolitan populations that, because of poverty or other reasons, do not take advantage of metropolitan medical services;

2) the impact of health care services on social and economic indices, including demographic indices such as mortality, morbidity, nutrition, and epidemiological trends;

3) the relationships between health care systems and other community organizations and services, such as schools and agricultural extension programmes, and community participation in health care systems; and

4) staffing of health care systems: the functions of different personnel, particularly paramedical personnel, their training (curricula), distribution, and utilization.

Discussions of basic clinical medicine or biomedical research are not included in this bibliography. Nor are references to literature on population and family planning programmes, except in instances where family planning forms an integral part of health services, or where auxiliaries are utilized. However, the reference works, bibliographies, guides, directories, news bulletins, and other special sources of information listed in section I may be scanned for literature dealing with the above-mentioned topics and with public health. In addition, most of the items included in this bibliography contain their own bibliographies; in each case, the number of references is noted, and the reader is advised to refer to them for additional information.

A great deal more material was received than has been input into the data base, and only those items that were considered to be most useful to persons involved in community health work were selected for annotation. The 700 references that make up this volume were the first items selected for inclusion in the data base. So far, no attempt has been made to sort the literature we have received according to importance, urgency, or timeliness.

The five broad sections (or 31 sections and subsections) into which entries have been arranged and the title of the bibliography will remain the same throughout the series. Readers interested in finding literature on a particular subject should first consult the Table of Contents and only afterwards the indexes included at the end of the bibliography. Items relevant to more than one section have been cross-referenced by a "*See also*" entry at the beginning of each section, with the bibliographic citation and abstract appearing in the section to which the work is most relevant. Similarly, individual entries that bear any relationship to each other have been cross-referenced by a "*See also*" within the entry itself. Furthermore, teaching aids and manuals for all categories of health workers have been grouped together in sections IV.7.1 and IV.7.2, and then cross-referenced to the section concerning the type of worker for whom they are intended. For example, item 0573, a manual entitled *Simple Dental Care for Rural Hospitals* is abstracted under section IV.7.1, but appears as a "*See also*" at the beginning of section IV.4.2, which concerns the training and utilization of nonprofessional dental auxiliaries.

Bibliographic entries have been arranged alphabetically in order of the principal authors', editors', or compilers' surnames. Anonymous articles are placed alphabetically in order of the corporate bodies sponsoring the document.

Articles such as "A" and "The" have been deleted where they appear as the first word in a title. Non-English titles are given in either the original language or a transliterated version, whenever possible, with the English translation in parentheses. Diacritical marks have had to be omitted from foreign words as the bibliography is computer-generated.

The source information, given in full without any abbreviations, is arranged as follows: for journals — journal title, place of publication, volume number and/or issue number (with only the issue number appearing in parentheses), date of publication, pagination, and language(s) of publication; for books and monographs — the place of publication, name of publisher, date of publication, pagination, identifying document numbers, if any, and language(s) of publication.

All bibliographic information, including abstracts, has been stored in the ISIS (Integrated Set of Information Systems) computer system presently in operation at IDRC. The material was indexed using a combination of controlled vocabulary and free text that makes possible custom searches for people with an interest in a very specific topic, e.g., the utilization of mobile health services in Kenya. The subject index at the end of the bibliography was computer-generated from the keywords assigned to each entry.

IDRC unfortunately is not able to supply copies of all the materials listed in the bibliography.

However, every effort has been made to ensure that publisher information is complete and accurate, so that the reader should have no difficulty in identifying and obtaining commercially available material.

We realize that some of the fugitive literature may be more difficult to locate. If local bookshops and libraries are unable to supply this material, interested persons in developing countries may apply to *Rural Health Care Bibliography, c/o Library, IDRC, Box 8500, Ottawa, Canada K1G 3H9*, using the coupons at the back of the bibliography. It is assumed this service will be used only to procure a few papers of special importance to the requestor. Anyone seeking to build up a comprehensive collection of the material should make use of local sources of supply.

I wish to express my appreciation to the many individuals and institutions who assisted me in the collection of material for this bibliography. Without the efforts of the Multilingual Services Division of the Secretary of State Department, Ottawa, and especially Mr Manual Brandres of that Division, the wealth of foreign literature included in this edition could not have been abstracted.

This bibliography could not have been completed without the support of the staff of the IDRC Library. In addition, thanks are due to Frances Delaney, Kate Wild, Faye Shaver, and Sheryle Clifford for handling the computerization; to Wendy McRae, Hope Cadieux, and Lynette Yip Young for abstracting, research, and editorial assistance; and to Heather Webster for her general collaboration and efficient typing.

SHAHID AKHTAR
International Development Research Centre,
Ottawa

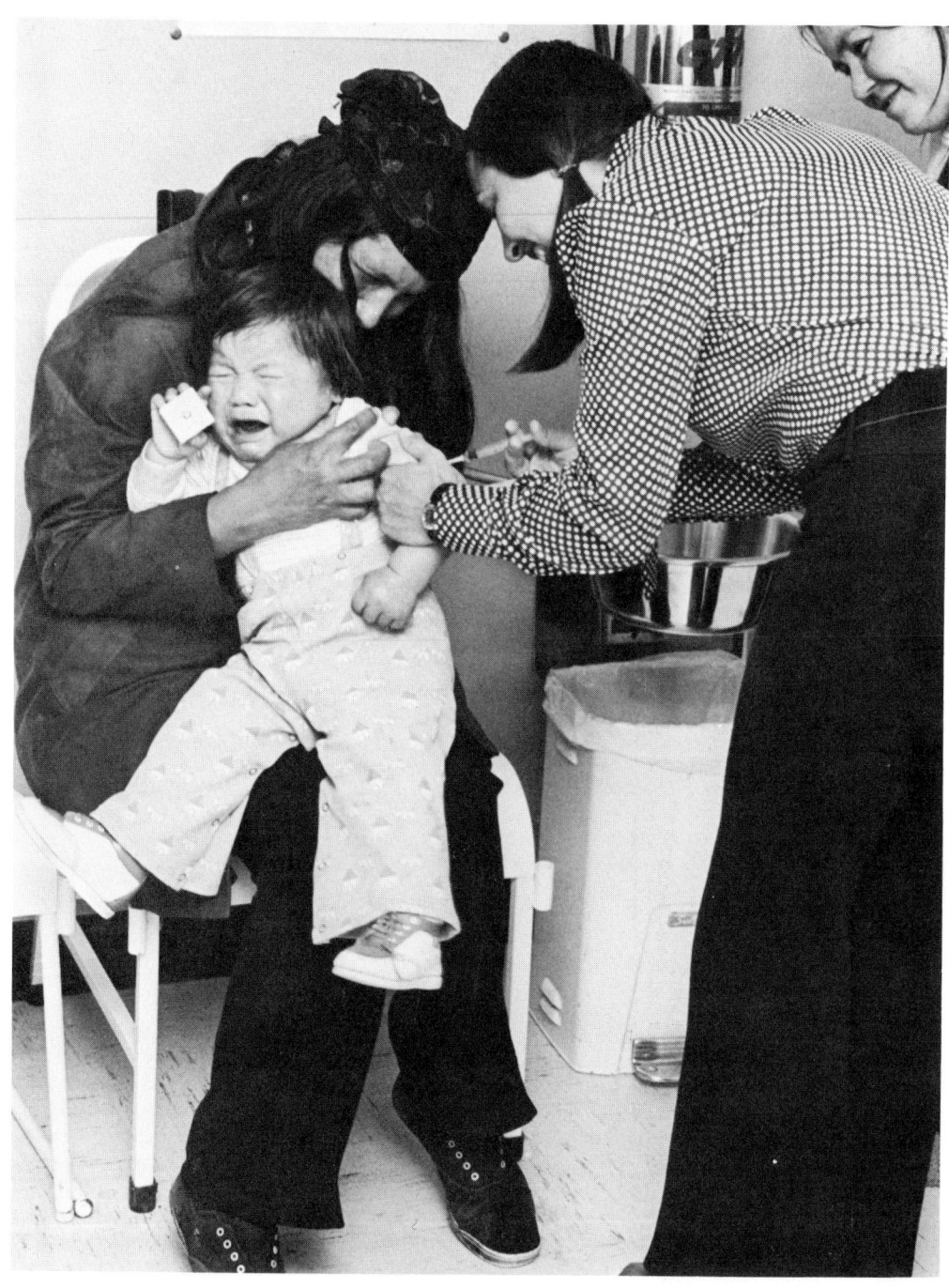

Inoculation of children, Rupert House, Quebec, Canada.

Introduction
Rural Health Care: Issues and Alternatives

Universal Problems — National Issues

It is becoming clear that medicine as practiced in developed countries, which stresses curative rather than preventive treatment and relies upon large numbers of physicians, is inappropriate to the needs and scarce resources of less-developed countries. This fact has only recently been grasped by the industrialized world. Rising costs and continuing inequalities in health services are leading more and more countries to seek alternative models of health care delivery. "Good for the many," rather than "best for the few" is becoming the byword in health services, as nations consider the relative merit of outpatient vs. inpatient care, health centres vs. hospitals, preventive vs. curative treatment, and lower- and middle-level trained health workers vs. physicians.

There is much to admire in the courage and resolve shown by a number of developing country governments in adopting innovative health programmes in recent years. It is hoped that leaders in industrialized countries will show equal courage in taking the necessary political risks to make long overdue changes in their health care systems.

Even more important, developing countries should have an opportunity to learn from one another. Health workers are often unaware of innovative health programmes being carried out in their own countries, let alone in others'. Much of the reluctance to adopt new approaches is based on limited information. This series of IDRC bibliographies hopefully will stimulate discussion, experimentation, and wider implementation of appropriate health care, by making known to the community of developing nations those innovative programmes and alternatives in this field that have been carried out in their own and other parts of the world.

Emphasis — Developing Countries and Rural Peoples

Since it is the policy of the International Development Research Centre (IDRC) to work for the benefit of developing nations, these bibliographies will address themselves primarily, though not exclusively, to literature concerning Africa, Asia, and Latin America, and only incidentally to other parts of the world.

One of the main concerns of IDRC is the "well-being of rural peoples." It is recognized that self-reliance in the agricultural sector is a prerequisite to economic and social development in other sectors. As populations increase, however, demands on each country's resources to maintain or improve the standard of living for rural peoples become challenges of enormous magnitude. A strong productive agricultural sector is the cornerstone upon which further development can be built. A productive people must of necessity enjoy the highest possible level of health, since those who are debilitated or chronically ill are less able to meet the physical demands of agricultural labour and production. It follows that investment in low-cost effective health care is an investment in national agricultural self-sufficiency as well as an issue of social justice and concern. However, with few exceptions (the People's Republic of China being one), little attention has been devoted to the health of rural peoples. Although every nation can point to some effort in rural health, few have made major commitments in this field.

In nations with socialist economies, rural health programmes have received somewhat greater attention. The administrative and political structures of these nations permit more rapid implementation of national decisions. A real challenge exists, however, for non- and semi-socialist countries to develop health care systems that reach a majority of their rural peoples through an appropriate mixture of public and private resources. Participation at the central, provincial or state, and local levels has maximized the viability, cost-effectiveness, and local support necessary to such systems within the limitations imposed by available funds, supplies, and trained personnel.

Health and Productivity

Western economists have insisted for many years that health is a "consumption" expenditure rather than a "production" investment. The Chinese on the other hand have insisted that sick people are less productive people, that sick people require attention, and this in turn interferes with the productivity of others. Although it does not automatically follow that better health contributes directly to productivity in all situations, there is no question that good health contributes to human welfare and ill health results in economic costs to society.

Labour availability is affected by morbidity and work absenteeism. The manager of a hotel in Malawi pointed out that it was necessary to hire about one-quarter more people than would be required if malaria were less prevalent. A careful study of tuberculosis control in Korea reached the conclusion that a return of U.S. $150 would accrue from each $1 spent in an optimal control programme.[1] The benefits of such programmes would be most noticeable in decreased absenteeism and increased work life. A Colombian study estimated that 5% of total annual man-days of work were lost through accidents, injuries, and illness.[2]

Substitutions of skilled, semiskilled, or even unskilled workers are necessary because of frequent illness in the regular labour force, and although this substitution relieves the high underemployment in developing countries, it results in an economic loss. As well, poor health of the labour force may result in productivity losses without worker absenteeism.

The World Bank recently carried out a study among construction and rubber workers in Indonesia.[3] Of the group studies, 85% suffered from hookworm and 45% from iron-deficiency anemias. A 60-day treatment with iron supplement resulted in a productivity increase of 19%. The cost of the treatment was U.S. $0.13 per person. It was calculated that correction of iron-deficiency anemia among rubber workers has a benefit : cost ratio of 280:1. Studies now in progress in several parts of the world will likely demonstrate similar economic benefits from health care investment. It is only recently that studies have been designed that can demonstrate the economic benefits associated with targeted cost-effective health care.

Infections and parasitic illness make extra demands on the body's metabolism through nutrient wastage. Fevers, parasites, and diseases such as tropical sprue, which result in malabsorption, all require additional nutritional intake. A study by the U.S. Office of International Health suggests that in Panama in 1972 the cost of excess food consumed in each case of enteric infection approached U.S. $10.[4] Such studies reveal that labour availability, labour productivity, and food resource requirements are all negatively affected by illness.

The Health Situation in Developing Countries

The disease pattern of a nation is often a direct reflection of its standard of living. As a nation improves its economic health, ordinarily the balance between communicable and noncommunicable disease shifts towards noncommunicable diseases, resulting in an increase in life expectancy and a reduction in child mortality. This change in the disease balance is usually due to the effects of the availability of safe water, more hygienic disposal of human and animal excretion, and other sanitary improvements.

In the developing world, the majority of deaths and illnesses are caused by communicable diseases. Whether in Asia, Latin America, or Africa, health conditions and disease patterns among poverty groups are similar. The core pattern includes nutritional deficiency diseases (i.e., those resulting from the synergism between malnutrition and infection) and those carried by air, excrement, vectors, and parasites whose elements are omnipresent in the environment.

As the economic level improves, so do the sanitation and water supply. Fecally transmitted diseases are reduced through improved sanitation facilities, and air-borne diseases are reduced through better housing and less crowding. Clearly, major reductions in disease incidence

---

[1] Feldstein, M.S., Piot, M.A., and Sundaresan, T.K., *Resource Allocation Model for Public Health Planning: A Case Study of Tuberculosis Control*. Geneva, World Health Organization, 1973.

[2] Mejia, A., and Paredes, R., *Health Planning for Colombia: Part 2*. The Millbank Memorial Fund Quarterly (New York), 46(2), April 1968. 276-289.

[3] Basta, S.S., and Churchill, A., *Iron Deficiency Anemia and the Productivity of Adult Males in Indonesia*. IBRD Staff Working Paper No. 175, 1974.

[4] Wooley, P.O., Perry, B.A., Eccles, R.N., eds., *Syncrisis: The Dynamics of Health. An Analytic Series on the Interactions of Health and Socioeconomic Development. Volume I: Panama*. Washington, D.C., Department of Health, Education and Welfare, Office of International Health. 1972.

can be made through cost-effective "impersonal" improvements in water supplies, excrement disposal, and vector control. In most instances it is cheaper in the long run to prevent disease than to treat it. It is also more effective to eliminate foci of infection than to prescribe expensive antibiotics and medication to patients who are returning to environments where reinfection is almost inevitable. Such an approach, however, requires a commitment to community health rather than to individual cures. However, due to the existing training, reward structures, and manpower patterns of most health systems, logical high priority approaches such as this receive little encouragement in terms of financing and staffing.

The "Enough Doctors" Myth

There is a prevailing myth that urban solutions to health care delivery are equally applicable to rural, remote, and sparsely populated areas. For many years governments and professionals believed that to solve health care delivery problems, the highest priority is "enough" doctors. The Government of the United States of America, for example, has over the past decade, increased its spending on health manpower programmes from $65 million to $536 million annually, totalling $3.5 billion for this period. Much of this money was spent on medical education and physician training. What has been the return on this investment? Dr Charles C. Edward's conclusions are sobering:

If you regard the last decade of federal support of health manpower training as having the goal of turning out more physicians, dentists, nurses and allied health professionals, then you would have been highly successful.

But if you look at health manpower development efforts as part of a broader national purpose — namely, to make health services available to everyone at a cost that both the individual and the society can afford — then it is clear that all of us . . . have to reassess our priorities in the manpower field and perhaps adopt some fundamentally different ones.

. . . simply increasing the aggregate supply of doctors has not and will not solve the problems we face in making health services available to the people . . .[5]

A well-known medical educator once jokingly made projections to show a point in time where one-half of the people of the United States would be physicians treating the other half; but health statistics would not reflect much improvement, since 90% of the residents of cities would be physicians treating one another, with the countryside remaining inadequately served.

The production of physicians alone cannot solve such problems as the inability of patients to pay for services, the availability of physicians where they are needed, or the lack of general practitioners versus the plethora of specialists. Having "enough doctors" is not enough, if health care is to be delivered to rural peoples, especially when developing countries have limited amounts to spend on health care. John Knowles, President of the Rockefeller Foundation, has put it quite bluntly: "The next major advances in the health of both developed and developing countries will result from a marked increase in public health programmes, and not more doctors practising acute, after-the-fact, curative medicine."[6]

Options and Alternatives

This bibliography is about low-cost health care for rural people. The physician is not a low-cost item, and the experience of many developing, and, more recently, developed nations, suggests that there are valid alternatives. A health system that incorporates well-trained, well-supervised primary care workers with a well-organized system of providing drugs and supplies on a regular and dependable basis, can benefit the majority of the people of a nation at a fraction of the cost of providing those same services through physicians.

Primary care workers (PCW's) is a generic term for nonphysician health personnel who carry out many of the primary medical tasks, and it has been proved that they can supply most health care when appropriately trained and equipped. PCW's have many names, such as feldsher, dai (midwife), nurse practitioner, medex, medical assistant, physician assistant, clinical officer, health extension officer, health assistant, or auxiliary, but all perform primary health and medical care functions, usually within a structured system. Greater or lesser degrees of supervision and control are exercised by more highly qualified PCW's and other professionals. This bibliography contains many citations and abstracts of training programmes that involve the use of PCW's, emphasizing the practical

---

[5]Edwards, C.C., *A Candid Look at Health Manpower Problems*. Journal of Medical Education (Washington, D.C.), 49(1), Jan 1974. 19-26.

[6]Knowles, J.H., *The World of Health and the American Physician*, Journal of Medical Education (Washington, D.C.), 49(1), Jan 1974. 50-56.

rather than the theoretical, and provides readers with information on alternatives that have been tried in different places.

Ruth Freeman of Johns Hopkins School of Hygiene and Public Health was fond of advising: "In life and public health, it is usually a matter of choosing the 'least worst' alternative." No matter what the state of a country's economic health or well-being, the ideal will always, perhaps, remain just that — an ideal to work and hope for. In the meantime, selection of the "least worst" alternatives to meet the harsh demands of the realities of rural health care seems not only a prudent but also a humane and socially just course to follow.

The Chinese Model

As an example, it is important to recognize the moral and ethical impetus associated with the Chinese model rather than focus exclusively on the political or ideological context in which it is found. Irrespective of political beliefs or attitudes, in matters of rural health care there is much to be learned from the Chinese experience.

Wendell MacLeod summarizes a number of salient principles worthy of consideration in any rural health care scheme.[7] Iran, a profoundly different society, has found elements in the Chinese experience worthy of incorporating into her own health care system. The "White Revolution" of Iran is of a quite different nature than the "Red Revolution" of the People's Republic of China; yet even now Iran is in the process of adopting the health strategy of the *behvarz* and *behdashtyar*, village health workers not unlike "barefoot doctors" of China, adapted to the needs of Iran's 55 000 remote and scattered villages. If there is a moral in this somewhere, it must be that of Halfdan Mahler, Director-General of the World Health Organization, who urges countries of the world: "Don't adopt — adapt! Or if that is unacceptable — I would add 'improvise'."[8]

PCW's and Health Care Costs

In many regions and in many countries, appropriately trained PCW's can and do deliver almost total health and medical care. Unfortunately, medical conditions that they are unable to diagnose or treat have little chance of being treated by a private physician or in a hospital due to great distances. However, this is an improvement over the situation in several developing countries, which have advocated "first class physician care or nothing," where the bulk of rural residents receive either nothing or only what untrained indigenous traditional practitioners can supply.

Many of those who have worked with PCW's have come to realize that 80-90% of patients' needs do not require the time and attention of a person trained to the level of physician. Common and recurring ailments, e.g., sore throats, respiratory infections, constipation, diarrhea, rashes, conjunctivitis, and many more, can be handled, in most instances, properly, safely, and effectively by PCW's under minimal supervision. In addition, the cost per man-hour for a PCW is approximately $5 as compared to $25 per man-hour for a physician, and the total cost of training a PCW is between $3000 and $5000 as compared to $25,000-84,000 for a physician.[9] A country has to consider whether it is better to spend the bulk of its health manpower budget on a few, costly physicians, who might only practice in rural areas if compelled by the state, and then for a short time only, or to train a cadre of PCW's selected from rural areas who might find relative satisfaction in serving in areas like their own. Even in many urban areas, financial necessity is forcing governments to reconsider their approaches to such medical care.

Infrastructure: Some Choices

Many countries have chosen the large hospital as the cornerstone upon which to build a health care system. Although theoretically attractive, in practical economic terms the results are far from satisfactory. This "edifice complex" results in the construction of large national hospitals that serve only the 1-2% of the country's population living within a small radius of the buildings. In a survey of Ghana's five major hospitals, Sharpston[10] reported that 80% of the inpatients came from the same urban area in which the hospital was located.

---

[7]MacLeod, J.W., *The Significance of the Chinese Experience in Health Care.* In, Akhtar, S., *Health Care in the People's Republic of China: A Bibliography with Abstracts.* Ottawa, International Development Research Centre, (IDRC-038e), 1975. 8-12.

[8]Geneva, WHO, *Report of the Director-General to the 1973 World Health Assembly.* Mimeo. A27/VR/3. 12-16.

[9]Fendall, N.R.E., *Auxiliaries in Health Care: Programs in Developing Countries.* Baltimore, Johns Hopkins Press, 1972. 184-186.

[10]Sharpston, M.J. *Uneven Geographical Distribution of Medical Care: A Ghanian Case Study.* Journal of Development Studies (London), 8(2), Jan 1972. 205-222.

A south-central African country is now committed to building a $37 million hospital.[11] Since experience in several developing countries suggests that recurring operating costs in such institutions amount on an average to one-quarter of the capital costs, the government can expect to expend $9 million annually on this one institution for many years to come. This hospital, if experience elsewhere is a guide, will tend to have first call on the national health budget, irrespective of needs in other regions. The country's approximate per capita expenditure on health was $2.10 per person in 1970. This hospital alone can be expected to absorb an amount equal to public sector health care funds for 4.4 million citizens. This amounts to a case of the best for the few rather than the good for the many.

A related question that must also be considered concerns the much-discussed health care pyramid. If financial and human resources are concentrated on the apex of the pyramid (e.g., specialist-professionals and large hospital complexes), little will be left for the base or foundation made up of PCW's at the community level.

To bring the discussion from theory to practice, Gish[12] compares investing 6 million Tanzanian Shillings either in one regional hospital or in 15 health centres in Tanzania. The comparative benefits are illustrated below:

	Investment Option	
	1 Regional Hosp.	15 Health Centres
Capital cost†	6.0	6.0
Operating costs†	2.0	2.0
Inpatient admissions‡	9	15
Outpatient visits‡	400	1000
Population covered‡	10–30	300–500

† Millions of Tanzanian Shillings
‡ Thousands

Tanzania has opted for the "good for the many" and now has an extensive health centre programme and a high-priority scheme to train rural medical aides to staff them.[13]

Options and the IDRC Bibliography

Whether in programmes, personnel, institutions, or structures, many options confront those responsible for and concerned with the health systems of their countries. Clearly there are no universal prescriptions, although a number of principles seem deserving of "near-universal application."[14]

The primary interest of this IDRC series of bibliographies is to bring to the attention of decision-makers and interested workers annotated citations of literature relating to issues and problems relevant to them. It is our desire to share with developed and developing country health workers the benefits of this work and experience.

DONALD C. E. FERGUSON

*Associate Director
Population and Health Sciences
International Development Research Centre*

---

[11]Morley, D., *Paediatric Priorities in the Developing World.* London, Butterworths, 1973. 19.

[12]Gish, O., *Resource Allocation, Equality of Access and Health.* World Development (Oxford), 1(12), Dec 1973. 37-44. Table constructed from data in D. Morley, *op.cit.* 31.

[13]Gish, O., *Planning the Health Sector: The Tanzanian Experience.* London, Croom Helm, 1975.

[14]King, M. ed., *Medical Care in Developing Countries: A Primer on the Medicine of Poverty.* Nairobi, Oxford University Press, 1966 and D. Morley, *op.cit.*

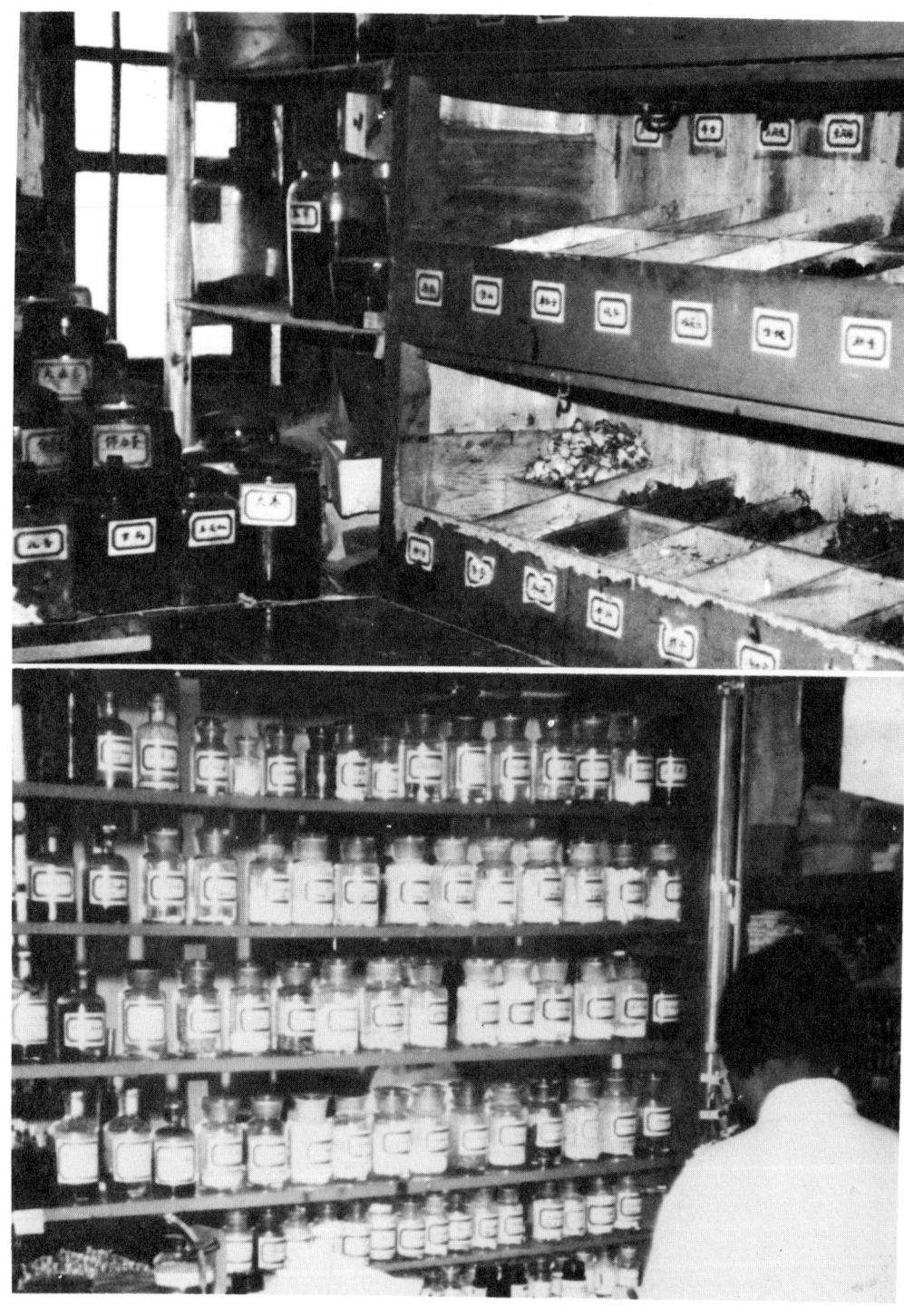

Herbal medicine dispensary (top) *and Western medicine dispensary* (bottom), *commune hospital, Lo-Kang Commune, Kwangchow municipal district, People's Republic of China.*

I Reference Works

See also: 0136

0001 American Medical Association, Chicago. *Medical socioeconomic research sources.* Chicago, American Medical Association. Engl.

See entry 2 for information on "Medical Socioeconomic Research Sources, Annual Cumulation."

Monthly issues of this reference source provide information on the social and economic aspects of medicine and health. Entries are listed according to subject categories, e.g. Abortion, Ambulatory Care, Child Health Services, Nursing, Periodicals, Rural Health, School Health, etc. For most references there is a very brief indication of the article's content. Pamphlets, books, journal articles, selected newspapers, and unpublished documents are included, and an author index is provided. Although most references pertain to the United States, the papers on community health problems, paramedical personnel, and rural health may be of value to health planners in developing countries. Subscription rate for 12 monthly issues and annual cumulation is U.S. $20.00 ($25.00 Foreign). The publisher's address is the American Medical Association, 535 North Dearborn Street, Chicago, Illinois 60610, USA.

0002 American Medical Association, Chicago. *Medical socioeconomic research sources: annual cumulation.* Chicago, American Medical Association. Engl.

See entry 1 for "Medical Socioeconomic Research Sources."

This annual cumulation lists journals, serials and subject headings used in the preceding monthly issues. The subject index lists under subject headings all documents indexed for the year. Citations in the author index are listed under the name of the first author; second and third authors are referred to the first author. Publishers are also listed in the author section. In addition to the published format the cumulation is also available on machine-readable tape. Subscription rate for annual cumulation and 12 monthly issues is U.S. $20.00 ($25.00 Foreign).

0003 Association of American Medical Colleges, Washington, D.C. *Journal of medical education.* Washington, D.C., Association of American Medical Colleges. Engl.

This monthly publication is designed as an international medium for the exchange of ideas in medical education. In addition to articles related to medical education each issue contains a bibliography of citations obtained through the National Library of Medicine's MEDLARS Programme. Entries are listed according to subject categories such as Accreditation, Certification, Licensure, Continuing Education, Curriculum, Medical Education in Other Countries, Teaching Hospitals, Teaching Methods and Materials, and Libraries and Information Centres. Published by the Association of American Medical Colleges, the journal is available at U.S.$15.00 per annum from the Business Office, Association of American Medical Colleges, One Dupont Circle, N.W., Washington, D.C. 20036, U.S.A.

0004 Bureau of Hygiene and Tropical Diseases, London. *Tropical diseases bulletin.* London, Bureau of Hygiene and Tropical Diseases. Engl.

See entry 5 for the complementary issue, "Abstracts on Hygiene."

This bulletin contains abstracts of papers and reviews of reports, conference proceedings, and books published in all parts of the world. Entries are listed according to the particular disease they deal with, e.g. malaria, trypanosomiasis, leishmaniosis, cholera, etc. There is also a section for book reviews of recent publications in tropical medicine. An annual subscription for 12 monthly issues is available from the Bureau of Hygiene and Tropical Diseases, Keppel St., London WC1E 7HT, England, at a cost of U.S. $26.00.

0005 Bureau of Hygiene and Tropical Diseases, London. *Abstracts on hygiene.* London, Bureau of Hygiene and Tropical Diseases. Engl.

See entry 4 for the complementary issue, "Tropical Diseases Bulletin."

This reference source abstracts papers, reports, conference proceedings, and books published in all parts of the world. Contents are grouped in such categories as Community Medicine, Environmental Hygiene, Non-Communicable Diseases, and Communicable Diseases. There is a special section for book reviews. The reader is directed to the *Tropical Diseases Bulletin*, which is the complementary publication of *Abstracts on Hygiene*. The annual subscription rate for 12 monthly issues is U.S. $40. Orders should be sent to the Bureau of Hygiene and Tropical Diseases, Keppel St., London WC1E 7HT, England.

0006 **Colombia, Ministry of Public Health.** *Estudio de instituciones de atencion medica: directorio nacional. (Directory of national health care facilities).* Bogota, Ministry of Public Health, Institute of Special Health Programs, Series II, No. 5, Jul 1972. 980p. Span.
See also entry 623.

This publication lists all institutions engaged in health care delivery in Colombia, and includes government, semi-government, and private organizations. Information on the services provided by each institution, professional and paramedical staff, budgets, etc. is included. Similar information is provided for rural health posts, which may be attended by a full- or part-time physician or by an auxiliary health worker.

0007 **Commonwealth Bureau of Nutrition, Aberdeen, Scotland.** *Nutrition abstracts and reviews.* Aberdeen, Commonwealth Bureau of Nutrition. Engl.

Annotated references are presented for such topics as Physiology of Nutrition and Human Diet in Relation to Health and Disease. Aspects of human diet that are represented include Feeding of Infants and Children, Assessment of State of Health, Diet in Etiology of Disease, Malnutrition, Disorders Associated with Foods, Clinical, Therapeutic, and Preventive Studies, etc. Subject and author indexes are provided. The journal appears monthly and is available at U.S. $117.00 per annum from Central Sales Branch, Commonwealth Agricultural Bureaux, Farnham Royal, Slough, SL2 3BN, England.

0008 **de Glanville, H., ed(s).** African Medical and Research Foundation, Nairobi. *AFYA: a journal for medical and health workers.* Nairobi, African Medical and Research Foundation. Engl.

The monthly issues of *AFYA* feature articles on diagnostic methods and treatment procedures for lower and middle-level health workers. Articles on topics such as nutrition, hygiene, integrated health projects, and health centres are written in very simple instructional terms with appropriate illustrations. Although comments and articles deal with epidemiological conditions peculiar to East Africa, the journal is of interest to medical and health workers in other developing regions. *AFYA* is available at a cost of Sh.10/- (for 12 issues) from the Editor, P.O. Box 30125, Nairobi, Kenya.

0009 **Excerpta Medica Foundation, Amsterdam.** *Public health, social medicine and hygiene.* Amsterdam, Excerpta Medica Foundation, Section 17. Engl.
For additional information on the abstracting journals published by Excerpta Medica see entries 10 and 11.

More than 3 500 international biomedical journals, consisting of 20 000 individual issues each year, constitute the source material for Excerpta Medica Foundation's data bank and its literature abstracting journals. Approximately 200 000 citations are computer-stored annually, and about 80 000 of these contain abstracts. Since 1968, 1 200 000 citations and about 700 000 abstracts have been stored in the Excerpta Medica's data bank. As of 1969, Excerpta Medica is publishing 33 English-language abstract journals in its regular series, all of which are completely computer-processed. Subject and author indexes are cumulated annually in each journal. Some of the relevant abstracting journals include: *Health Economics and Hospital Management, Pediatrics and Pediatric Surgery*, and *Public Health, Social Medicine and Hygiene*. In the *Public Health, Social Medicine and Hygiene* section, topics such as the following are included: Medical Education, Demography, Communicable Diseases, Nutrition, Hygiene, Water Supply, Environmental Sanitation, etc. For individuals interested in a special literature search the total information input into the Excerpta Medica data bank can be searched and the results are available to the requester in the form of a computer printout. Literature searches can be ordered at any desired frequency intervals. Further information can be obtained by contacting Mr B.T. Stern, Excerpta Medica Foundation, P.O. Box 1126, 119-123 Herengracht, Amsterdam, The Netherlands.

0010 **Excerpta Medica Foundation, Amsterdam.** *Health economics and hospital management.* Amsterdam, Excerpta Medica Foundation, Section 36. Engl.
For more complete information on the Excerpta Medica Foundation's automated storage and retrieval programme see entry 9.

This section of Excerpta Medica abstracts literature on topics such as: Health Care Organization, Ambulatory Health Care, Health Systems Running Costs, Manpower, Output of Health Care Systems, Prevention, Insurance, and Hygiene. Author and subject indexes are provided in each issue.

0011 **Excerpta Medica Foundation, Amsterdam.** *Pediatrics and pediatric surgery.* Amsterdam, Excerpta Medica Foundation, Section 7. Engl.
For more complete information on the Excerpta Medica Foundation's automated storage and retrieval programme see entry 9.

This section of Excerpta Medica abstracts literature on topics such as: Mental and Emotional Development, Newborn Infant, Nutrition, Feeding Problems, Sudden Unexpected Death, etc. Author and subject indexes are provided in each issue.

0012 **Gish, O., ed(s).** *Health manpower and the medical auxiliary: some notes and an annotated bibliography.* London, Intermediate Technology Development Group, 1971. 65p. Engl.
Individual articles have been abstracted separately under entries 34 and 145.

This publication arises from the Intermediate Technology Development Group's discussions about rural health. It is intended as a guide for those who plan and administer health programmes in developing countries. Included are articles on health planning in developing countries, the use of intermediary medical personnel, and medical auxiliaries as physician substitutes. There is also an annotated bibliography (134 entries) presenting most of the significant published material from 1960 to 1970 that is concerned with medical manpower and particularly medical auxiliaries. The first part of the bibliography lists sources on health planning; the second part deals with health manpower; and the third concerns medical auxiliaries. Each of the three sections is divided into two parts: the first includes material such as books or reports that have been published as independent documents; the second includes articles available as parts of larger publications. All entries are listed alphabetically by author.

0013   Gray, G.L. *Health services research and development abroad: a selected bibliography.* Bethesda, Md., Capital Systems Group, Jul 1971. 161p. Engl.

This bibliography was developed from a project entitled, "Systematic Inventory of Active Non-U.S. Information Sources and Preparation of Bibliography of Foreign Literature in Health Services Research and Development in 1965-1970." It describes a sample of literature selected from the larger mass of documentation identified and examined during the course of this study. The sources were: a search of approximately 100 different indexing/abstracting journals and bibliographies; literature provided or suggested by health specialists in the USA and abroad; special computer searches using the MEDLARS system of the National Library of Medicine and the Excerpta Medica automated Biomedical Data Bank; and direct searching of the contents of specific journals considered to be most important in the field of health services research. Non-English documents are annotated in English. Author and subject indexes are included. There are 521 annotated references listed under the following headings: (1) economics and planning; (2) health care services; (3) manpower and training; (4) methodology and technology; and (5) bibliographies and services. (Revised book abstract.)

0014   Heald, K.A., Cooper, J.K. RAND Corporation, Santa Monica. *Annotated bibliography on rural medical care.* Santa-Monica, The RAND Corporation, Document No. R-966-HEW, Apr 1972. 35p. Engl.

This bibliography on rural health care has been compiled for persons interested in health problems of rural America. A total of 180 annotated references are categorized according to the following subject areas: manpower supply and distribution; demand for health services; factors affecting physician placement; physician shortage; and related topics.

0015   Kohn, R., Radius, S. *International comparison of health services systems: an annotated bibliography.* International Journal of Health Services (Westport, Conn.), 3(2), Spring 1973, 295-309. Engl.

References to selected publications facilitating cross-national comparisons of health services systems are listed. Originally assembled for a graduate level seminar, the bibliography grew to its present scope through a series of literature searches, including the Medical Literature Analysis and Retrieval System (MEDLARS) search of the National Library of Medicine. Currently, this bibliography presents only English language sources. It consists of an annotated bibliography of selected books, including both national and cross-national studies. Because of limitations imposed by size, selectivity was necessarily exercised in choosing subject areas as well as individual entries within the bibliography. The bibliography will be kept up to date, and in the future it will be expanded to incorporate new publications, non-English sources, and suggestions from readers. (Author abstract.)

0016   Malawi, Health Extension Service. *MOYO: a health extension service publication.* Blantyre, Malawi Health Extension Service. Engl.

MOYO features articles for personnel associated with the health and community development programme in Malawi. Articles on topics such as malnutrition, maintenance of hospital equipment, under-five clinics, and maternal and child health are written in very simple instructional terms. Reports from primary level health and community workers on their work in Malawi are included in each issue. Although content of the journal focusses on maternal and child health and nutrition programmes, it occasionally includes articles concerning hospital maintenance, laboratory procedures, accident prevention, etc. *MOYO* is available from the Editor, MOYO, Health Extension Service, P.O. Box 3, Blantyre, Malawi.

0017   National Library of Medicine, Bethesda, Md. *Selected references on environmental quality as it relates to health.* Bethesda, Md., National Library of Medicine. Engl.

This bibliography, a product of the National Library of Medicine's computer-based retrieval system (MEDLARS), cites selected articles from 2 200 biomedical journals. Each monthly issue includes references cited in the monthly *Index Medicus* for the corresponding month. Citations are arranged under subject headings, which appear in alphabetical order. These subject headings are index terms selected from *Medical Subject Headings* (MESH). In the subject section, subject headings such as the following are included: Air Pollution, Childcare, Community Health Services, Comprehensive Health Planning, Delivery of Health Care, Environmental Health, Family Planning, Infant Mortality, Nutrition, etc. In the author section, senior authors' names receive full citations whereas second and third authors' names are cross-referenced. Published on a monthly basis, the periodical is available from the Superintendent of Documents, U.S. Government Printing Office, Washington D.C. 20402, at U.S. $4.00 per annum.

0018 **National Library of Medicine, Bethesda, Md.** *Current bibliography of epidemiology: a guide to the literature of epidemiology, preventive medicine, and public health.* Bethesda, Md., National Library of Medicine. Engl.

The purpose of this bibliography is to provide a comprehensive and continuing index to the current periodical medical literature for practitioners and investigators in community medicine and for others concerned with the etiology, prevention, and control of disease. The bibliography is divided into two parts, each arranged in alphabetical order. Section One, Selected Subject Headings, includes references related to some 200 topics, e.g. Birth Rate, Child Health Services, Communicable Disease Control, Environmental Health, Hygiene, Nutrition Surveys, Preventive Dentistry, Sanitation, World Health Organization, etc. Section Two, Diseases, Organisms, and Vaccines, includes the current references related to the etiology, prevention, and control of specific diseases. Topics here include Abortion, Birth Injuries, Deficiency Diseases, Gynecologic Diseases, Kwashiorkor, Trypanosomiasis, etc. Since each reference cited here appears at least once in *Index Medicus*, a separate author index is not required. Each volume consists of 12 monthly issues accompanied by an annual cumulation at the end of the year. Subscriptions can be ordered from the Superintendent of Documents, U.S. Government Printing Office, Washington D.C. 20402, at U.S. $22.50 per annum.

0019 **Ohio Medlars Center, Columbus.** *Recurring bibliography: education in the allied health professions.* Columbus, Ohio State University, The College of Medicine, Ohio Medlars Centre. Engl.

This annual recurring bibliography includes those articles listed in *Index Medicus* from April through March of the following year. References cited focus primarily on education in the health professions and the reader is referred to the following related recurring bibliographies developed by the National Library of Medicine, Washington, D.C.: *Bibliography on Medical Education, Index to Dental Literature, International Nursing Index,* and *Bibliography of Epidemiology.* In this recurring bibliography citations are listed, in subject categories such as Allied Health Personnel, Community Health Aides, Dental Assistants, Dietetics, Health Manpower, Hospital Administration, Nutrition, Physicians' Assistants, Psychiatric Aides, Public Health Administration, etc. An author index is provided. Copies are obtainable from The Ohio Medlars Center, The College of Medicine, Ohio State University, Columbus, Ohio, or from the National Library of Medicine, Washington, D.C.

0020 **WHO, Geneva.** *Reference material for health auxiliaries and their teachers: Remaha.* Geneva, WHO, 1973. 41p. Engl., Fren.

A preliminary list with an introductory note.

Reference material suitable for use by health auxiliaries has been organized under the following subject categories: nursing, midwifery, maternal and child health, family planning, health education, nutrition, diagnosis and treatment, first aid, and environmental health. Entries have complete source information and a brief annotation indicating the usefulness of each book or manual. The selection includes approximately 200 items in three languages: English, French, and Spanish. In addition to training manuals designed specifically for use by auxiliary health workers, source books for teachers of auxiliaries are included.

II Organization and Planning

II.1 Health manpower

See also: *0012, 0080, 0111, 0115, 0123, 0196, 0244, 0312, 0440, 0446, 0479, 0613*

0021 Akinkugbe, O.O. *Identifying the health needs of the nation.* Nigerian Nurse (Lagos), 4(1), Jan-Mar 1972, 19-21. Engl.

This paper, which was delivered by the Dean of the Medical School, University of Ibadan, to the Professional Association of Trained Nurses of Nigeria, concerns the role of nursing in the Four Year National Development Plan. The plan makes provision for the training of various types of health personnel. The role of the nurse is bound in with that of the other members of the health team. The nurse must adapt to local situations and serve a polyvalent function, moving easily from urban to rural settings. Preventive medicine, health education, and the gathering of accurate morbidity statistics are also given high priority.

0022 Bactat, J.L. *Rural health: its implications to public health nursing.* Newsette (Makati-Rizal, Philippines), 8(2), Apr-Jun 1968, 23-29. Engl.

The public health nurse in rural health service works as a member of the health team. She participates in diagnosis, treatment, and health planning. The Philippine Department of Health is legally responsible for safeguarding the health of rural people through rural health units. However, most deaths between 1920 and 1965 are those due to preventable causes. BCG vaccination and health education in the barrios (districts) is called for. It is noted that health officers hold nurses back by discouraging home visiting. Evidence reveals present services to be inadequate. No study has yet been conducted that would show the most satisfactory number of physicians, nurses, and sanitary inspectors required by the population. There is a significant lack of nurses in the rural areas. Priorities must be reassessed. Defects in basic nursing education have definitely limited the effectiveness of nurses on the job. Nurses must participate in policy formation to correct these deficiencies.

0023 Badgley, R.F., Bloom, S., Mechanic, D., Pearson, R.J., Wolfe, S. *International studies of health manpower: a sociologic perspective.* Medical Care (Philadelphia), 9(3), May-Jun 1971, 235-252. Engl.

This report reviews past inadequacies of health manpower planning and traditional approaches to manpower study in the health field. After reviewing the more common approaches, a sociologic framework is suggested for the analysis of health manpower. Finally, the paper presents various areas of study that will be useful in expanding and developing this perspective. Forty-five references are listed.

0024 Badgley, R.F. *Studies in planning health manpower: the Varna meeting.* Journal of Health and Social Behavior (Washington, D.C.), 12, Mar 1971, 4-10. Engl.

Sessions at a symposium of researchers in medicine and sociology convened in Varna, Bulgaria, in 1970, dealt with problems of cross-national research in the sociology of health services, public responses to medical services, planning medical manpower, and the organization of health services. This review summarizes issues raised at the session of planning medical manpower. All of the researchers agreed that a health service system includes all formal and informal activities centred on the provision of health services, and their utilization by a population. In terms of health manpower this includes all health personnel (formally trained and indigenous workers), their recruitment and training, a range of health facilities, the work behaviour and values of health workers, etc. In the papers presented at the symposium more attention is paid to students than to faculties, to patients than to doctors, and to the social and demographic attitudes of practitioners than to their working conditions or standards of medical practice. They often project a sense of unreality for they seldom refer to government planning agencies or educational institutions. Nevertheless they represent a useful contribution toward the development of a comparative sociology of health.

0025 Baker, T.D. *Health manpower planning.* In Reinke, W.A., ed., Health Planning: Qualitative Aspects and Quantitative Techniques, Baltimore, Md., Johns Hopkins University, 1972, 179-198. Engl.

Health manpower planning is a means of trying to make sure there will be enough health workers to meet, but not exceed, future economic demands. Effort must be put into making more use of effective planning since it takes time to train people. An analytic framework was developed for health manpower planning after being put into practice in studies carried out by Johns Hopkins University's Department of International Health in Taiwan, Turkey, Peru, and Nigeria. The framework included: (1) supply analysis (measuring current supply of all types of health workers in detail); (2) analysis of projected supply; (3) analysis of effective economic demand for services; (4) analysis of projected demand; (5) estimation of worker productivity; (6) analysis of the anticipated gap between future supply and future demand; and (7) constraints that will limit any recommendations. Each factor in the framework is discussed in terms of its component parts. The importance of health manpower planning is established and processes involved in it are clarified. Fifteen references are listed, with additional recommended readings.

0026 Baker, T.D., Perlman, M. *Health manpower in a developing economy: Taiwan, a case study in planning.* Baltimore, The Johns Hopkins Press, 1967. 203p. Engl.

This study was the first in a series of four Johns Hopkins' health manpower surveys; the others were carried out in Turkey, Peru, and Nigeria. The book is designed to assist planning in Taiwan and to develop methods of health manpower analysis. The conceptual framework of the study is in six parts: (1) qualitative and quantitative analyses of the supply of health workers; (2) projection of this supply to the future; (3) analysis of current public and private sector demands for health services; (4) projection of these demands; (5) trial balance of supply and demand; and (6) corrective measures for any imbalances. Health workers considered here are physicians, herbalists and quacks, nurses and midwives, dentists and pharmacists, and environmental sanitation workers. Supply of nurses and midwives is a crucial problem in health manpower planning in Taiwan. There is a shortage of nurses but there are twice as many physicians as qualified nurses. Consequently, physicians perform inappropriate tasks better delegated to trained nurses. Untrained nurses' aides assume responsibilities for which they are not qualified. One causal factor is that nursing is not a high prestige occupation in Taiwan. Midwives outnumber nurses but the number of new entrants is falling, not even keeping pace with the increase of population or replacing the retiring midwives. Demand for medical care is examined considering the biological basis and the private and public sectors. Two appendices provide the statistical analysis and the household survey sampling design.

0027 Braga, E. *New concepts in medical education.* In Wolstenholme, G., O'Connor, M., eds., Teamwork for World Health, London, J. and A. Churchill, 1971, 143-155. Engl.
See also entry 198.

Countries should adopt an ecological approach toward their health services. Education and training should be adapted to local circumstances, as part of each national health plan. This pattern is difficult to carry out in countries undergoing rapid socioeconomic changes. Although training and education of personnel occurs mostly in isolation from the institutions that absorb these personnel, traditional schools of medicine and allied health services are gradually trying to cooperate.

0028 Collis, W.R., Nicholson, T.F., Audu, I.S. *Medical education in Nigeria.* Lagos, Lagos University Medical School, n.d. 7p. Engl.
Unpublished document.

A solution to Nigeria's physician shortage is training of auxiliary health workers. Their basic training should be similar to that of a nurse, but specialized so as to relieve the medical doctor. A new orientation is necessary for all medical teachers and medical personnel; medical courses will stress the advisory/supervisory role of the physician to a group of ancillaries.

0029 Colombia, Ministry of Public Health. *Recursos humanos para un Servicio nacional de salud. (Manpower for a national health service).* Bogota, Ministry of Public Health, Administration of Human Resources Bureau, Dec 1971. 32p. Span.

Manpower requirements and cost of a national health service for Colombia, projected to 1975, are established at national, regional, rural, local, and university levels. Tables showing existing resources and estimated requirements at different development stages are included. The usefulness of auxiliary health workers and rural health promoters, who can be delegated a wide range of duties, is comparatively great, in view of the low outlay of time and money required to train them. Estimates for health personnel other than physicians are seen to decrease considerably when the rural service makes use of this manpower source. Priority should therefore be given to training such workers.

0030 Cooper, E.S. *American Health Education for African Development, Inc. (AHEAD).* Journal of the National Medical Association (New York), 59(4), Jul 1967, 233-237. Engl.

The American Health Education for African Development, Inc., (AHEAD) was founded in 1963. It is a voluntary, nonprofit, nonsectarian organization whose aim is to lead the campaign to banish major debilitating diseases from Africa. Its first major project is the establishment of a Nursing Education Centre in Freetown, Sierra Leone, West Africa. The new nursing school will be a self-contained unit connected with a new teaching hospital group consisting of five Freetown hospitals. Duration of the course will be 3 1/2 years, including 6 months of introductory work. State registered nurses will be graduated there. Other AHEAD projects are planned. Since funds for health education in Africa are limited, the service offered by AHEAD does not duplicate other programme efforts.

0031 Fountain, D.E. *Primary health professionals in developing countries.* n.p., 10 Jan 1972. 14p. Engl.
Unpublished document.

Progress in delivery of health care is impeded by prejudice against nonphysician medical personnel. Terms such as "subprofessional" should be supplanted by functional titles that describe the roles of each category of personnel. The term "primary health professional" would describe personnel who see a patient first, whereas "secondary health professional" would describe those who provide specialized treatment. The primary health professional should be a multipurpose worker. In contrast to popular opinion among health leaders, primary health professionals need to be decision-makers rather than subordinates; thus their training should provide experience in decision-making. Modern teaching methods must be applied to improve all aspects of training and strengthen teamwork for effective health care. Five references are listed.

0032 Ghana, Ministry of Information. *Ghana medical facilities.* Accra, Ministry of Information, Feb 1971. 28p. Engl.
Statistical data describe availability and location of hospital facilities, rural health centres, health posts, dental health services, private practitioners, and maternity homes in Ghana.

0033 Goswami, A.L. *Deployment of medical officers in rural areas.* Journal of the Indian Medical Association (Calcutta), 52(8), 16 Apr 1969, 399-400. Engl.
Letter to the editor.
In India, though the number of primary health centres continues to grow, more and more of them go without qualified medical officers. One solution, rather than unceremoniously dumping young doctors in rural areas, would be to introduce these physicians to rural service through a district civil hospital. District hospitals in West Bengal, for instance, are well equipped and well manned by qualified young doctors. Working in these hospitals can help attune young physicians to health problems in the area where they are posted. Each trainee could serve for a period of time in a primary health centre in the district. After this training, health service administrators would have some experienced workers to select from in staffing primary health centres. It is clear too that some experienced older health staff would like to remain in service rather than retire at retirement age. They should be given a choice to retire or not retire, according to their own choice.

0034 Hill, K.R. Intermediate Technology Development Group, London. *Intermediate technology in medicine.* In Gish, O., ed., Health Manpower and the Medical Auxiliary, London, Intermediate Technology Development Group, 1971, 24-29. Engl.
See also entries 12 and 145.
In 1965, WHO established an objective for the following decade of training one doctor for each 10 000 population. The situation in Northern Nigeria, where by 1971 there was one doctor to 150 000 people, is similar to that in other developing countries. One reason is that the number of secondary school graduates has not reached expectations and those who graduate are in demand not only in medicine but in other fields such as agriculture and engineering as well. Physician education should be innovative rather than a duplication of Western models: training should be designed in the context of local problems. The physician's training in this context must include orientation toward the practice of preventive medicine and public health; training in the instruction and leadership of auxiliaries; instruction in handling mass campaigns; a sympathetic appreciation of local culture and resources, etc. Given the lack of resources or the educational infrastructure required to produce the needed number of doctors through university training, a well-trained and disciplined corps of intermediary personnel is essential.

0035 Journal of the Indian Medical Association, Calcutta. *Rural medical practitioners in Andhra Pradesh and West Godavary district.* Journal of the Indian Medical Association (Calcutta), 55(8), 16 Oct 1970, 293-294. Engl.
Letter to the editor.
In a letter to the Indian Medical Association, an anonymous rural practitioner denounces the lack of clear-cut legislation governing the retirement of practitioners working under the Rural Medical Scheme. This scheme, introduced in 1925, provided a fixed subsidy for independent medical practitioners who would settle in a village and work for a fixed number of hours every morning. The position was nontransferable. As long as their duties were efficiently discharged, they would continue to receive the subsidy. Pay rates for practitioners, assistants, and other trained personnel are quoted, as are various memos varying in their recommendations as to the age at which the practitioner should retire. The author objects to the practitioner being dismissed at age 60 on 3 months notice, "without gratuity, pension, compensation, or consideration", and recommends that rural medical practitioners who produce a physical fitness certificate be permitted to continue.

0036 Karefa-Smart, J. *Health and manpower: interrelationship between health and socioeconomic development.* Israel Journal of Medical Sciences (Jerusalem), 4(3), May-Jun 1968, 586-598. Engl.
Fourth Rehovoth Conference on Health Problems in Developing States, Rehovoth, Israel, 15-23 Aug 1967.
See entry 96 for complete proceedings.
Health and economic development are interrelated. Health protection of workers is important in assisting production. Malaria, chronic diseases, malnutrition, and tuberculosis are some of the conditions affecting development. Developing countries need to consider whether they can afford to sustain the heavy economic losses resulting from lack of health services. Auxiliary health manpower is essential, especially in rural areas. Social reform and economic development as well as health care must focus on the development of human potential.

0037 Kleinbach, G., Rapoport, M., Hays, C. *Training of health manpower for the developing world: a policy seminar, Part I, II and III.* Boston, Harvard School of Public Health, Spring 1973. 2v.(various pagings). Engl.

II Organization and Planning

This document includes materials prepared for the policy seminar on training of health manpower for the developing world, which took place at the Harvard School of Public Health in the Spring of 1973. Directed toward the concept of community medicine rather than curative medicine, attempts are made to resolve issues related to manpower development. Included are resumes of seminar session papers, seminar questions related to topics discussed, and lists of reading materials recommended for each session.

0038 Lyman, K. *Basic nursing education programmes: a guide to their planning.* Geneva, WHO Public Health Papers No. 7, 1961. 80p. Engl.

This is a guide prepared on the basis of consultations with many nursing authorities to suggest a method of approach to planning basic nursing education programmes at local, state, or national levels, and intended to be of particular use in countries where nursing education programmes are developing. It comprises a part devoted to an extremely detailed questionnaire for use in preliminary fact-finding, and a part discussing the factors involved in planning a basic school of nursing. A select bibliography is included. (WHO abstract.)

0039 Majekodunmi, M.A. *Medical education and the health services: a critical review of priorities in a developing country.* Lancet (London), 1(7429), 15 Jan 1966, 142-144. Engl.

First priority in Nigerian health services should be to satisfy the health needs of the whole community. The lack of physicians, nurses, and auxiliary health workers hinders progress. Highest priority has been accorded to the training of physicians and not to training medical assistants on a crash basis. Experience showed the shortcut method of producing doctors led to abuse of chemotherapeutic drugs and lowered ethical standards. The author recommends building a medical service of "highest quality" and rejects emphasis stressed elsewhere on quantity of care for a developing nation.

0040 Malawi, Ministry of Finance. *Proposed new training school for clinical officers and medical assistants in Lilongwe.* Zomba, Malawi, Ministry of Finance, Jul 1971. 13p. Engl. Unpublished document.

A proposal for the construction and establishment of a Medical Auxiliary Training School in Lilongwe, Malawi, to train workers for rural health work, indicates that morale among rural medical auxiliaries is low. Limited opportunities for promotion, the uncertainty of auxiliaries' future role, and their vulnerability to public criticism are problems confronted by this cadre of workers in Malawi. As it is realized that they will continue to be the backbone of the health system for a long time, attention is being given to solving these problems and to expanding training.

0041 Mann, K.J. *Family physician and the general hospital.* Reprint; source unknown, 137-140. Engl.

Incorporating the family physician as a member of the medical centre staff involves changes in administration as family physicians working in isolation are brought in as full members of the internal medicine department and granted free access to and use of hospital resources. Appropriate changes in teaching methods bring medical students into contact with patients early in their studies and provide experiences in community health centres and hospital departments. A pilot project implementing these suggestions was initiated near Jerusalem, Israel. Observations suggest that the objective and subjective status of the integrated physicians has risen and that the quality of health care has increased. It is suggested that this pattern of community health care be introduced in other countries through similar pilot projects. Nine references are listed.

0042 Ong, G.B. *Problems of population explosion: staffing structure related to service and educational needs.* Journal of the Royal College of Surgeons of Edinburgh (Edinburgh), 16(1), Jan 1971, 196-202. Engl.

Population has increased greatly in Hong Kong since 1841. Facilities are stretched to their maximum capacity. Influxes of refugees strain the system and many people live without sanitation facilities or good water supplies. Because of crowded living conditions certain diseases have become prevalent, i.e. tuberculosis, waterborne diseases, and parasitic infestations. Demand for hospital beds overwhelms supply. Training of surgeons is described.

0043 Ramalingaswami, V. *Unfulfilled expectations and the third approach.* British Journal of Medical Education (London), 2, Dec 1968, 246-248. Engl.

The most peripheral yet most vital outpost in India's health service organization is the primary health centre. Ideally, the physician at the primary health centre is responsible for total health care of the community, but in many cases the physician's education does not prepare him for the task. In follow-up home visiting, deployment of health assistants in preventive work, and in generating health consciousness in the community, he has not succeeded. A large gap exists between the needs of individuals in the environment of their homes and farms and the capabilities of modern medicine. To fill this gap a new type of physician is needed — a social biologist who can communicate effectively with patients, who will be an effective leader of health programmes, and who will use his knowledge to stimulate other community building programmes. Training of this new type of physician should be accompanied by community research. Five references are listed.

0044 Razaq, A.A. *Speech delivered by Alhaji Abdul Razaq, Commissioner for Health and Social Welfare.* Nigerian Nurse (Lagos), 4(1), Jan-Mar 1972, 14-15. Engl. Conference of the Professional Association of Trained Nurses of Nigeria, Lagos, 28-29 Oct 1971.

This paper records a speech delivered by the Commissioner for Health and Social Welfare, Kwara State, to the Professional Association of Trained Nurses of Nigeria. He proposes that, due to an acute shortage of doctors in Nigeria, nurses be trained and licensed to perform tasks normally left to doctors. These "midi" or "maxi" nurses will man rural health centres in the absence of a medical doctor, and will play an important role in the implementation of the Four Year National Development Plan, to provide new health facilities and improve old ones in Nigeria.

0045 Reiff, R., Reissman, F. *Indigenous nonprofessional: a strategy of change in community action and community mental health programs.* New York, National Institute of Labor Education, Mental Health Program, Report No. 3, Nov 1964. 48p. Engl.

This is a report discussing a strategy to meet the manpower and programme crisis that faced new U.S. community action and community mental health programmes. The need for and use of indigenous nonprofessional workers in such programmes is systematically analyzed. The nonprofessional worker is recognized for his capacity to interact easily with his social community because of his social position, life style, motivation, language, and knowledge of the community. The nonprofessional indigenous worker expedites programmes by relating as a link between the programme's clients and the community resources that exist to aid the client. He or she acts as interpreter, negotiator, lay attorney, educator, instructor, helper, companion, counselor, supporter, intervener. Mental health services have been able to use these workers as community action aides, housing service aides, home manager, child care aides, parent education aides, home service aides, child service aides, case work aides, or research aides. Each type represents a new or different way agencies have used to provide services employing nonprofessional-type indigenous workers. Issues in training indigenous nonprofessionals are discussed and include the need to be assured these workers do not lose touch with their communities after they are trained. In conclusion the use of indigenous nonprofessionals is likely to be effective in helping community action programmes of various types meet their objectives of community interaction with the programme. Fifty-five references are listed.

0046 Smith, R.A., Onuaguluchi, G.O., Pratt, K.A., Ojo, O.A., Bankole, M.A., Manuwa, S. *Manpower planning.* In Akinkugbe, O.O., Olatunbosun, D., Esan, G.J., eds., Priorities in National Health Planning: Proceedings of an International Symposium, Ibadan, Caxton Press (West Africa) Ltd., 1973, 141-179. Engl.

See entry 123 for full report of symposium.

The chapter covers six papers on health manpower planning. The first paper explains the Medex System of the United States and emphasizes that it can be modified to the needs of a particular country. The second paper proposes a university training program (in Nigeria) for medical assistants with opportunities for postgraduate training following a period of field experience in the rural areas. It lists problems of expansion of undergraduate medical education, such as scarcity of teachers in the basic medical sciences; concentration of teaching facilities in teaching hospitals; inadequate numbers of consultants and teachers to train the teachers; and lack of funds. Paper three observes that nurses in Nigeria comprise the largest single professional group of health manpower; hence they should have representation at all levels of health planning operation. The fourth paper emphasizes the need for biostatisticians and other health statistics personnel to provide vital statistics for health manpower planning in Nigeria. Paper five proposes a survey to identify the specific health problems in Nigeria, to be followed by an operational programme according to the health plan. The final paper emphasizes that the medical assistant cadre was meant as a temporary feature, which should later be absorbed into the appropriate hierarchy in the Nigerian health delivery system. Subsequent discussions centred on medical assistants, cheaper construction of hospital structures, task analysis, improving the environment and housing conditions, establishment of a planning unit in each ministry of health, preventive and curative medicine, coordination of medical activities to make adequate use of existing personnel, and the need to pay more attention to dental care.

0047 Sofoluwe, G.O. *Assessment of the health administration in Ibarapa district council area with some suggestions on the methodology of rural health planning.* West African Medical Journal (Ibadan), 15, Feb 1966, 33-39. Engl.

An analysis of the areas served by Nigeria's Ibarapa District health workers and a description of available manpower and of health auxiliaries' functions lead to the following suggestions for planning methods: workers must have specific tasks; there should be two levels of teamwork, i.e. health centre and health dispensary; specialists must make periodic visits to rural areas; a division of rural health should be established within the Ministry of Health; etc. No attempt is made to suggest an increase in staff but rather to make existing staff more useful. Eight references are listed.

0048 Stewart, W.H. *Health problems of rural communities.* In Long, E.C., ed., Health Objectives for the Developing Society: Responsibilities of Individual, Physician and Community, Durham, N.C., Duke University Press, 1965, 24-32. Engl.

Health problems in rural communities are discussed regarding both the newly developing areas and the developed nations. Health problems in the former arise from malnutrition (which in turn arises as a result of scarce resources), parasitism (the solution for which is environmental sanitation and immunization), accidents, the expectations of the rural population, and the existing system that the society has developed for contending with disease and illness, i.e. traditional medicine. Rural health problems in the developed regions differ in that they relate to bringing high quality medical care to the rural dweller or bringing the rural dweller to the medical care. The USA is discussed as an example.

0049 Waddy, B.B. *Rural health services in the tropics and the training of medical auxiliaries for them.* Transactions of the Royal Society of Tropical Medicine and Hygiene (London), 57(5), Sep 1963, 384-391. Engl.

Since most people in developing countries are agriculturalists living in rural areas, rural welfare should be of the greatest importance and attacks on ill health must go beyond providing treatment for those who come and ask for it. Administrative deficiencies make building more hospitals in developing countries a defeating task. Health centres and appropriate training of well-placed auxiliaries promise to work best. Examples from African countries are given. Selection of trainees and help for them on the job are two important considerations when planning rural services. Five references are listed.

0050 Wade, C.C., Farmer, S.K. *State of Bahrain, hospital service: manpower study.* Bahrain, Ministry of Health, Jul 1973. 75p. Engl.

A report to the Minister of Health, Bahrain.
A study was conducted to assess the staff establishment and work pattern of hospital and rural health centre services in the State of Bahrain, and to make recommendations for staffing requirements and possible training schemes for a new hospital. Detailed observations and questionnaire-based evaluation of manpower point up difficulties arising from the administrative set-up both for conducting the study objectively and for the achievement of work goals by health service staff. Difficulties encountered included expatriate staff, language barriers, salary anomalies, lack of a fixed national pension age, indiscipline, and what is described as "more than a hint of a non-dismissal policy." A selection of job descriptions is included.

0051 WHO, Alexandria. *Health manpower planning.* Alexandria, WHO, May 1971. 22p. WHO/EM/RC21/4. EMRO/71/615. Engl.
Unpublished document.

Future health manpower needs will be determined by future trends in diseases, technological advances, and the future organization of health services. Prediction is based on a quantitative analysis of data on present disease patterns and achievement rates. Factors to be taken into consideration include: demographic data; disease statistics by demographic characteristics; and data on the work load capacity of physicians and other health personnel. Once the components entering into the calculation are established, a mathematical formula indicates the projected future manpower needs. The paper discusses in some detail what type of statistics should be included in data gathering, and includes some general forecasts on disease trends. Five references are listed.

0052 WHO, Brazzaville. *Methodology of health team manpower planning: report of a symposium, Brazzaville, 29 May-3 June 1972.* Brazzaville, WHO, 1 Sep 1972. 166p. WHO/AFR/PHA/99. Engl., Fren.

This report of a symposium on the methodology of health team manpower planning summarizes discussions on the following: patterns in the constitution and management of health teams in the African region, duties of health team members, definitions of the health team according to the needs of the region, operation and administration of health teams, and educational objectives for training of health teams. The concept of the health team is universally accepted but difficulties are encountered in putting it into practice. Functional description of individual team members' duties requires continuous study since health workers' duties change with advances in health service technology and administration.

0053 WHO, Geneva. *Development of studies of health manpower: report of a WHO scientific group.* Geneva, WHO Technical Report Series No. 481, 1971. 56p. Engl.

A WHO expert committee reports on key issues related to the research of health manpower needs in developing countries. It provides a basic checklist of the questions that health manpower studies should answer, and reviews methods of research currently used to evaluate manpower needs.

0054 WHO, Geneva. *Education and training of health personnel in Africa, 1960-1970.* WHO Chronicle (Geneva), 15, 1961, 374-381. Engl.

Most Africans live at the subsistence level and have little education. Since most health services are curative and exist in urban areas there is an urgent need for the training of local health personnel. The number of medical and paramedical personnel in Africa as of 1960 and projections of personnel requirements for 1960-70 are given. It is suggested that health education be incorporated into the curriculum of school programmes as an alternative to specialized premedical and health/technical training. Since no single African language predominates enough to be used in medical schools, English and French remain the languages of instruction. Other problems in nurse and sanitary staff training are discussed. Training for all categories of health personnel should stress public health. The training of professional staff in methods of utilizing auxiliaries is essential.

II.2 Organization and administration

See also: 0032, 0189, 0192, 0195, 0234, 0280, 0292, 0356, 0643

0055 African Medical and Research Foundation, Nairobi. *Health care for remote areas.* Nairobi, African Medical and Research Foundation, Jul 1973. 24p. Engl.

Positive measures to meet health needs, which can be taken within the limited resources of a developing country, are in the areas of: (1) training; (2) administration and communication; (3) public health; (4) curative medicine; and (5) family planning. It was recommended that at the village level in southern Sudan the Village Midwife, Village Health Auxiliary I (preventive emphasis), and Village Medical Auxiliary II (curative emphasis) be trained to provide easily accessible health care for the rural population. Training in rural settings is planned for Nairobi health professionals, since training in hospital settings leaves many trainees at a loss when confronted by actual situations in the bush. Experience at Gondar, Ethiopia, proves that rural service workers must have supportive supervision to ensure flow of drugs, pay, equipment, etc., and to keep auxiliary worker morale high. Communication in East African rural areas is facilitated by radio contact between hospitals and mobile units. Transportation of the very ill and treatment for remote groups is made possible by air transport. In countries where over 50% of the population is under 15 years of age, it is essential to reserve beds for children in hospitals.

0056 African Medical and Research Foundation, Nairobi. *Basic medical services for the whole population of Botswana.* Nairobi, African Medical and Research Foundation, n.d. 11p. Engl.
Unpublished document.

Medical services in developing countries fail because they emphasize hospital services and professional training. The greatest needs are for readily accessible maternal and child health care and sanitation services. The goal for Botswana should be the provision of trained health personnel to meet these needs, so that within 10 years 90% of the population would have access to basic health services without having to travel more than 2 miles. Once trained, staff would be expected to work on a voluntary basis. Short courses for village sanitarians, mothers' aides, medical auxiliaries, and rural specialists are outlined.

0057 Akin-Deko, G., Osuntokun, B.O., Akinkugbe, O.O., Kirfi, M.B., Jose-Williams, A., Na Oruwariye, T.O. *Integrated approach in health care delivery.* In Akinkugbe, O.O., Olatunbosun, D., Esan, G.J., eds., Priorities in National Health Planning: Proceedings of an International Symposium, Ibadan, Caxton Press (West Africa) Ltd., 1973, 237-275. Engl.
See entry 123 for full report of symposium.

This chapter deals with six papers presented on integrated approach in health care delivery. The first paper calls for an important consideration to be given to food and nutrition in national health planning. The second paper discusses the inadequacy of medicare in Nigeria; the role of the doctor in the formulation of policy in medicare; the training of medical personnel; the need for medical auxiliaries; and the special role of teaching hospitals and medical schools. It then calls for an integrated development of the country's educational, socioeconomic, and agricultural potentials towards adequate medical care delivery. Paper three deals with the role of the pharmacist in the health team, as an expert on medicinal products in an advisory capacity to both the doctor and the patient. It then emphasizes the importance of giving mutual respect to the functions of each team member. The fourth paper examines problems facing health care administration in Nigeria and calls for research into specific areas to facilitate policy decisions. Paper five asks for more government financial support to enable existing facilities in medical schools, state hospitals, and health centres to be used to train more doctors and other health personnel. The final paper emphasizes the important role of the general practitioner in reducing the cost of medical service as compared to government-sponsored service: his training is simpler and he has extensive experience in dealing with all minor human and health problems in rural areas. An increase in the number of general practitioners would reduce the urgency of the need for medical auxiliaries. The main points of discussion were: (1) control of health centres; (2) increasing doctors' responsibility to extend to rural areas; (3) expanding existing teaching hospitals; (4) providing basic school amenities in the rural areas to enable doctors to work there; and (5) the need for all health personnel to present a unified front in solving the country's health problems.

0058 All India Institute of Hygiene and Public Health, Calcutta. *Three decades of progress.* Calcutta, All India Institute of Hygiene and Public Health, 28 Jan 1963. 63p. Engl.

The All India Institute of Hygiene and Public Health was established in 1932, with the prime objective of providing postgraduate training in the principles and methods of public health and preventive medicine in the Indian perspective. The Institute has been involved in training, research, communicable disease control, environmental sanitation, food and nutrition projects, maternal and child health programmes, and public health practice through the Rural Health Unit and Training Centre at Singur and the Urban Health Centre at Chetla. It has been involved in direct service through emergency, specialist, and community services and in national planning. The staff members of the Institute have published over 700 articles, the most important of which are listed.

0059 Arbona, G. *Rural health.* Israel Journal of Medical Sciences (Jerusalem), 4(3), May-Jun 1968, 553-561. Engl.
Fourth Rehovoth Conference on Health Problems in Developing States, Rehovoth, Israel, 15-23 Aug 1967.
A discussion follows the paper. See entry 96 for complete proceedings.

II Organization and Planning

Health centre experiments in Venezuela, Canada, and Central America illustrate the advantages of several different systems. Perhaps the most important factor for successful regional health systems is a programme of continuing education for health workers. Other issues discussed here include communication, participation, planning, and evaluation.

0060 Arole, R.S., Arole, M. *Comprehensive rural health project, Jamkhed.* Journal of the Christian Medical Association of India (Mysore), 47(4), Apr 1972, 177-180. Engl.

The 80% of India's population living in villages remain neglected. In some areas the qualified physician-to-population ratio is 1 to 30 000. In southeast Ahmednagar, facilities were inadequate or lacking, population was increasing rapidly, infant and under-five mortality and morbidity rates were high, and tuberculosis and leprosy were prevalent; thus it was decided to start comprehensive medical work in this area. The actual area for the project was chosen after visits with community leaders. The selected area qualified because of its need for services, because an invitation to proceed was provided by the Panchayat Samitit and Minister of State for Rural Development, and because the community was willing to donate land, provide a rent-free building for a clinic, provide housing for the staff, and take an active part in the project. A main health centre was established in Jamkhed and provided an under-five nutrition and immunization programme, family welfare planning programme, and a leprosy control programme. Service to villages in a 5-10 mile radius from the centre was provided by subcentres. Multipurpose mobile clinics visit more isolated villages on a regular schedule.

0061 Australia, Department of Health. *Rural health services in Australia.* Canberra, Australian Government Department of Health, n.d. 9p. Engl.
Unpublished document, prepared in response to a request by WHO.

Medical service to remote areas of Australia is at present inadequate. Few medical school graduates enter general practice and fewer still rural practice. Health care delivery is complicated by great distances, sparse population, and high morbidity rates, particularly among the Aborigines. Medical care is currently provided by private practitioners, the Royal Flying Doctor Service, and the Northern Territory Aerial Medical Service. A team of medical officers, nursing sisters, and field health inspectors visits outlying settlements at 3-6 week intervals. Physicians are difficult to recruit and services need more continuity. Resources could be better organized to provide multipurpose front line personnel, well-planned preventive services, local institutions for first aid, diagnoses, and public health, and more effective transportation — changes that would require only a marginal increase in the number of doctors.

0062 Bisley, G.G. *Some aspects in the prevention and treatment of blindness in Kenya.* Transactions of the Opthalmological Societies of the United Kingdom (London), 84, 1964, 55-65. Engl.

Among 1 093 Africans examined for blindness in a survey, 43% were blind due to senile cataract, and 36.9% due to infection traced to the trachoma virus. A comprehensive country-wide programme of prevention and treatment would be difficult to implement in Africa, due to lack of manpower, money, and materials. However, certain steps have been taken. The Kenyan Ministry of Health has engaged African Health Assistants and Health Visitors to provide health education to village groups. The teaching is reinforced in the primary school curriculum. Medical assistants administer treatment of eye infections and cataracts in schools and among pastoral tribes through the use of a Mobile Eye Unit. The Unit is preceded by adequate publicity and spends about 4 days in one place. However, preventive and educative measures for pastoral tribes are unlikely to become effective without a social revolution.

0063 Boletin de la Oficina Sanitaria Panamericana, Washington, D.C. *Servicios de salud en areas rurales. (Health services in rural areas.)* Boletin de la Oficina Sanitaria Panamericana (Washington, D.C.) 64, Jan 1968, 6-28. Span.

Poor quality of life in rural Latin America has led to mass migration to the cities. In 1965, 47.6% of the total Latin American population lived in rural areas; by 1970 the percentage had dropped to 42.6%. If the current trend continues, by 1980, only 31.2% of the population will be rural. Accurate statistics are hard to come by as countries differ in their opinion of what population density constitutes a rural area. However, they agree that the rural population has an important role to play in the economic and social development of the country and that steps must be taken to ameliorate the conditions, such as malnutrition, high infant mortality rates, and infectious disease, that lead to this exodus. Difficult access to rural areas is a prime obstacle to rural health promotion. Attempts have been made to overcome this difficulty by training auxiliaries, or even primary school teachers and policemen, to take on various health related duties. Procedures whereby doctors make the rounds of the rural zones in mobile units are also discussed. Two major problems encountered in these attempts are inadequate supervision of auxiliaries and the gravitation of professional workers toward the urban centre. As a result, a number of countries have started special health programmes in rural areas as part of their national economic and social development plans. Thirty-six references are listed.

0064 Bomgaars, M.R. *Family folder: a community health care aid.* Journal of the Christian Medical Association of India (Mysore City), 47(5), May 1972, 222-227. Engl.

Samples of records contained within the family folder designed for a rural Punjab (India) community are presented. This type of folder is advantageous in that all family members are recorded together, and staff are informed of the social, economic, and health status of family, etc. Any family folder should be adapted to social conditions of the area being served.

0065 Brodie, A. *World health scandal.* New Internationalist (London), Apr 1973, 14-17. Engl.

Developing countries often spend more than half their entire health budget on modern hospitals and medical centres in capital cities, i.e., on expensive, individualized curative services for a small urban elite. Consequently, among rural populations, millions suffer from preventable disease. Inequality is further perpetuated by the prevalence of private practice and the draining of doctors from the developing to the developed world. A 1969 survey in Pakistan showed 55% of its medical school output had left the country. Viable auxiliary health systems do, however, exist. In Sri Lanka care is equitably distributed through a system of auxiliaries. Health services in centres manned by auxiliaries tend to be more dedicated to the interests of the communities they serve.

0066 Castano, A.A., de Martinez, V.G. *Simplified system of health services in Candelaria.* Candelaria, Colombia, Universidad del Valle, Department of Public Health and Preventive Medicine, Health Division, n.d. 13p. Engl.

A simplified system of health services, allowing a total coverage of the population, has been proposed for the district of Candelaria, Colombia. The health services offered have a family and community focus, the three basic activities being prevention of illness, care of the sick, and rehabilitation. The primary health unit, or unit of education and information, relies on a health almanac with health messages for the whole family, a health card for each child under 5 years of age, and a health volunteer or promoter who visits homes every 2 months, educates the family through the health card and the health almanac, collects information on vital statistics, etc. Volunteers are supervised through the intermediate or service unit by auxiliary nursing personnel. A physician and a nurse compose the supervisory and programming unit. Job descriptions for volunteers, auxiliaries, and physicians are provided.

0067 Chang, K.K. *Intensive village health improvement program in Taiwan, Republic of China.* Chapel Hill, N.C., University of North Carolina, School of Public Health, 1 May 1969. 10p. Engl.
Unpublished document.

An intensive village health improvement programme was begun in Taiwan as part of a community development programme. Its goal is to have the county or city provide the budget and personnel for mobilizing township manpower resources for intensive village health improvement. The programme includes personal hygiene, home sanitation, fly control, environmental sanitation, and family planning. Beginning in one village the programme is extended to other townships, one by one. Village health education nurses work closely with county advisory committees and with the township in organizing resources and training local workers. Details of instructions for families, training and conducting group meetings, and means used to maintain records and activities are given. Instructions are designed to be easily followed by local workers. Nine references are listed.

0068 Chang, W.P. *Development of basic health services in Ethiopia.* Addis Ababa, Haile Selassie I University, Faculty of Medicine, Department of Preventive Medicine and Public Health, 1967. 26p. Engl.
Unpublished document.

In developing countries, basic health services are recognized as the foundation of health programmes. They consist of permanent long-range programmes, within a country-wide system. Progress in developing these around the world has been very slow, despite continuing efforts over the past decade. With aid in various forms, international and governmental, Ethiopia's services have shown successful development; this serves as an example of a practical, realistic approach. International help accounts for a great deal of the progress made. The Public Health College in Gondar is an institution of high standards that trains health workers for rural health service within this decentralized system. Efforts need to be made to keep its training from becoming too academic and isolated from the real problems graduates will face in their daily work in rural health centres. Recent efforts concentrate on improving the quality of care and the kind of care offered at these centres, rather than on increasing the number of centres. Supervision of staff in rural health centres is a task of great importance. A supervisory team assists the Ministry of Health to reorient work in centres toward preventive measures. A special evaluative project has been initiated to study the function of health centres under technical supervision. Twenty-eight references are listed.

0069 Corsa, L. *Health implications of population planning.* Ann Arbor, Michigan, University of Michigan, School of Public Health, Department of Population Planning, Population Reprint Series, Reprint No. 31, 1970. 19p. Engl.

The principal factors determining the extent to which health services and family planning services are or should be integrated at the point where service is directly provided to people are the following: the extent to which the contraceptive technology being used requires the same kinds of skilled manpower and specialized facilities that health services require, the extent to which health services are available in rural areas, the extent to which combination of health services and family planning services most efficiently provide their combined services, particularly in rural areas, the relative benefits to a given country at a given time of preventing an unwanted birth compared to postponing a death, etc. The implication that seems most certain in the long run is that health services and family planning services will be united.

0070 Dehne, E. *Health programs in the Ryukyu Islands.* Archives of Environmental Health (Chicago), 14, Feb 1967, 355-360. Engl.

Since the beginning of American administration in the Ryukyu Islands in the western Pacific the death rate has declined from 8 per 1 000 before World War II to 5 per 1 000 in 1967. Malaria has been eradicated. Maternal and child health problems remain, however, due to a lack of qualified medical and health personnel. The government aims at upgrading the existing dispensaries on the small islands and in remote areas by raising the competence of the local professional personnel, improving communication and transportation facilities, and setting up clinics to treat people on a scheduled basis. Problems unique to this area are identified and discussed.

0071 Elliott, J. *Health in Hong Kong.* Nursing Times (London), 65, 7 Aug 1969, 1003-1005. Engl.

Hong Kong's greatest asset is its people. Health services are therefore indispensable as there is so much overcrowding in Hong Kong. The Queen Elizabeth Hospital is described. Floating clinics visit the many small islands around Hong Kong and there is a flying doctor service for isolated villages.

0072 Fendall, N.R. *Primary medical care in developing countries.* International Journal of Health Services (Westport, Conn.), 2(2), 1972, 297-315. Engl.

Common to all developing nations are lack of financial resources and trained manpower, illiteracy, high fertility, a traditional society based on the soil, and diseases related to undernutrition, infections, and vector-borne illnesses. Most diseases are not of the exotic, tropical kind but common diseases of the respiratory and digestive tracts. There is much less self treatment than in industrialized nations, but many complaints could be treated by nonphysicians. The distribution of scarce physician resources is poor. Most physicians seek to live and work in capital cities and not in the rural areas where most people live. There are too few paramedical workers to support the physicians. The growth of the population constantly exceeds the increase in the number of physicians, some of whom are lost through the brain drain to more developed countries. Although there is no lack of knowledge or understanding of what to do about these problems, there is insufficient application of such knowledge toward practicable solutions. More realistic planning for primary care is necessary in the future. The only hope lies in greater use of nonprofessional workers operating from planned centres. Among the priorities are: screening for early major abnormalities, better emergency care and transport services, and birth control. More emphasis must be given to child care in rural areas, where children under 15 account for more than half of the population. Five references are listed. (Author abstract).

0073 Fendall, N.R. *Comparison of family planning programs in Iran and Turkey.* HSMHA Health Reports (Rockville, Md.), 86(11), Nov 1971, 1011-1024. Engl.

Turkey and Iran differ substantially in their family planning programmes. Iran has a highly visible programme supported by a resourceful organization, whereas the programme in Turkey maintains a low profile and its organizational structure is less flexible. Neither programme has had an appreciable impact on the birth rate, and abortion is prevalent in both countries. Educational programmes on all levels have developed faster in Iran than in Turkey. The Iranian programme is integrated with maternal and child health care. Twenty-seven references are listed.

0074 Fisek, N.H. *Example of an integrated approach to health care: the Turkish national health services.* In Wolstenholm, G., O'Connor, M., eds., Teamwork for World Health, London, J. and A. Churchill, 1971, 55-77. Engl.

See also entry 198.

In 1960 a new system of health services, called "socialized health services," was accepted by the Turkish government. The design of the Turkish National Health Service is based on team work and cooperation. The characteristics of the Turkish National Health Services, the status of the health services before nationalization, and the results of a field study on the National Health Service are given in this paper. A discussion is included.

0075 Gale, G.W. *Some factors affecting rural health services in developing countries.* Lancet (London), 1(7387), 27 Mar 1965, 696-697. Engl.

In rural areas of developing countries each village should have its own health centre or subcentre. Health education should aim toward making each household head the effective medical officer of health for his domain, by protecting water supplies, disposing of wastes, growing protective foods, etc. Success along these lines can be achieved if every member of the health team incorporates health education into all his work, and demonstrates in his own home life what he teaches in the community.

0076 Ghana, Ministry of Health. *Health services in Ghana.* Accra, Ministry of Health, 1967. 47p. Engl.

This paper surveys the important aspects of curative and preventive health services available in Ghana as of 1967. Included are statistical data and descriptive information on the following: environmental control, maternal and child health services, health education, immunization, etc.

0077 Graham, R.G. *Services medical team in Vietnam.* New Zealand Medical Journal (Wellington), 67, Jun 1968, 631-632. Engl.

Forty-two military and civilian medical teams operated in South Vietnam in 1967. These teams helped local Vietnamese operate hospitals and dispensaries. They taught and assisted in immunization and preventive medicine programmes. Rural dispensary work was backed up by help from the hospital-based teams. Dispensaries were staffed by two male nurses and maternity help was provided by Vietnamese midwives. The type of medical aid provided by the New Zealand team is likely to be needed for many years.

0078 Griffith, D.H. *Final report on public health programme, Andhra Pradesh, WHO Project: India-151, (Jul 1961-Nov 1962).* New Delhi, WHO, 1963. 30p. WHO/SEA/PHA/30. Engl.

A WHO team was engaged in the following aspects of a public health programme in Andhra Pradesh, India: the development of rural training areas for doctors, nurses, and auxiliary personnel; the development of rural training and orientation programmes for doctors, nurses, and auxiliaries; the organization and conduct of courses in rural health work for doctors, nurses, and auxiliary personnel; and the study of primary health centres. Practice fields were established at four health centres. Existing orientation courses were stimulated with seminars, group discussions and simulation experiments. Problems confronting the primary health centres were the shortage of trained personnel in the face of a wide range of diseases requiring specialist attention, and the lack of interest shown by many young medical officers. Four demonstration districts that were functioning lacked sufficient administrative integration with public health centres. Recommendations have been offered for improving the status of rural training areas, continuing evaluation of the orientation courses, reorganization of the administration of rural medical facilities, conducting village surveys, and transferring greater administrative authority to officers in charge of the demonstration districts.

0079 Gupta, S.C. *Family health care at the urban health centre, Alambagh.* Journal of Family Welfare (Bombay), 12(3), Mar 1966, 37-45. Engl.

An urban health centre at Alambagh, India, provides health care for 500 families plus training for undergraduate and postgraduate students in community health. Composition of the health team and the family health care programme are presented. Local agencies in urban areas should organize existing dispensaries and hospitals to provide a family health programme. Seven references are listed.

0080 India, Department of Health Services, Kerala. *Health services in Kerala: a brochure, 1968.* Trivandrum, Department of Health Services, 1968. 32p. Engl.
See also entry 81.

This report describes the organization of, and programmes provided by the Department of Health Services, Kerala, India. Campaigns against leprosy, malaria, tuberculosis, and cholera, and programmes in environmental sanitation, maternal and child health services, family planning, public health education, and state insurance are outlined with respect to objectives, coverage, and staff.

0081 India, State Health Education Bureau, Trivandrum, Kerala. *Health services in Kerala: a brochure.* Trivandrum, India, Government Press, 1968. 35p. Engl.
See also entry 80.

This brochure describes the history and organization of health service programmes in Kerala State, India, and provides statistical data on medical and health facilities. There are 162 public health centres that provide rural health care and function in the control of communicable disease. Midwives register expectant mothers, and professional care is provided for problem pregnancies. Prenatal and child care clinics are conducted weekly at health centres and subcentres. Family planning programmes have expanded since the establishment of 70 family planning clinics and 35 sterilization institutions in 1959. Other aspects covered in the article include the following: methods of gathering vital statistics, school health services, health training schemes, public health and government analysts' laboratories, and a programme of applied nutrition.

0082 Institute of Rural Health and Family Planning, Gandhigram. *Administrative and financial code for the Institute of Rural Health and Family Planning, Gandhigram.* Gandhigram, Institute of Rural Health and Family Planning, 1965. 1v.(various pagings). Engl.
Unpublished document. See also entries 454 and 542.

A detailed procedural code for the financial and administrative affairs of the Institute of Rural Health and Family Planning, Gandhigram, India, is presented. The Institute was built up from the Pilot Health Project that began in Gandhigram in 1959. The regulations cover details related to the merger of the Pilot Health Project and the new Institute. Objectives and activities of the new Institute centre around action research, demonstration projects, and training programmes for key personnel in the family planning and public health programmes of India.

0083 John, R., Kimmelman, D., Haas, J., Orris, P. *Public health care in Cuba.* Social Policy (New York), 1, Jan-Feb 1971, 41-46. Engl.

Cuba's health care system is well organized, decentralized, and citizen-responsive, even reaching people in remote areas. Since 1959, the government has built 47 rural hospitals and 260 linked polyclinics, providing outpatient treatment, dental services, and community health education. Health care personnel, including physicians, share in local agricultural work, while medical students are regularly assigned to poor families who become their personal medical responsibility. Doctor-patient relationships rest on "common goals and familiar bonds" and are not "culturally alienated." Steps have been taken through nonformal educational programmes to prepare large numbers of paramedical personnel and volunteers, whose training has focussed on health education and disease prevention. The success of the system and the high regard in which it is held by the Cuban people, is attributed to citizen participation in

II Organization and Planning

planning and modifying health policy. Citizens participate through health commissions at every level of the Public Health Ministry.

0084 Journal of Tropical Pediatrics and Environmental Child Health, Kampala. *Report on the seminar on health services in rural areas, Tunis, Tunisia, 7-16 Oct 1968.* Journal of Tropical Pediatrics and Environmental Child Health (Kampala), Mar 1971, 26-30. Engl.

Participants in a seminar on rural health services agreed that the provision of health care for rural populations is a neglected issue. Rural people themselves are insisting on the right to health care. Discussion focussed on the preparation, training, and utilization of staff and on the organization, administration, and financing of health services in rural areas. Participants recommended the integration of curative and preventive care, regional administration for peripheral health services, effective supervision and communication with rural health personnel, and recruitment and training of auxiliary personnel locally, under conditions similar to those in which they will work.

0085 Judy, M. *Lone hospital in the mountains.* Association of Operating Room Nurses (Englewood, Colo.), 7, Mar 1969, 57-62. Engl.

The author describes conditions in an isolated Guatemalan hospital and its developing resources, i.e. a laboratory, professional and auxiliary personnel, and hospital equipment.

0086 Kafuko, G.W. *Organization of health services with limited professional manpower.* Israel Journal of Medical Sciences (Jerusalem), 4(3), May-Jun 1968, 599-604. Engl.
Fourth Rehovoth Conference on Health Problems in Developing States, Rehovoth, Israel, 15-23 Aug 1967.
A discussion follows the paper. See entry 96 for complete proceedings.

On the attainment of independence in developing countries there has been a tendency to decentralize health services and place major responsibility in the hands of local authorities for the administration of rural medical and health services. Ministries have become advisory agencies, but retain inspectorial duties under the law. Although auxiliaries take over a great deal of the medical duties, professional workers are needed to guide auxiliaries. Relations between professional and auxiliary workers will necessarily be determined by tasks and priorities of the health programme. In Uganda, the great majority of diseases are preventable. Domiciliary midwifery and home nursing are top priority tasks for paraprofessionals in developing countries.

0087 Mann, K.J. *Summary of recommendations of the Israel Medical Association Committee on the Organization of Health Services in Israel.* Israel Journal of Medical Sciences (Jerusalem), 6(1), Jan-Feb 1970, 168-175. Engl.

A committee investigation in 1970 revealed that major dissatisfaction with medical services in Israel arises from the following: the lack of a single national authority to plan and execute health policies; fragmentation of existing health services; lack of integration between various branches of medicine; specialists' isolation from corresponding hospital departments; family physicians' separation from the hospital; lack of paramedical staff; and concentration of undergraduate medical education in the large hospitals, isolated from family clinics. All patients should be referred to the family physician who is assisted by a health team and associated with a regional hospital. Regional health authorities should be established under a single national health authority. Further committee recommendations focus on the role of the family physician.

0088 Mann, K.J. Hadassah Medical Organization, Jerusalem. *Administration, Organization and Finance: an experiment in community health within the framework of a university hospital.* London, Eighth International Hospital Congress, 25-30 May 1953. 4p. Engl.

In 1947, the Hadassah Medical Organization of Israel opened, in its hospital area, five district medical stations staffed by public health nurses and general practitioners. These are now expanding into community health centres whose development will depend on the results of a pilot project in Beth Mazmil. Here a health centre with two teams, each made up of a general physician, two public health nurses, an health educator, and psychiatric social worker, functions on the following principles: one agency is responsible for all aspects of community health; personal and environmental health are interdependent; the whole family is the subject of medical care, which continues throughout life; and health is positively promoted. The project is to be used as field training for undergraduate students and for research in the relief of family and community tensions.

0089 Mathews, M. *Report on team work during flood relief operation.* Nursing Journal of India (New Delhi), 59(2), Feb 1968, 46-47. Engl.

In 1967 the author participated with student nurses in flood relief operations conducted from the Rural Health Training Centre, Najafgarh, India. The training centre is near New Delhi and serves the health needs of 72 villages through three primary health centres and subcentres. For flood relief work, teams of 9-10 workers were created, directed by medical officers. Cholera and typhoid inoculations were provided and nutritional supplements were available for mothers and children. Since sanitation in the villages had been disrupted by the floods, health education on sanitation was provided and wells were disinfected. The programme continued until the water receded. Organization of this flood relief work made it possible to control water-borne diseases during flooding.

0090 Medical Research Centre, Nairobi. *Medical Research Centre, Nairobi, Kenya: annual report*

1972. Amsterdam, Royal Tropical Institute, 1972. 139p. Engl.

The scope of the Medical Research Centre's activities in Kenya has widened beyond the biomedical research field and now includes behavioural and social science studies. Projects are outlined. Among these projects are a study of modern and traditional forms of maternity care among the Akamba; a cross-sectional study of attitudes of Akamba people toward the concept of modern medicine in relation to childhood diseases of measles, whooping cough, and acute diarrhoea; a study of feeding of young children in rural areas of Kenya; and many other projects. Disease entities as well as health behaviour and the organizational aspects of health care delivery are researched by the Centre.

0091 Navarro, V. *Editorial: health and health services in People's China and Cuba.* International Journal of Health Services (Westport, Conn.), 2(3), Aug 1972, 327-329. Engl.

Although numerous publications on rural health care in developing countries are available, accounts of the experience of socialist countries, such as the People's Republic of China and Cuba, are underrepresented. Experiences in China and Cuba put to question the widely held beliefs that due to lack of resources, developing nations cannot provide comprehensive care to all their people. Socialist countries' experiences indicate that failure to deliver care to the majority of people is simply a matter of poorly distributed resources. Both China and Cuba demonstrate in health services their commitment to minimizing inequalities between social classes, between cities and rural areas, and between regions. Redistribution of resources must be accompanied by development of new resources. In this sense socialist countries are defining the people as their resource and are deploying them to create health services for rural and urban population. Massive popular participation in the health sector is required rather than the training of a few to care for the majority.

0092 Ordonez-Plaja, A. *Teamwork at ministry level.* In Wolstenholme, G., O'Connor, M., eds., Teamwork for World Health, London, J. and A. Churchill, 1971, 167-176. Engl.
See also entry 198.

Experts cannot agree on common definitions of "disease" and "health." The best resolution of cultural, social, and political differences in these areas arises when experts pool approaches. Latin American people at all levels are used to the "strong-man" concept, and acceptance of the team approach will come only with successful experiences in using it. A Colombian health project provided such an experience, although the team approach developed is presently in jeopardy.

0093 Otiende, J.D. Kenya, Ministry of Information and Broadcasting. *Development of health services in Kenya.* Nairobi, Kenya News Agency, Handout No. 290, 7 Sep 1969. 6p. Engl.

Transcript of a speech delivered at the National Conference on Social Welfare, University College, Nairobi.

This paper outlines development of health services in Kenya and major recent advances in rural health centres, health personnel training, and preventive medicine.

0094 Patino, J.F. *Education in the health professions to meet the needs of the nations.* Journal of Medical Education (Chicago), 43(2), Feb 1968, 221-231. Engl.
See also entry 95.

Man's health and well-being are not just one goal of economic development, but are actually its foundation. Some countries, like Colombia, have recognized this interrelationship in health policies. Only a health team can solve problems common to developing areas. Universities need to be active in teamwork for community health. Medical and health education is a powerful instrument of national development, but first medical education must be reoriented; it must familiarize itself with important social and economic factors. Research is needed to help develop services related to field problems. Developing countries need to create programmes based not on models used in industrial countries but on their own needs. University efforts and government programmes should be coordinated. Ways in which Colombia is reorienting medical education are discussed.

0095 Patino, J.F. *Education in the health professions to meet national needs.* World Medical Journal (New York), 14, May-Jun 1967, 84-88. Engl.
See also entry 94.

Not only should medical education in developing countries be based on the needs of those countries, but also the medical practitioner should be trained to play his part in the process of social readjustment that a national development plan represents. Medical and health education are not ends in themselves; when integrated with other national development efforts they become the means by which social well-being and productivity are increased. Responsibility for programme development should be shared by those providing services: educators, administrators, professionals, etc., and the consumers of the services: the members of the community. Research and training, closely related to field needs, are an important part of the programme directed to overall national health goals, which the Colombian Association of Medical Colleges has embarked on in collaboration with affiliated institutions such as the National Institute of Nutrition, and with the Colombian Association of Universities, and governmental bodies. International cooperation and strengthening of national and regional organizations will help medical educators play a more meaningful role in developing their societies.

0096 Prywes, M., Davies, A.M., ed(s). *Proceedings of the fourth Rehovoth conference on health problems in developing states.* Israel Journal of Medical Sciences (Jerusalem), 4(3), May-Jun 1968, 326-778. Engl.

Fourth Rehovoth Conference on Health Problems in Developing States, Rehovoth, Israel, 15-23 Aug 1967.

Individual articles have been abstracted separately under entries 36, 59, 86, 120, 125, 131, 158, 173, 268, 271, 272, 410, 416, 440, 479, and 554.

Seventy-one delegates participated in the Fourth Rehovoth Conference on Health Problems in Developing States, held in Rehovoth, Israel, in August 1964. The keynote address by Dr M.G. Candau stressed that developing countries must find their own solutions to the future rather than follow the mistakes of the more developed countries. Of the 32 papers presented, most related to issues of health care delivery in developing countries.

0097 Pugh, A.O. *New patterns of African rural health in Rhodesia.* Central African Journal of Medicine (Salisbury), 15(6), Jun 1969, 125-128. Engl.

As disease patterns in Rhodesia change rapidly, so must methods of health care delivery. Measles, bronchopneumonia, and gastroenteritis have replaced smallpox and poliomyelitis as the most common causes of death. Malnutrition contributes significantly in these deaths, however, and often goes unrecognized as the true killer. The cooperation of the people must be enlisted in combatting malnutrition. Traditional diets must be modified, personal and domestic hygiene learned, and safe water used. Health education has a major role to play in attaining these objectives. In this respect, the work of the rural nurse in the maternal and child welfare clinic is important, since she has the advantage of being close to the villagers and is in a position to promote disease prevention and health and family planning education.

0098 Reinke, W.A. *International comparative aspects of health delivery systems.* In Attinger, E.O., ed., Global Systems Dynamics, New York, John Wiley & Sons, Inc., 1970, 306-320. Engl.

Global Systems Dynamics International Symposium, Charlottesville, USA, 1969.

A conceptual framework for comparing health delivery systems in various countries is outlined. Health services draw upon resources in response to certain health problems to produce improved health status; but higher health status is dependent on more than per capita expenditure. Within this framework, health problems, resources and expenditures are broken down for an analysis of their interrelationship. Such models are useful in planning health services. This one is currently being applied in the development of a national health plan in Chile. A project directed by the Department of International Health, Johns Hopkins University, is using this model in a functional study of health workers in two provinces in India and three in Turkey, to discover how much activity can be shifted onto workers with the lowest level of skill commensurate with adequate care. The objective of these studies is to be able, eventually, to predict the impact of certain system interventions on the magnitude of problems, distribution of functions and requirements for training health workers. Seventeen references are listed.

0099 Ronaghy, H.A., Nasr, K. *Medical problems of developing nations: an attempt to bring medical care to rural communities in Iran.* British Medical Journal (London), 31 Jan 1970, 295-296. Engl.

As a solution to the problem of delivering medical care to rural communities, the government of Iran drafted medical and paramedical personnel into a Health Corps rather than into military service. After 6 months training in public health and rural medicine, draftees spent 18 months in the villages. Members of the corps were assigned to stationary units or to mobile units consisting of a doctor with two high-school graduates serving as assistants, and a vehicle for transportation. Each mobile unit visited two villages a day, and each village once a week. In 4 years over 13 million patients were seen by a doctor. With the health corps functioning at the village level, hospitals in nearby towns have to provide more advanced services and continue to be the link with the university medical centre. Ten references are listed.

0100 Sansarricq, H. *Principes d'evolution rationnelle des services de sante pour la lutte contre les grandes endemies dans les pays d'Afrique au sud du Sahara. (Development of health services in the fight against endemic diseases in Africa south of the Sahara).* Annales des Societes Belges de Medecine Tropicale de Parasitologie et de Mycologie Humaine et Animale (Anvers), 51 (4-5), 1971, 505-519. Fren.

Mass campaigns still play a role in the fight against endemic diseases in Africa, and, due to lack of funds and resources, must continue to take precedence over other forms of medical care in African countries south of the Sahara. However, techniques of organizing more campaigns, such as the use of auxiliary health worker teams, could be applied to the organization of future basic health services in rural areas of Africa. The irregularity of visits by mobile teams has limited the effectiveness of health education and preventive medicine. Local populations should be assured services when a team of multipurpose or polyvalent workers under appropriate supervision keep a known schedule at a fixed spot. Mass health campaigns of the past will provide a model for future rural health care in Africa.

0101 Shah, N.K. *Development of health services in Nepal.* Chapel Hill, N.C., Carolina Population Centre, Dec 1971. 18p. Engl.

Unpublished document.

The article outlines Nepal's progress in the following areas of health care: preventive services (i.e. a family planning and maternal and child health project, malaria eradication, leprosy control, etc.); training institutions for nurses, auxiliary health workers, assistant nurse-midwives, and physicians; curative services of hospitals; and education.

0102 Singh, K. *Outline of the medical services in Malaysia.* Medical Journal of Malaya (Singapore), 25(2), Dec 1970, 79-82. Engl.

Paper read at the 5th Council Meeting of the Commonwealth Medical Association in Kuala Lumpur.

Following independence in 1963, West Malaysia formed three 5-year development plans, each with increased budgets for rural health services. As a result, in the period 1963-70 a rural health service system was established, with maternity clinics for every 2 000 population, a health subcentre for every 10 000, and one main health centre (providing preventive and curative services) for every 50 000 people. Tuberculosis control and malaria eradication have received special attention. Population pressure and the need for economic development, are expected to constrain future public health expenditure. Development of institutes of medicine and expansion of family planning education and services are recommended for the next 5-year development plan.

0103 Stein, Z., Susser, M. *Cuban health system: a trial of a comprehensive service in a poor country.* International Journal of Health Services (Westport, Conn.), 2(4), Nov 1972, 551-566. Engl.

A travel report.

This article reviews Cuban health programmes in terms of six goals ostensibly adopted by the administration. Postrevolutionary Cuba has placed a high priority on health, and aims to create a health service that is comprehensive in scope and content, in population covered, and in organizational forms and levels of specialization. Within this service, the Cuban health administration has applied what is known about the major diseases that affect their society. This health programme has also focussed on human needs, has tried to measure the effects of its activities, and has responded to evaluation. Some trends in Cuban health patterns are described from available data. With preventable diseases under control, Cuba now faces problems similar to those of developed countries. The new phase will require new approaches, with emphasis on the research techniques of epidemiology and the social sciences to develop and evaluate possible preventive approaches to chronic disease. Eleven references are listed. (Author abstract.)

0104 Stoeckle, J.D., Candib, L.M. *Neighbourhood health center: reform ideas of yesterday and today.* New England Journal of Medicine (Boston), 280(25), 19 Jun 1969, 1385-1391. Engl.

The early health centres of the 1900's were meant to solve special out-of-hospital health problems of the poor, chiefly infectious disease, infant malnutrition, and infant feeding. The organizational ideas of centres, district location, community participation, bureaucratic organization, and centralization of community health and social services were derived from democratic, religious, and industrial ideas common to the era of progressive reform. In actual practice some of the organizational goals were contradictory. For example, although a goal such as community participation was important to bring services close to people, simultaneous pressures for efficiency in bureaucratic organization often conflicted. The new health centres, whether traditional or organized as private group practice, have a different and more complex set of health problems requiring social rehabilitation through personal health services. Although new definitions are being applied to the older organizational ideas, contradictions in dealing with modern problems are also being encountered. Seventeen references are listed. (Journal abstract.)

0105 Stone, B. *Health work in Masasi, Tanzania.* Saving Health (London), 12(3), Sep 1973, 48-50. Engl.

Development of Tanzania as a country depends on the development of agriculture. Recent health efforts have focussed on improving the health of rural populations, upon which agricultural progress depends. Despite governmental policy (supportive of village development and progress), it is clear that the farther one gets from urban areas the worse the living conditions become. Lack of medical facilities, not dire poverty, is the problem. Nearly 50% of children die before reaching age five. Mobile health teams recently were made part of rural health care delivery. Work of the Masasi Diocese Mission Hospital is described. It relates its planning to health plans made on the national level for the rural population.

0106 Tait, H.P. *Health services in India and Burma: their evolution and present status.* Medical History (London), 16, Apr 1972, 169-178. Engl.

The author outlines developments in the health field and indicates health objectives of the Government of India. He summarizes the structure of India's health administration and points out that India was the first country to adopt family planning as a national policy. Trained doctors and medical teachers are urgently needed. Distribution of doctors is uneven with most engaged in private practice. The Fourth Five Year Plan proposes further training and hospital facilities. Although there have been improvements in education of nursing and paramedical staff, much remains to be done. Construction of health facilities is being undertaken in rural areas. The fields of public health, general sanitation, nutrition, maternal and child health, school health, and communicable disease control are discussed. In Burma, the overriding problem is a financial one. Special programmes deal with malnutrition and communicable diseases. Burma's health organization unified curative, preventive, and social medicine; a system of rural health centres staffed by health assistants is well established. The author outlines Burma's health administration. There is only one doctor per 9 000 population and the shortage of nurses is acute. A school of paramedical science has been established at Rangoon to train health assistants and teaching programmes for other medical personnel are being expanded. Public health activities cover general sanitation, nutrition, maternal and child health, etc.

0107 Taylor, D., Thapa, R. *Nepal.* New York, Population Council, Country Profiles, Apr 1972, 1-8. Engl.

Health services in Nepal are inadequate and unevenly distributed. Traditional cures are sought for most illnesses; otherwise, a government doctor or paramedical worker is consulted. Inadequate training facilities and rugged topography hinder rural development programmes. The government has launched a national family planning and maternal and child health programme, relying on paramedical staff and using all available means of transportation. Thirteen references are listed.

0108 Thach, P.N. *Le service de sante de la Republique Democratique du Viet Nam face aux taches de la guerre. (Wartime health service in the Democratic Republic of Vietnam).* Sante Publique (Bucharest), 11, 1968, 3-22. Fren.

This article describes briefly the war of aggression undertaken against the Democratic Republic of North Vietnam (DRNV) and the increased tasks this imposes on the public health services. Mother and child health is the object of special care, given the fact that the women have to carry the burden of production. The health network of the rural cooperatives turned out to be the backbone not only of first aid services but also prophylactic measures against epidemics. This network took on increased importance due to the displacement of urban populations to the countryside due to the bombardments. Immediately above the village was the district health centre, with a 50-bed hospital, that was to become the pivot of all health activities. The evolution of health services during the war can be described as progressive and planned decentralization. Begun prior to the war, the process accelerated during the hostilities. Following the American bombardments of February 1965, a special effort was made to train surgical personnel at all levels, and continual bombing of hospitals led to the dispersion of the complex techniques of modern medicine; only the most efficient and simple were kept. This forced decentralization, despite the huge problems it raised, enabled the health services to extend their activities, associate clinical medicine to "realistic grassroots medicine," unify inpatient and outpatient care and preventive and therapeutic medicine. It turned the medical doctor not into the doctor of the patient or the illness, but into "the real doctor of man in all his somatic, psychic, ecological, family, social, and economic complexity." The discovery and use of the traditional pharmacopoeia enabled the creation of new medicines. The decentralized pharmaceutical production thus rendered possible was most useful until hostilities interrupted communications. Increased efforts in the field of training of medical personnel enabled the country to pass from one medical doctor per 150 000 inhabitants and one health officer per 85 000 to one medical doctor per 8 700 and one health officer per 1 850. Despite the efforts, the immense ravages of the war in terms of wounds inflicted upon the civilians forced the auxiliary medical personnel to take on many new tasks. Mortality declined in 10 years from 20-30% to 7%. Constant research into new medical and surgical techniques enabled the DRNV to restrict mortality to tolerable levels and occasionally even decrease it. Family planning efforts were also continued. Thus, faced with a quasi superhuman challenge, the medical services of the DRNV responded with amazing efficiency and finally reached a much higher level of services by the end of the conflict.

0109 Torrey, E.F. *Health services in Ethiopia.* Milbank Memorial Fund Quarterly (Boston), 45, Jul 1967, 275-285. Engl.

Traditional medicine is still commonly practiced in rural Ethiopia, although modern medicine has been present since 1900. In 1947 the Public Health Proclamation established the legal basis for a modern health system. This was followed in 1954 by the foundation of the Gondar Public Health College and Training Centre designed to train staff for provincial health centres. This fit in with a newly emerging emphasis on generalized, decentralized health services. There is still a great need for health education to counterbalance harmful folk medicine practices. Five references are listed.

0110 Vogel, L.C. *Implications of the transfer of basic health services from county councils to central government in Kenya.* East African Medical Journal (Nairobi), 47(5), May 1970, 242-246. Engl.

In Kenya until the end of 1969 basic health services in rural areas were provided by county councils through health centres and dispensaries. In January 1970 these health services were taken over by Central Government, i.e., the Ministry of Health. Some of the possible implications are: vastly increased responsibilities for the Ministry of Health; the need for the Ministry to provide the additional means and to set up the additional administrative machinery for these responsibilities; the need to review priorities; reformulation of training objectives and educational curricula for all grades of personnel in basic health services; revision of the relationship between the District Medical Officer of Health and the county council; and more equitable distribution of health facilities.

0111 Ward, J.P. *Surgery in the provinces of Nepal.* Annals of the Royal College of Surgeons of England (London), 44, Apr 1969, 224-227. Engl.

The establishment of surgical centres in Nepal's Kosi Zone began with the zonal hospital in Biratnagar. From here a main foothills surgical station, completely self-sufficient, was set up at Dhankuta. It is recommended that a surgical team in isolated areas should consist of four persons, have essential equipment and drugs, place responsibility on experienced personnel only, and remain stationary.

0112 WHO, Alexandria. *Integration of maternal and child health and family planning activities in the general health services.* Alexandria, WHO, 20 Aug 1971. 32p. WHO/EM/RC21/Tech. Disc./2. Engl.
Unpublished document.

Integration of maternal and child health and family planning activities with general health services in member countries of the WHO's Eastern Mediterranean Region is discussed. Even if some justification is made for promoting family planning through separate services initially, there should be a clear plan to integrate them with basic health services at some appropriate time. Prolonged separation of family planning services, with their large annual budgets, weakens health services through adverse competition for trained personnel and other resources. Important aspects of integration are considered.

0113   WHO, Alexandria. *Health examinations and screening procedures for chronic non-communicable diseases.* Alexandria, WHO, 1 May 1968. 11p. WHO/EM/RC18/5. Engl.
Unpublished document.

The role of periodic medical examination and health surveillance in preventive medicine is reviewed. Screening procedures for ischaemic heart disease, breast cancer, cancer of the cervix uteri, chronic bronchitis, diabetes mellitus, intraocular tension, and unreported mental illness are indicated. Choice of the method for organizing screening and health surveillance services depends on a multitude of factors that vary from country to country. Accepted principles for organization of services are: the necessity of including health education; the importance of involving primary health services, general practitioners, and health centre doctors; supporting the programme through medical records maintenance, and adequate laboratory and special diagnostic facilities; repetition of screening at periodic intervals; using screening procedures during routine hospital admission. Nonhospital screening schemes are illustrated. Multiple screening for whole populations is financially beyond the reach of even the most affluent societies. An alternative is the progressive introduction of relatively simple medical surveillance based on periodic medical checkups. Such surveillance would also contribute valuable data for research of disease prevalence and the natural history of chronic disorders.

0114   WHO, Alexandria. *Integration of mass campaigns into the national basic health services.* Alexandria, WHO, 18 Aug 1967. 46p. WHO/EM/RC17/Tech. Disc./2. Engl.
Unpublished document.

Integration of mass health campaigns into basic health services demands reconsideration of priorities. Demographic and epidemiological variables need to be examined during planning, since health care has an impact on these. In countries of the WHO's Eastern Mediterranean Region the population is predominantly rural with a high proportion under 15 years of age. The services developed over the past 20 years are mostly in urban areas. Integration of health services to produce basic services requires creative reorganization; old structures must be coordinated with new orientations. This is often difficult and demands a high level of cooperation among interest groups that have been accustomed to fighting among themselves for scarce financial resources. Organizational, technical, administrative, and training aspects of this process are outlined.

0115   WHO, Geneva. *Rural health services in Latin America.* World Health Chronicle (Geneva), 22 Jun 1968, 249-253. Engl.

Latin America's rural population has inadequate housing, sanitary services, educational facilities, etc. Besides illiteracy and isolation, other factors, such as the population's traditional concepts of health and disease, the interpretation of disease in terms of magic, and social differences between the population and the health workers, are related to health problems of rural areas. It would be of value to hire social scientists to pioneer programmes acceptable under these conditions. Public health programmes in rural environments are supported by the population if auxiliary health workers are recruited from the population itself and trained to carry out specific duties. General aspects of disease control, health resources, and rural public health services in several Latin American countries are discussed.

0116   WHO, Geneva. *Health education in the USSR.* Geneva, WHO Public Health Papers No. 19, 1963. 70p. Engl.

The USSR's health system relies heavily on health education, which is outlined in this report under the following headings: objectives, planning and organization, research, training of personnel (physicians, feldshers, health education specialists), and health education activities in rural and urban areas, factories, and schools. The system is characterized by free medical service, both curative and preventive, negligible private practice, and obligatory participation of all medical and paramedical personnel in dissemination of mass health information.

0117   WHO, Geneva. *Participation of health centres in ambulatory health care.* Geneva, WHO, 11 Feb 1959. 8p. WHO/OMC/33. Engl.

A WHO expert committee defines the health centre as "a place where the appropriate basic services are rendered." These should be linked with other services such as education and agriculture. Different countries have defined these units according to their own needs, some emphasizing geographic range of service, others proximity to a hospital. Differences exist in emphasis on curative, preventive, or integrated care. Historically the trend seems to be from the provision of preventive services to rural areas to the provision of comprehensive health care for the whole population.

0118   WHO, Manila. *Work of WHO in the Western Pacific Region: twenty-second annual report (1 July 1971-30 June 1972) of the regional director to the regional committee for the Western Pacific.* Manila, WHO, Jul 1972. 145p. WHO/WPR/RC23/3. Engl.

II Organization and Planning

This is a report on projects supported by the World Health Organization in the Western Pacific. The Regional Committee for the Western Pacific has consistently suggested that member countries formulate national health plans. In response to this request, efforts were made to formulate a planning methodology emphasizing in-country training. The report is divided into three parts: (1) a general statement of WHO activities in the realm of disease control and prevention, family health, education, the organization of health services in various countries, etc.; (2) evaluation summaries of selected projects; and (3) a list of ongoing WHO-supported projects.

0119 Zaghloul, A.Z. *Rural health services in U.A.R.* Journal of the Egyptian Public Health Association (Cairo), 38(5), 1963, 217-224. Engl.

In 1960, 61.8% of the Egyptian population was rural. Even in some urbanly defined districts, work is agricultural. Typical developing country conditions threaten health of rural people; these are poor housing, poor sanitation, polluted water, communicable disease, poverty, ignorance, traditions that impede change. Bilharzia, ancylostoma, and malaria are related to agriculture. Disease is influenced by migration patterns resulting from land reclamation and labourer migration. Funds are lacking for development of services, and there is a shortage of medical staff and hospital facilities. Rural health programme efforts for the country began in 1936 with the founding of a Ministry of Health and an Undersecretary for Rural Affairs. Organization of service structures in 1963 are described.

II.3 Planning

See also: 0049, 0057, 0068, 0072, 0109, 0220, 0227, 0445, 0507

0120 Abel-Smith, B. *What priority health? Tasks and priorities in the organization of medical services.* Israel Journal of Medical Sciences (Jerusalem), 4(3), May-Jun 1968, 350-355. Engl.
Fourth Rehovoth Conference on Health Problems in Developing States, Rehovoth, Israel, 15-23 Aug 1967.
A discussion follows the paper. See entry 96 for complete proceedings.

All over the world countries are in search of criteria for development planning. The priority that different countries give to health does not appear to be explicable by any simple formula. Breakdown of budgets for health in developing countries produces depressing results since many countries only give lip service to preventive medicine. The relative prestige given curative work is one of the worst legacies of colonialism. Economic data are not the only data to consider in deciding the value of various plans. One great potential contribution health services may make for people in developing countries is the capacity to limit family size. Eleven references are listed.

0121 Abramowitz, J. *Planning for the Indian health service.* Journal of Public Health Dentistry (Raleigh), 31(2), Spring 1971, 70-78. Engl.

In setting up its Indian Health Service to improve the health of its native Indian and Alaskan people, the United States Public Health Service has the unique opportunity to plan and implement one of the most comprehensive community health care programmes in the country. To ensure provision of the greatest level of dental care for each Indian community in the face of a shortage of dentists and limited resources, all available methods are employed; preventive care is stressed, dental assistants are trained, and equipment and clinical floor plans are designed for maximum efficiency. Careful preliminary planning with the active participation of the recipients, the setting up of an information system to identify problems, a long-range goal and plan of action for efficient use of resources, and ongoing evaluation all contribute to sound management and assure the effectiveness of the programme. Thirteen references are listed.

0122 Adedeji, A., Akenzua, S.I., Ogunlesi, T.O., Okediji, F.O., Dada, B.A. *Economics of health care.* In Akinkugbe, O.O., Olatunbosun, D., Esan, G.J., eds., Priorities in National Health Planning: Proceedings of an International Symposium, Ibadan, Caxton Press (West Africa) Ltd., 1973, 81-137. Engl.
See entry 123 for full report of symposium.

The chapter covers five papers on the economics of health care. The first paper maintains that the best strategy for health development in Nigeria would be to give the highest priority to preventive health programmes and then immediate attention to the problems of medical and paramedical manpower and financing of health services. The second paper offers proposals for the improvement of the Nigerian national health plan, i.e. establishment of cheaper hospitals and more health centres, development of a cadre of intermediate technologists to compensate for the shortage of doctors, and increasing government contributions to health care financing. Paper three observes that health care is a complex subject involving economic, political, and philosophical considerations especially in Nigeria. It discusses the economic value of good health to the country. The fourth paper discusses the consistency of health objectives and problems of health care delivery in Nigeria, and suggests guidelines for tackling them. Paper five presents some detailed statistics on health services in Nigeria, including recurrent expenditures by state governments on health and social welfare, and health manpower and facilities. Final discussions centred on the size of the financial allocation to health, the gap between allocation and actual expenditure, the relative emphasis between preventive and curative medicine, the training of medical assistants, and the need for health care delivery to rural areas.

0123 Akinkugbe, O.O., Olatunbosun, D., Esan, G.J., ed(s). *Priorities in national health planning: proceedings of an international symposium.* Ibadan, Caxton Press (West Africa) Ltd., 1973. 331p. Engl.

Individual articles have been abstracted separately under entries 46, 57, 122, 126, 408, 617, and 639.

The main topics discussed during a symposium held in Nigeria include priorities in health care, preventive and curative care, economics of health care, manpower planning, medical education and planning, systems of health care delivery, and the provision of health manpower for Nigeria. The proceedings covered all disciplines and professions involved in health care delivery in Nigeria. Major decisions are influenced by the shortage of manpower in all sectors of the health field; economic appraisal of major health problems; acceptance of the basic tenet that the unit of consumers in the health industry is the community, not the individual; and the establishment of a national health planning commission.

0124 Argentina, Department of Social Welfare. *Pautas de programacion y normas de atencion programas: de salud para areas rurales. (Health plan for rural areas: programmes and standards of care).* Buenos Aires, Department of Social Welfare, 1969. 153p. Span.

The purpose of this plan is to improve and broaden the delivery of health services to rural communities. Specific technical objectives are: to provide care during pregnancy and maternal and child care, prevent communicable diseases by immunization and environmental sanitation, and promote community participation as a preventive mechanism against disease. The plan provides for the administrative regionalization of the health services and health manpower, and details the measures to be taken for prevention, control, and care of communicable diseases. The duties of all involved in rural health care, their interdependence within the regional administrative plan, incentives, etc. are described and a training manual for auxiliary health workers is appended.

0125 Barzilai, I. *Some reflections on developing health services.* Israel Journal of Medical Sciences (Jerusalem), 4(3), May-Jun 1968, 382-389. Engl.

Fourth Rehovoth Conference on Health Problems in Developing States, Rehovoth, Israel, 15-23 Aug 1967.

See entry 96 for complete proceedings.

Lacking sufficient numbers of skilled medical personnel, developing countries need help from developed countries in construction of medical schools and medical, administrative, educational, and organizational training for young people at all levels. It is as important to ensure that half the children born do not die before the age of 5 as it is to bring down the rate of infant mortality. While waiting for the full-fledged health service to come into being, it is imperative that developing nations be helped in organizing and utilizing their human resources, particularly in the fields of sanitation and disease prevention, where intermediate medical personnel can perform basic services along the lines of successful experiments made in other countries.

0126 Bassir, O., Ogunlana, A., Adadevoh, B.K., Pearson, C.A. *Systems of health care delivery.* In Akinkugbe, O.O., Olatunbosun, D., Esan, G.J., eds., Priorities in National Health Planning: Proceedings of an International Symposium, Ibadan, Caxton Press (West Africa) Ltd., 1973, 279-298. Engl.

See entry 123 for full report of symposium.

The chapter deals with four papers presented on systems of health care delivery. The first paper lists a number of problems in the medical care delivery system: shortage of doctors; inadequate laboratory facilities; shortage of drugs; poor feeding procedures; poor surgical facilities; environmental infection; and bribery from the porter to the consultant. It discusses methods of training medical personnel in addition to remuneration for work done. Paper two calls for a concerted effort of health educators in designing, planning, and effecting an appropriate, coordinated, and fully integrated training programme to meet the demand for health personnel in Nigeria. The third paper emphasizes the need for the development of a comprehensive laboratory service for health care delivery in developing countries. And the final paper draws attention to the operations of the Under Fives Clinics, which treat children under 5 years of age, as well as the basic requirements for such a clinic: buildings, equipment, staff, and supporting services. It indicates that with the aid of such clinics child mortality was reduced from 49 to 11% in 10 years. Subsequent discussions centred attention on: (1) classification of health problems into short-term and long-term ones; (2) setting up of planning committees at State and Federal levels; (3) the need for social participation; (4) the need to have specific conclusions of the symposium for Nigeria's Third Development Plan; (5) making better use of the "native doctors" and the traditional midwives in social health delivery; and (6) relieving doctors of excessive and often unnecessary responsibilities.

0127 Bennett, F.J. *Health care systems in Africa for the delivery of services to the family.* Dar es Salaam, University of Dar es Salaam, Faculty of Medicine, 1973. 18p. Engl.

Unpublished document. Paper presented at the Parenthood Association of Sierra Leone Conference on the Health of the Family, 17-21 Sep 1973.

Family health services are organized and operated at two main levels, a rural district and a moderate-size town. Health care systems in the rural area presently include: (1) district hospital-health centre-dispensary system, in which the health centre is most attuned to family care; (2) traditional medical system, with diviners, herbalists, traditional midwives, etc., who if trained, could be incorporated within government health care plans; (3) mobile health services, delivering

II Organization and Planning

a variety of services (immunization, child nutrition, family planning, etc.), in some instances working outward from the health centre; (4) voluntary agency or mission hospital, charging for services, and separate from the government system; (5) self-help village services, where villagers are highly motivated to build and staff a health centre or dispensary; (6) multiple single-purpose services; (7) cooperative services; and (8) private practitioners. In urban areas, systems such as: (1) the large regional referral hospital; (2) home visiting services; and (3) city health departments are in operation. In some African countries coordination of systems for the benefit of families should be a priority; if the family is taken as the unit of health care, services can become very effective. Fourteen references are listed.

0128 Boletin de la Oficina Sanitaria Panamericana, Washington, D.C. *Atencion medica en las areas rurales. (Medical care in rural areas).* Boletin de la Oficina Sanitaria Panamericana (Washington, D.C.), 64, Jan 1968, 29-38. Span.

Medical care services advance in direct relation to the progress made in industry, agriculture, and trade in any given country or area. But scientific advances, in addition to helping attain high calibre medical services, also tend to increase the cost of such services. It often happens that when institutions defray the costs of medical care, it tends to be of inferior quality, particularly in rural areas. Also, there is usually a large concentration of physicians in the cities whereas the surrounding rural areas lack even the most elementary care services. In some countries Social Security medical care services have attempted to solve the problem by offering ambulatory services in out-patient clinics and on occasion by renting hospital beds in establishments belonging to health ministries or charitable institutions, but these measures have not succeeded in meeting the needs of the people. The health ministries have also offered medical care services on an even more extensive scale than Social Security institutions. Although such care is far from sufficient, it has become an established right of the rural community. Improvement of rural services is indicated in the infant and child mortality curves, the availability of drinking water, indexes of immunization against communicable diseases, etc. The lack of satisfactory financing and qualified personnel has led to agreements between Ministries and other institutions in such countries as Peru, Venezuela, Mexico, and Chile, for the purpose of protecting the rural communities. In Chile, for example, 76 rural hospitals and 461 rural posts were built to provide health care services to the rural population. In view of the difficulty of obtaining sufficient numbers of qualified personnel, the building of regional hospitals is recommended in order that they may collaborate closely with rural hospitals and these may benefit from all scientific advances and would give economic protection to the patient and his family. Twelve references are listed. (Journal abstract.)

0129 Bright, M. *Demographic base for health planning.* In Reinke, W.A., ed., Health Planning: Qualitative Aspects and Quantitative Techniques, Baltimore, Md., Johns Hopkins University, 1972, 138-157. Engl.

Demography is the study of the size, territorial distribution, and composition of the population. It includes the components of population change, i.e. fertility, mortality, migration, and the changing characteristics of population. Specific data needed for health planning include statistics on the crude death rate, the age-specific death rate, the age-sex-cause specific death rate, and the infant mortality rate. This information is incomplete at present. Appropriate methods for various types of planning, from local health services to a national analysis of health service distribution, are discussed. Examples are taken from developing countries. Eleven references are listed, with additional recommended readings.

0130 Campbell, E.P. *Health and development: Brazil.* n.p., Sep 1967. 24p. Engl.
Unpublished document.

In Brazil, goals set for health development are not being achieved because of a shortage of trained health manpower and the absence of investment in human resources. Of the total population, 60% occupy one-third of the territory. There are strong currents of internal migration with attendant health and economic problems. The population is growing at a rate of about 3.1% per year. Efforts are being made to improve the number and distribution pattern of physicians. There is less than one-third the necessary auxiliary personnel to back up the physicians. Brazil's northeast and southeast are compared with respect to human resource potential. Life expectancy and maturity and literacy variables are discussed, with the conclusion that the difference between the economic potentials of the two areas is very great, the GNP for the average southeast family being five times that of a northeast family. Brazilian families invest in their children, but in the northeast, returns are small, the tremendous loss from infant mortality, disease, and malnutrition creating a precarious social and economic structure. It is recommended that Brazil: (1) emphasize disease prevention; (2) train prevention-minded health personnel; (3) employ modern planning processes to develop health objectives; (4) stimulate the investment concept in health development; (5) use medical technology to eradicate and control communicable diseases; and (6) take advantage of bilateral and multilateral technical assistance. Statistical data on various aspects of health and manpower are presented. Thirteen references are listed.

0131 Candau, M.G. *Keynote address: knowledge, the bridge to achievement.* Israel Journal of Medical Sciences (Jerusalem), 4(3), May-Jun 1968, 343-349. Engl.
Fourth Rehovoth Conference on Health Problems in Developing States, Rehovoth, Israel, 15-23 Aug 1967.
See entry 96 for complete proceedings.

The keynote address of the Fourth Rehovoth Conference on Health Problems in Developing States stresses that health problems in developing countries are complex and varied and that innovative solutions are required. An "ecological" approach of an interdisciplinary nature must be used to solve health problems. Developmental projects do not solve problems in isolation from one another, but require coordinated planning so that solutions to one problem do not create new hazards.

0132   Chakravarti, D.N., Bhattacharjee, B.N. *Pattern of health service in a developing economy.* Indian Journal of Public Health (Calcutta), 11(1), Jan 1967, 23-24. Engl.

Comments from a group of speakers on the delivery of health care in a developing country (India) are reported. Although various speakers emphasized comprehensiveness of care, economic determinants that limit care, planning and political processes, and personnel training, conclusions by the rapporteur suggest rural Bengal's population is making specific demands for modern specialized medical care in preference to indigenous care. There is evidence that rural people are willing to organize to pay for such care at the local level.

0133   Chang, W.P. WHO, Alexandria. *Assignment report: supervisory team for health centres in the Empire of Ethiopia, October 1962-February 1967.* WHO, Geneva, Mar 1967. 23p. WHO/EM/PHA/115. Ethiopia 25/R UNICEF. Engl.

Supervision of health centres in Ethiopia has become an urgent problem. A team of coordinated specialists was established to supervise health centres and to advise the Ministry of Public Health concerning development of basic health services. The team makes short field visits and advises rural health centre staff. Health stations or subcentres are operating poorly due to isolation. Data collected at centres is uneven, making evaluation difficult. However, data indicate that in isolated centres, costs for services are high in relation to benefits derived. Site selection for centres needs to be carefully considered. Manuals of procedures for health centre operations are described and recommendations for future supervisory team work are presented.

0134   Corsa, L., Oakley, D. *Consequences of population growth for health services in less developed countries: an initial appraisal.* Ann Arbor, Michigan, University of Michigan, School of Public Health, Department of Population Planning, Population Reprint Series, Reprint No. 45, 1971. 36p. Engl.

Consequences of population growth for health services in less developed countries are appraised, pointing out the lack of adequate data on mortality, morbidity, and utilization of health services. Planners in developing countries need this kind of data to estimate need for services. Investment in the reduction of natality in most countries will enable these countries to invest in other aspects of development, beyond basic maternal and child care. The value of reducing natality is so great that the WHO together with individual governments should invest in such programmes with efforts equal to those shown in earlier years to eradicate such diseases as malaria. Reduced birth rates have implications for school planning, industrialization and jobs, housing, food, agriculture, national income, and income distribution. Forty-eight references are listed.

0135   de Silva, D.M. *Public health and sanitation measures as factors affecting mortality trends in Ceylon.* New York, United Nations, 1954. 28p. UN/E/CONF.13/413. Engl.

Fertility and mortality trends in Sri Lanka are examined in light of the health and sanitation measures that have most affected them. These public health efforts have reduced death rates from cholera, smallpox, plague, malaria, tuberculosis, and endemic disease. Prenatal clinics started in Colombo in 1921 have helped reduce maternal and child mortality. Future attention on malnutrition in Sri Lanka could be expected to favourably affect mortality trends.

0136   Deshaies, J.C., Seidman, D.R. *Health information systems.* Socio-Economic Planning Sciences (Elmsford, N.Y.), 5(6), Dec 1971, 515-533. Engl.

The purpose of this article is to describe the definition and scope of health information systems. Specifically, the article seeks to identify the types and sources of data for health information systems; to present a sample of useful indicators derived from these data; to describe some techniques that may be used to portray and analyze these indicators and to discuss various categories of uses of health information systems. The health information system subject matter contact is limited to five broad areas: (1) status of community health; (2) utilization of health services; (3) general population and housing characteristics; (4) inventory of health facilities and health service manpower; and (5) status of community environment. Seventeen references are listed. (Journal abstract.)

0137   Elebute, E.A. *Problem of under-doctored areas: the place of surgical aides and of services ancillary to surgery.* Journal of the Royal College of Surgeons of Edinburgh (Edinburgh), 16(1), Jan 1971, 177-184. Engl.

Health services in Nigeria are unevenly distributed, with wide differences in doctor/population ratios from state to state. Herbalists and native doctors predominate because of a lack of modern medical facilities. Although the UN suggests that medical assistants be developed to relieve medical problems in developing coutries, this recommendation presupposes the existence of an organized health service and qualified supervising physicians. This is especially an important consideration if surgical medical assistants are to be developed for a country like Nigeria. The need for qualified supervisory physicians necessitates rapid development of medical doctors. At present, almost all African surgeons are trained in Europe or America. The author

II Organization and Planning

recommends support for in-country training of surgeons and development of more adequate medical facilities in general.

0138 Fendall, N.R. *Organization of health services in emerging countries.* Lancet (London), 11 Jul 1964, 53-56. Engl.

Four essential components of the Ministry of Health in a developing country should be a research and evaluation unit, a planning and policymaking unit, a personnel training unit, and a health service unit. Since developing countries are primarily agricultural, top priority must be given to health services for the 80% of the population who live on the land. Training and its planning, especially for auxiliary health workers, should be adapted to local needs. There is a need to develop flexible health workers for remote posts who are trained to deliver comprehensive preventive and curative services rather than specialized care.

0139 Fendall, N.R. *Planning health services in developing countries.* Public Health Reports (Washington, D.C.), 78(11), Nov 1963, 977-988. Engl.

Limited economic resources, scarce technological manpower, and population growth need to be considered in planning health services for developing countries. In Kenya, integrated curative and preventive care is provided through a structure of rural health centres. Hospitals serve populations within a 10-mile radius, whereas health centres serve greater numbers of persons at greatly reduced costs per illness. Lack of long-term health planning for developing areas, and reliance on short-term pilot projects that are not applicable nationally, hinder progress. Unquestioned application of health service practices from developed countries leads to programme failures. Preventive and curative approaches to care need to be balanced and integrated to provide universal low cost health care. Sixteen references are listed.

0140 Ferrand, G.J. WHO, Manila. *Report on a field visit to Korea, 24 February-7 March 1969.* Manila, WHO, 15 Jul 1969. 10p. WHO/WPR/CHS/FR/7. Korea - 0025 (WP) P7/76/2. Engl.

Following a field visit to South Korea, a WHO consultant recommends that the staffing pattern be completed with the recruitment of assistant sanitarians. Local training should be organized to enable all the health personnel doing single-purpose work to become multipurpose health aides. A detailed schedule of work for the health aides should be prepared; a checklist of activities would cover tuberculosis, maternal and child health, family planning, and malaria active case detection. Supervision by trained public health nurses is recommended. Demonstration areas should be developed in each province and activities should be evaluated to estimate the health service's impact on the population.

0141 Fisek, N.H. *Health planning in Turkey: as an example for planning in developing countries.* Annales de la Societe Belge de Medicine Tropicale (Brussels), 48(3), 1968, 381-392. Engl.

A discussion follows the paper.

The master plan of developing countries has to be designed at the national level and regional and local plans should be drawn up within that framework. Turkey's health plan is presented here as an example for health planning in developing countries. Priority has been given to expansion of the national health service, which is to extend to even the smallest communities and to lay stress on home and outpatient treatment rather than on a more extensive system of hospitalization. A compulsory health insurance system for nonagricultural workers will help finance the programme. Before the final document is drafted, technical decisions concerning organizational pattern, manpower problems, priorities, targets, etc. have to be made. These depend on the availability to planners of accurate statistics on resources. Drafting of the final phase of a plan also requires decisions on timing and location of organizational units. Execution of plans is as important as their formulation, the ultimate aim being to give maximum service to the people at minimum cost. As a result of health planning in Turkey, the health budget rose from around 3% prior to planning, and reached 15% in the plan period. Prior to the plan there were few medical doctors practicing in rural areas; by 1968 there were nearly 600. The number of nurses and midwives graduated annually used to be around 500. During the plan period the number of graduates increased three times and is expected to double in 5 years.

0142 Gale, G.W. *Health service problems in developing countries.* Royal Society of Health Journal (London), 93, Jan 1973, 17-18,28. Engl.

Western sanitary health measures have helped reduce mortality and increase populations in developing countries. Modern curative health services from the West are now attractive to non-Western populations, who actively demand them. Because population continues to increase rapidly, it becomes less and less possible to meet citizens' demands for health care. A large part of the blame for failure to meet rising demands must fall on the "hospital fixation" of Western medical training now applied in developing countries. Hospital-trained medical personnel are not trained to deal with the many kinds of illness that are not seen in hospitals. It is necessary to train physicians in medical sociology and to provide them with practical experiences in health centres and with auxiliary health workers.

0143 Gilbert, D.N., Greenberg, J.H. *Vietnam: preventive medicine orientation.* Military Medicine (Washington, D.C.), 132(10), Oct 1967, 769-790. Engl.

Awareness of disease hazards in the environment and contact with the native population helped U.S. Army medical personnel in South Vietnam diagnose, treat, prevent, and control disease among the troops. Sixty-eight references are listed.

0144 Gill, P.S., Prasad, B.G. *Some thoughts on school health service for rural areas of India.* Journal of the Indian Medical Association (Calcutta), 53, 1 Aug 1969, 156-158. Engl.

Although a 1961 School Health Committee recommended developing school health service through supplementing the staff of the primary health centre with four auxiliary nurse-midwives and one medical officer, the scheme has not proved practical. A study of 810 children in Lucknow illustrates typical problems that the children may have. Most were from large, rural, poor families. They were poorly dressed and without shoes. Families of the children used the open field for latrines and water was typically drawn from open wells. Standards of personal hygiene were poor although the children's knowledge of health was better than their urban contemporaries. Military recruitment records at a recruitment centre in Uttar Pradesh showed a rejection rate, on the basis of health defects, of 93.8%. Most defects were preventable. The problem of reaching rural school children is a difficult one simply in terms of the size of the problems alone. School health services for rural children will have to rely on paramedical workers for a long time to come. A scheme for developing a programme in stages is described. It is suggested that one or two volunteer teachers from each primary school be trained to work as part-time paramedical workers and health guides. Similarly one or two teachers could be selected from a group of 10-15 primary schools to be trained and attached to primary health centres for work in schools. Eleven references are listed.

0145 Gish, O. Intermediate Technology Development Group, London. *Towards an appropriate health care technology.* In Gish, O., ed., Health Manpower and the Medical Auxiliary, London, Intermediate Technology Development Group, 1971, 11-23. Engl.
See also entries 12 and 34.

The mere existence of advanced techniques does not assure their successful application to the problems of developing countries. There are three basic reasons why planning for health care must be radically different in rich and poor countries: (1) there are different levels of resources (money and skilled manpower) available to rich and poor countries; (2) the population structures and distributions differ; and (3) poor countries have drastically different disease patterns from rich ones, with half or more than half of all deaths occurring in children under five. Health centre service, or a system of aid stations and mobile clinics run from health centres, is required in poor countries. Health centres can be operated by a variety of paramedical staff, including the medical assistant. Doctors must be trained to lead teams of medical auxiliaries. Maternal and child health care must be an integral part of the health centre's activities.

0146 Gish, O. *Health planning in developing countries.* Journal of Development Studies (London), 6(4), Jul 1970, 67-75. Engl.

Health care in poor countries with limited resources and trained manpower must rely heavily on small rural health centres that can reach the majority of people; large hospitals with costly equipment and specialized personnel should be deemphasized. Many of the diseases prevalent in these countries can be effectively countered by this approach.

0147 Gonzalez, C.L. WHO, Geneva. *Mass campaigns and general health services.* Geneva, WHO Public Health Papers No. 29, 1965. 87p. Engl.

Two possible approaches to the problem of health in developing countries are discussed, i.e. building up a framework of general health services able to deal in due course with the prevalent diseases, or attacking the principal diseases by mass campaigns. The role of general health services in mass campaigns, and suggested approaches to conducting mass campaigns are considered. Specific examples are given from India, Taiwan, Togo, and Thailand.

0148 Gourley, G. *Helping the client use health care services.* n.p., Feb 1966. 15p. Engl.

Although the incidence of communicable and chronic disease is higher among low income groups (in the USA) than in the rest of the population, these groups do not take advantage of available health resources. Social workers should give more attention to medical aspects of health problems. The social worker must first have some basic medical knowledge. The way medical services are provided must be changed so that families can follow medical recommendations. Clinics and other services must be psychologically as well as physically available, i.e. health personnel must be positive toward clients. Social scientists can point out how cultural values affect attitudes toward medical care. There must be a team approach in medical social work, with doctor and social worker sharing in patient care. The integration of these services is essential to family welfare. Six references are listed.

0149 Haraldson, S. *Appraisal of health problems and definition of priorities in health planning.* Ethiopian Medical Journal (Addis Ababa), 8, 1970, 37-44. Engl.

This paper explores the relationship between health planning and general national and socioeconomic planning in developing countries (the author is writing from Ethiopia but seems not to mention that country by specific reference). Evaluation and reporting are necessary for effecting planning and decision making. In countries with limited resources the importance for careful ordering of priorities and of health planning is stressed. Even where statistics are lacking, observational information and data from personal experience should take precedence over political pressure as a tool in decision making. Political favouritism conflicts with objective information and ordering of priorities.

0150 Hilleboe, H.E., Barkhuus, A., Thomas, W.C. WHO, Geneva. *Approaches to national health* *planning.* Geneva, WHO Public Health Papers No. 46, 1972. 108p. Engl.

Various approaches to national health planning are considered, including the experiences of India, the USSR, Sweden, the USA and PAHO-CENDES (Pan American Health Organization – Centre for Development Studies). Health manpower planning in Peru, Taiwan, and Turkey is discussed.

0151 Hilleboe, H.E. WHO, Geneva. *Mass health examinations as a public health tool.* In Mass Health Examinations, Geneva, WHO Public Health Papers No. 45, 1971, 28-39. Engl.

Like relatives who have come for an indeterminate visit to your home, mass health examinations are here to stay. Let us make the most of them. There are values in and limitations to mass health examinations as a public health tool; however, it is possible to increase the values and decrease the limitations. In this brief presentation, some remedies are suggested from the point of view of a health administrator. Firstly, the use of modern planning processes is indispensable in developing the role of mass health examinations in projects, programmes, and delivery systems. Secondly, evaluation, which relates results to goals, is essential in both the planning and the implementation of mass health examinations. Thirdly, research on a broad basis in the public health aspects of mass health examinations is the key to unlocking the mysteries that still baffle us as we extend and diversify the use of this public health tool with the hope of improving human health and social well-being. (Author abstract.)

0152 Hinman, E.H. *Health and economic development in tropical Africa.* Archives of Environmental Health (Chicago), 10(3), Mar 1965, 481-492. Engl.

Africans in the 1960's expressed a desire for national independence and freedom from poverty, hunger, ignorance, and disease. The rural character of the populations and limited transportation have restricted health care improvements. Malaria is being tackled by preventive measures such as semiannual residual spraying. For a number of years programmes have been underway for control of schistosomiasis, trypanosomiasis, onchocerciasis, and other prevalent diseases. Scarcity of trained personnel is a major factor impeding progress; funds need to be used to develop health manpower. Investments in the health improvement of rural agricultural people is necessary for economic development. Seven references are listed.

0153 Horwitz, A. *Health, population, and development in Latin America.* In Sobrero, A.J., Lewit, S., eds., Advances in Planned Parenthood, New York, Excerpta Medica Foundation, 1969, vol 4, 3-8. Engl.

Sixth Annual Meeting of the American Association of Planned Parenthood Physicians, San Antonio, Texas, 16-17 Apr 1968.

Health care cannot be organized as a separate entity in a society. Health issues are related to the demographic and socioeconomic profile, which, in Latin America shows a young, predominantly rural population, a birth rate of over 40 per 1 000 population, a life expectation of 50-60 years, high illiteracy, low productivity, low and unevenly distributed income, chronic underemployment, and poor nutrition. Population dynamics is obviously a key issue in health care. WHO and PAHO are prepared to support family planning programmes, once the governments of these countries have established independent policies on the subject. Six references are listed.

0154 Hughes, J.P. *Economic development and the health planner: opportunity or handicap?* In Hughes, J.P., ed., Health Care for Remote Areas: An International Conference, Oakland, Kaiser Foundation, 1972, 7-24. Engl.

See entry 155 for complete proceedings.

Work projects frequently begin without plans for the health of the workers involved. The Volta River dam project provided the setting for a model health system in a work environment. Experiences of the Kaiser Foundation in providing health care for workers in Jamaica, Ghana, Ivory Coast, and Nigeria are given.

0155 Hughes, J.P., ed(s). *Health care in remote areas: an International Conference.* Oakland, California, Kaiser Foundation International, 1972. 163p. Engl.

Proceedings of an International Conference sponsored by Kaiser Foundation International, Bellagio, Italy, May 1972.

Individual articles have been abstracted separately under entries 154, 241, 253, 256, 285, 414, 476, 498, and 608.

This publication is a collection of papers concerning health care for remote areas and contains discussions on various issues related to specialized health care, maternal and child health, and auxiliary health worker training.

0156 Janer, J.L., Arbona, G. *Place of demography in health and welfare planning in Latin America.* Milbank Memorial Fund Quarterly (New York), 42(no. 2, pt. 2), Apr 1964, 328-345. Engl.

A discussion follows the paper.

Demography constitutes nowadays one of the most useful tools in planning properly for actions directed at the promotion of any aspect of the collective well-being of human populations. Therefore, it must be considered an essential tool in planning for health and welfare. Demography's role in planning is even more important when the object of the action programmes involved is an underdeveloped country. Consequently, it has become imperative to include social demography as a required subject in any course intended to train individuals for professional work related to the promotion of collective well-being in human populations. Twenty-six references are listed. (Author abstract.)

0157 Johnson, G.Z. *Public health activities as factors in levels and trends of mortality and morbidity in developing countries.* New York, United Nations, 1965. 6p. UN/WPC/WP/418. Engl.

United Nations World Population Conference, Belgrade, Yugoslavia, 30 Aug-10 Sep 1965.

This paper attempts to show what role health services have played in reducing mortality and morbidity in developing countries. Infant and early childhood mortality rates have been found to be the most sensitive indicators of community living standards. Decreases in mortality in this group can be largely accounted for by public health measures. Prenatal care, improved urban water supplies, and disease control campaigns have had a marked effect on lowered death rates for this age group. Mortality rates do not vary systematically with rural or urban residency, for countries in which the data were examined. More progress has been made in supplying good water to urban than to rural areas. Twenty references are listed.

0158 Kesic, B. *Rural health problems and some aspects of their solution.* Israel Journal of Medical Sciences (Jerusalem), 4(3), May-Jun 1968, 544-552. Engl.

Fourth Rehovoth Conference on Health Problems in Developing States, Rehovoth, Israel, 15-23 Aug 1967.

See entry 96 for complete proceedings.

Medical protection for rural populations is primarily a social and economic problem. Much of the per capita spending on health in developing countries goes to developed countries for purchasing drugs and equipment, for education of health workers, etc. Administrators should realize health problems can be tackled by rural people themselves. Health activities should be an integrated part of a unified plan for development of the rural area. Total health care coverage through health centres and substations should be the goal, and teamwork should be the basic tenet for carrying out all health activities.

0159 King, M. *Personal health care: the quest for a human right.* In Elliott, K., Knight, J., eds., Human Rights in Health, Amsterdam, Elsevier, 1974, 227-243. Engl.

Delivered at the CIBA Symposium on Human Rights in Health Care, London, Jul 1973.

A discussion follows the paper.

A health care package is defined as an integrated set of components promoting the application of a particular group of "interventions" — a convenient name for such medical procedures as administering a polio vaccine or penicillin, or even transplanting a kidney — for the improvement of health care under specific socioeconomic conditions. Such interventions, which constitute health care, can be simple or complex, expensive or cheap, but many are closely clustered or associated, so that if one is available, another can be provided at little extra cost. Hierarchical scales of interventions can be constructed for clinical pathology, surgery, radiology, etc. in terms of what health units in developing countries are capable of doing. The well-designed health care package is one that augments scarce technical, administrative, and educational skills. Priority needs for developing countries are delivery of outpatient rather than inpatient care, maternal and child care, simple surgical and laboratory services, such as blood transfusion. The contents of such packages by their nature define basic rights in personal health care and establish a basis for judging quality as well as quantity of services provided. Five references are listed.

0160 King, M. *Standard technology - the health care package.* Surabaya, Indonesia, The Lembaga Kesehatan Nasional, n.d. 6p. Engl.

Unpublished document.

With a view to reducing the need for each country to design standard service systems, health care "packages" to fit health centre and staff needs in about 50 countries, where their relevance is guaranteed by similarity of socioeconomic conditions, are proposed. Packages, including manuals with a "how-to-do-it" approach, must be applicable, easily comprehensible, translatable, and technique-oriented. Although not a panacea for poor services, indiscipline, and indifference, such packages may go a step further toward defining basic rights to health care. Three references are listed.

0161 Kpedekpo, G.M. *Planning and design of sampling surveys with particular reference to the epidemiological survey of the Danfa project in Ghana.* Ghana Medical Journal (Accra), 11(4), Dec 1972, 377-382. Engl.

Planning a sample survey begins with consideration of survey objectives, geographical coverage, methods of data collection, questionnaire design, sample design, selection and training of interviewers, etc. Consultation at the planning stage is essential. Possible sample designs include simple random, systematic, stratified, cluster, and multistage designs, or a combination of these. The author describes a sample design for an integrated multisubject health survey.

0162 Lathem, W., Newbery, A., ed(s). *Community medicine: teaching, research, and health care.* New York, Appleton-Century-Crofts, 1970. 342p. Engl.

Individual articles have been abstracted separately under entries 184, 376, 379, 384, 385, 386, 401, and 402.

This book records a conference on community medicine, at which medical educators, health administrators, government officials, and foundation executives from five continents discussed health needs, health systems, educational institutions, and the development of community medicine in their respective countries. In one section, programmes in community medicine at six universities in developing countries are described; in the other, the following aspects of community medicine are examined in detail: objectives, development of improved health care systems, the education, training, and utilization of health personnel, influence of cultural attitudes, relationship between universities and the government, etc.

0163 Long, E.C., ed(s). *Health objectives for the developing society: responsibility of individual, physician and community.* Durham, N.C., Duke University Press, 1965. 163p. Engl.

This seminar report emphasizes the development of health programmes in rural communities. Papers presented by various authors discuss health problems in rural areas of developing and developed nations; the achievements of the World Health Organization in the Western hemisphere; the particular requirements of Brazil, Canada, and southeastern United States (rural areas); the role of the individual, the physician, and the community in rural health; and the future possibilities of comprehensive health services.

0164 Lucas, A.O. *Public health priorities and population pressure in developing countries.* In Caldwell, J.C., Okonjo, C., eds., The Population of Tropical Africa, New York, Columbia University Press, 1968, 376-378. Engl.

Successful application of public health measures in developing countries has resulted in rapid population growth. This paper examines the consideration health planners need to make to decide on future health priorities. Highest mortality rates are found among infants and during early childhood. These would seem to point to a need to reduce death rates among this group and also among pregnant women. Since 50% of the population in many of these countries is under 14 years of age, the maternal and child health priority would seem to be clear. However, it would seem necessary to balance the needs of this group against the needs of the rest of the community. Priorities in health must relate to needs for economic development. If lasting progress is to be made in the area of health, it is necessary to make comparable advances in the economic area. For this reason the health of the productive members of society should be protected while the health of dependent members is cared for. Occupational health measures in developing countries today reach only a very few workers connected with government or industrial projects. The health, productivity, and life expectancy of agricultural workers need to be considered in planning for adequate health services. Five references are listed.

0165 Medina, E., Kaempffer, A.M. *Metodologia de la planificacion de salud en Chile. (Health planning methodology in Chile).* Revista Medica de Chile (Santiago), 96, Apr 1968, 282-287. Span.

The authors discuss health care planning from an administrative viewpoint of preparing long-term plans to obtain larger budgetary allocations from government sources. They enumerate institutional health services provided by the National Health Service of Chile, presenting a breakdown of hospital costs as they relate to the number of patients treated in each illness group, establishing mathematical models to calculate efficiency ratios in terms of deaths prevented and the cost of each death prevented.

0166 Mehta, S.A. *Priorities in planning balanced national community development.* Journal of Medical Education (Chicago), 43, Feb 1968, 185-189. Engl.

In her Fourth Five Year Plan, India gave highest priority to agricultural and industrial production for exports and import replacement in order to achieve economic self-reliance as soon as possible. Following this were plans for price stability, an increase in the production of food and agricultural raw materials, and the rise of rural incomes. Other priorities included the production of fertilizers and pesticides, textiles, sugar, drugs, and other items for mass consumption. Social services were to be extended to develop human resources. The only valid generalization regarding the priorities of planning is that in developing countries social services such as health and education are important in making agricultural and industrial planning viable, and vice versa. Each country has to work out its own priorities.

0167 Messing, S.D. *Social problems related to the development of health in Ethiopia.* Social Science and Medicine (Oxford), 3, Jan 1970, 331-337. Engl.

The relationship between the development of public health programmes and "social problems" is of increasing concern to students of social and cultural problems. Health is obviously related to the availability of good nutrition, which is essential in building resistance to contagious diseases that form the bulk of preventable health problems in underdeveloped countries. Good nutrition, in turn, is dependent upon availability of agricultural products, basic income to buy them, and education to utilize them properly. This article attempts to trace, briefly, some of the etiology of these interrelated problems in a country in which traditional values have not been distorted by a foreign-established colonial period, and which has experienced only superficial change in modern times. This makes it possible to view relationships more clearly than in other underdeveloped countries where they may exist in more complex forms. Fourteen references are listed. (Journal abstract.)

0168 Meyer-Lie, A. Ethiopia, Ministry of Public Health. *Existing and planned public health services in Ethiopia.* Addis Ababa, Ministry of Public Health, Jan 1971. 8p. Engl.
Unpublished document.

Reorganization of health services in Ethiopia emphasizing improved quality of service is reported. Hospital building is progressing and the appointment in several provinces of Ethiopian physicians with public health training promises to have a good effect. Health centres are the major instruments in preventive work, but while preventive services are desirable, the demand for curative services is overwhelming and lack of understanding of prevention hinders progress. Furthermore, the policy being to decentralize rural health care, supervision becomes difficult; centres are understaffed and staff are cut off from contact with colleagues. Refresher courses are planned for staff based in the provinces. A maternal and child health programme is being studied. Outbreaks of sleeping sickness and cholera, relatively new diseases in Ethiopia, have so far been controlled. Mass immunization, protection of wells, sewage disposal, citizen awareness campaigns, international help in setting up clinics, and training in case recognition and treatment have done much to reduce the threat of further outbreaks. At current (1971) population growth rates, expanded and improved health services will be needed. To finance this, perhaps a national health insurance scheme could be developed, as current resources alone will not suffice.

0169 Navarro, V. *Health, health services, and health planning in Cuba.* International Journal of Health Services (Westport, Conn.), 2(3), Aug 1972, 397-432. Engl.

The profound changes that have occurred in the Cuban health services since 1958 are described and appraised in this article. The first part treats the main socioeconomic policies, particularly the urban and agrarian reforms, that have had an equalizing effect on the distribution of resources (including health resources) between regions and social classes. These socioeconomic developments have determined changes in mortality and morbidity patterns, particularly in the control of waterborne diseases, in the reduction of the level of malnutrition, and in the increasing prevalence of chronic conditions. The second part describes the main characteristics of the health services development in the last decade: centralization of inpatient facilities; decentralization of ambulatory ones; and the training of large numbers of physicians, paramedical personnel, and, especially, auxiliary personnel. The health services are structured according to a regional model that aims at the integration of preventive with curative services, personal with environmental, and medical with social services. Within this model, great priority is given to primary care, especially in the rural areas, where the greatest benefits of the restructuring of the system have been realized. The education and training of human resources, particularly of physicians, in response to the requirements of the system and the flight of nearly half the medical manpower after the Revolution, are also discussed in this section. The third part of the article describes the process of decision-making and planning in Cuba today, with special emphasis on the health sector. This process is highly centralized in plan preparation but highly decentralized in plan implementation. The medical profession has a definitive and decisive influence in the preparation of the plans, through the very powerful advisory planning task forces. The advantages and disadvantages of this active participation are discussed. Plan implementation is accomplished with massive participation by the population and its organs, the mass organizations, which partly explains the great achievements of the public health programmes. The relationship between decision-makers and planners, not always an easy one, is also analyzed. Forty-six references are listed. (Author abstract.)

0170 Navarro, V. *Systems analysis in the health field.* Socio-Economic Planning Sciences (Elmsford, N.Y.), 3(3), Oct 1969, 179-189. Engl.

This paper reviews the application of systems analysis to the planning of health services. Planning models that have employed a systems approach in the health field are critically examined, their strengths and limitations are considered, and areas where more research is needed are indicated. New approaches that attempt to eliminate these limitations are presented. The use of health indices as performance indicators and their use as intrinsic variables in the models of development are also critically examined. Sixty-two references are listed. (Journal abstract.)

0171 Nepal, Ministry of Health. *Nepal: general data relative to health services, 15 November 1971.* Kathmandu, Ministry of Health, 1971. 15p. Engl.

Unpublished document.

General data relative to health services, population distribution, hospitals, and the need for specialists in Nepal's Fourth Five Year Plan, 1971, are presented. A progress report for family planning and maternal and child health is included.

0172 Okediji, F.O. *Public health promotion in Nigeria: a sociological viewpoint.* Ibadan: A Journal published at the University of Ibadan (Ibadan), (26), Feb 1969, 25-29. Engl.

Four main social problem areas relate to ill health in Nigeria. First, a large number of illiterate Nigerians fail to see any correlation between health of their families and the overall environment in which they live and work. Secondly, public health officers emphasize curative rather than preventive medicine. Thirdly, persons living in crowded urban areas are unwilling to move to rural areas because family members see such a move as evidence of personal failure. Finally, public health has low priority with the federal government, and therefore local communities must themselves remobilize to finance and operate their own environmental sanitation and health projects. Health promotion at the individual, family, community, and federal levels must be coordinated.

0173 Otolorin, M.P. *Priorities in medical services.* Israel Journal of Medical Sciences (Jerusalem), 4(3), May-Jun 1968, 368-383. Engl.

Fourth Rehovoth Conference on Health Problems in Developing States, Rehovoth, Israel, 15-23 Aug 1967.

See entry 96 for complete proceedings.

Developing countries forced to make plans for health services in the absence of reliable statistical data and confronted by a bewildering number of patterns set by developed countries can follow three broad principles: (1) plans must be capable of being executed under the

II Organization and Planning

system of government of the land; (2) it must be recognized that certain basic services such as water supply, housing, education, and employment, which are not within the jurisdiction of health ministries, are essential to the development of medical and health services, and must be developed parallel with them; and (3) preventive measures must be emphasized since a great portion of deaths are attributable to preventable diseases, and the integration of curative and preventive services is desirable. Health services should be financed mainly from national resources or from outright foreign loans with generous conditions of repayment. Large external debt leads to the stunting of economic growth. Planners must review the organizational and administrative framework of medical services bequeathed by the colonial administrators, with the purpose in mind of integrating curative and preventive services. Plans must be made at an early stage for establishing local schools to train medical workers and mobile health teams to provide services in rural areas. A discussion follows the paper.

0174 Passos, C. *Organizacao de cozinhas hospitalares. (Planning of hospital kitchen services).* Sao Paulo, Associacao Paulista de Hospitais, 1972. 231p. Span.

The author deals with the planning, organization, and operation of hospital nutrition and dietetic services for small, medium, and large hospitals. Specifications of all kitchen utensils and equipment are detailed, as well as the necessary administrative records. Thirteen references are listed.

0175 Patel, B.P. *Health and population planning in India.* Participant Journal (New Delhi), 4(8), Feb 1970, 27-31. Engl.

The objectives of India's health plan are: control of communicable diseases, provision of institutional facilities for medical care, improvement of environmental sanitation, safe water supply, preventive health care for rural communities, mother and child health services, development of technical manpower, and family planning and population control.

0176 Rao, N.S., Marwah, S.M. *Health statistical unit for a township with illustrations from Banaras Hindu University campus.* Indian Journal of Public Health (Calcutta), 15(3), Jul 1971, 77-82. Engl.

Well-planned health services rely on accurate statistics. In India, new townships have been established that need health statistical units. Such a unit established within the health office of each township would improve health administration and facilities, and serve as a demonstration centre for medical students. The unit would maintain a folder for every family in the township; maintain and analyze reports of births, deaths and infectious diseases; assess morbidity rates for disease prevailing in the township; and analyze student health examination records. For a township of 5 000 people an experienced health statistician should have two statistical assistants and the use of two calculating machines. In smaller townships the unit can be managed by experienced assistants. Costs should be covered by the health budget of the township. At a health statistical unit established at Banaras Hindu University, maternal and child health care and family planning services were provided utilizing the family folders, and the disease pattern of the campus population was identified by analyzing dispensary and hospital records, etc. Eleven references are listed.

0177 Reyes, W.L. *Philippine population growth and health development.* In Proceedings of the First Conference on Population, 1965, Quezon City, University of the Philippines Press, 1966, 423-468. Engl.

First Conference on Population, University of the Philippines, Quezon City, Philippines, 1965.

Since the turn of the 20th century the people of the Philippines have gradually improved their health. Outstanding progress has been made in reducing mortality rates in the world as a whole since World War II. The result has been population increase. For the future, projected estimates of rates of growth for the Philippines vary from 1.7 to 3.7% per annum depending on the conditions expected to be affecting rates. Results from this growth will undoubtedly include increased expected demand on health services, increased expenditure for health care, increased varieties of types of health workers and training facilities, and increased special health problems. Estimates for the future costs of health care should be used with caution, since a number of influences on cost are difficult to foresee. Projected costs depend on the accuracy of population estimates, accuracy of items included in cost, unit cost estimates of materials, supplies, etc., understanding and appreciation of health needs and acceptance of types of service by the public, quality improvements in care, and competition for the health dollar among other sectors of the community.

0178 Rochac, A. *Aspectos economicos de los servicios de salud en las areas rurales. (Economic aspects of health services in rural areas).* Boletin de la Oficina Sanitaria Panamericana (Washington, D.C.), 64, Jan 1968, 52-68. Span.

The life of the rural inhabitant is subject to biological and physiological cycles over which he has no control. Progress in the rural environment is limited by the following: concentrated land ownership; monoculture; low yield; weak agricultural credit; no agricultural extension; deficient marketing; and no health service infrastructure. These factors often lead him to seek refuge in the city. Shanty towns have sprung up around large cities in which the rural worker is forced to seek work for which he is not equipped. Lack of suitable housing plus poor nutrition cause serious community problems such as poor sanitation and the consequent increase in diseases. International agencies such as the Pan American Sanitary Bureau, the International Development Bank, and others have in recent years taken an interest in environmental sanitation and in the building of first aid centres in the rural areas in the hope that such actions will raise living standards. Rural health services appear to be one of the most important problems in the field of public health in Latin America. The obstacles to be overcome include the limited availability of health professional and health auxiliary personnel; the limited quantity and quality of health centres, and the uneven geographical distribution of these centres. The document recognizes that rural inhabitants cannot pay for the necessary services, as they are alienated from the economic mainstream of the country. It proposes rather, that Governments should create the necessary economic infrastructure to employ these people to give them access to all health care facilities.

0179 Schultz, G.P. *Logic of health care facility planning.* Socio-Economic Planning Sciences (Elmsford, N.Y.), 4(3), Sep 1970, 383-393. Engl.
This study presents a logical model for the planning of health care facilities. The objective is an optimal facility pattern, that is, one that maximizes net social benefit for the population of a metropolitan region. Several orders of services are defined and a successively inclusive facility hierarchy assumed for the provision of these services. A method is stated for determining the optimal scale and service area for each order. Net social benefit is computed from a set of basic functions that describe the demand for services, the unit cost of services, travel cost, and benefits derived. The geometry of location and a region-wide view of the system are discussed. Twelve references are listed. (Journal abstract.)

0180 Taylor, C.E. *A new style of international health work.* Baltimore, Johns Hopkins University, School of Hygiene and Public Health, 25 Oct 1973. 18p. Engl.
Unpublished document. Paper presented at the International Health Conference, "Health Care Systems and Human Values," Washington, D.C., 27 Apr 1973.
Social issues are changing medicine. Although health is talked about as a basic human right, the disparity between services available to the rich and poor within developing countries increases. Factors shaping health care are population growth, increased life expectancy, adaptation of Western technology to varied cultures, nutritional problems, and new donor-recipient political relationships. Development must be concentrated at the local level and approached with greater mutual collaboration between voluntary groups and developing countries. Ten references are listed.

0181 Transactions of the Royal Society of Tropical Medicine and Hygiene, London. *Medical education, research and medical care in developing countries.* Transactions of the Royal Society of Tropical Medicine and Hygiene (London), 65(6), 1971, 709-721. Engl.
Conference organized by the Royal Society of Tropical Medicine and Hygiene and the Wellcome Trust, Ditchley Park, Oxfordshire, England, 26-29 Mar 1971.

A distinguished 1969 international group designed a blueprint for development work in developing countries. Health problems were glossed over. Little appreciation was shown for the relationship between health and productivity upon which development depends. There are good reasons to consider health more seriously. Health care delivery to rural populations needs particular attention. Communicable diseases too deserve research attention because of their impact both on developed and developing countries. Britain has contributed significantly to medicine in developing countries. The conference reported on here was convened to bring doctors and health care recipients together to discuss Britain's role in assisting medical education, medical research, and medical care in developing countries. Research and aid priorities for Britain abroad are sketched. Operational research into health care delivery is high priority. In the decade ahead emphasis should be placed on provision of basic health services to as many as possible of the people who lack them.

0182 Tyrer, F.H. *Problems of occupational health in Nigeria.* Transactions of the Society of Occupational Medicine (London), 18, Jul 1968, 105-109. Engl.
Visits to a number of Nigerian factories and groups of workers indicate the need for a massive public health campaign, improved distribution of medical personnel, and better housing. There is also a need for greatly expanded curative medical services. Occupational health problems should not be allowed to make more than minimal demands on the trained manpower available. The establishment of a modest Occupational Health Institute maintaining close liaison with other medical services and the factory inspectorate is recommended.

0183 Van Die Redaksie. *Health ignorance: an indictment.* South African Medical Journal (Cape Town), 42(8), 24 Feb 1968, 173. Engl.
Editorial.
While the privileged white population of the Republic of South Africa shows Western patterns of cardiovascular disease, cancer, and mental illness, in the underprivileged communities of the Republic malnutrition is the major cause of death. Such problems reflect the social and cultural makeup of the society, and solutions cannot be found if they continue to be tackled in isolation, as in the past; they must be dealt with realistically, within the developmental framework of the society. Curative and preventive medicine, and sketchy formal education, have been used in the fight against poverty, disease, ignorance, and overpopulation in developing communities; only recently has promotive medicine been used to combat these problems. Nutrition education programmes are much needed among the less privileged in South Africa. A team approach is called for; however, one of the most important members of the health team, the health educator, is missing in South African health programmes. The author advocates that a state programme be started to train health educators, who should preferably come from the racial and cultural groups they will serve.

0184 Velazquez, G. *Community medicine as an experiment in health care.* In Lathem, W., Newbery A., eds., Community Medicine: Teaching, Research, and Health Care, New York, Appleton-Century-Crofts, 1970, 121-140. Engl.
See also entry 162.

In its beginnings, the Universidad del Valle rural health care programme concentrated too much on training professional workers and on caring for the family rather than the whole community. Failure to define objectives made evaluation and constructive self-criticism difficult, and failure to establish a methodology for measuring the level of health in the community made it impossible to perform cost-effectiveness studies. Health care policies are often defined by vociferous individuals rather than by strict measurement of community health needs. The design of health service strategies and the preparation of health workers requires baseline study of needs and resources. University departmental involvement in pilot programmes throughout the country is recommended as an approach to health studies. These departments may then serve as a central coordinating and advisory group. Use of industrial operations research methods may assist comprehensive national health planning.

0185 Venezuela, Ministry of Health. *Informe de la comision programadora del Instituto Universitario de Tecnologia de la Salud. (Report of the Planning Commission of the University Institute for Health Technology).* Caracas, Ministry of Health and Social Welfare, Nov 1973. 18p. Span.
Unpublished document.

In Venezuela health manpower resources are divided into two broad sectors: the health professionals (physician, dentist, etc.) and the nonprofessional health workers, very frequently trained while in service. The former represent 36% (or 18 000 of 50 000) and the latter 60% (30 000 of 50 000) of those involved in health care delivery. Between these two groups exists a vacuum that could be filled by the health technology occupations. This report discusses the University Institute for Health Technology and describes the structure of the Institute, courses offered, time allotted to each subject, and human and economic resources available. Courses take 2 or 3 years following secondary education.

0186 Wennen, E.C. *Developing World: health as a business.* Tropical and Geographical Medicine (Haarlem), 21, Sep 1969, 341-347. Engl.

The author's basic premise is that disease and premature death are more costly than health care. In Nigeria, the government and voluntary agencies spend great amounts of money, primarily in the curative field, which seems far less able to improve the health of the people than money spent in the preventive field. The author recommends a taxation reform, a reallocation of government spending, and an imaginative self-help policy to encourage personal hygiene. Sectors of the population needing special attention are leprosy patients, victims of the guinea-worm parasite, victims of motor accidents, and cigarette smokers. Doctors could do more if patients were first screened by a nurse, and if a flying doctor service were established. Medical manpower at all levels could be used more efficiently. Operational costs could be cut by reducing senior staff salaries, and limiting the use of expensive drugs. Health education in Nigeria is not well developed, but those teachers who give health education classes are more important in the long run than doctors.

0187 WHO, Alexandria. *Problems of rural water supply.* Alexandria, WHO, 10 Jul 1967. 15p. WHO/EM/RC17/6. Engl.
Unpublished document.

Only during the last 150 years have water purification methods been used on any great scale. Whereas large cities can often afford to bring water from great distances, rural villages have had to relocate when water supplies were scarce. Few villages, especially in the member countries of WHO's Eastern Mediterranean Region, have had adequate water supplies. WHO has contributed to maintenance of rural water supplies in Pakistan, Sudan, Iraq, and Saudi Arabia. Urban water supply problems are somewhat easier to handle than rural ones, since rural people must first be educated to accept the value of clean water.

0188 WHO, Brazzaville. *Towards a philosophy of health work in the African region.* Brazzaville, WHO Afro Technical Papers No. 1, 1970. 38p. Engl.

Public health priorities in Africa are: (1) control of communicable diseases, i.e. massive use of vaccination and pesticides to eradicate and control yellow fever, malaria, small pox, etc. and the provision of safe water supplies; (2) development of national health services, e.g. redistribution of trained health workers; and (3) training of sufficient, qualified staff, conversant with local needs and resources, and provision of training centres.

0189 WHO, Geneva. *Organizational study on methods of promoting the development of basic health services.* Official Records of the World Health Organization (Geneva), 206, 1973, 103-115. Engl.

WHO has attempted all of the obvious solutions to the promotion of the development of health services over the past years. The realities behind the lack of effective change would appear to rest upon the low priority they have been given within country programmes and the consequences at the international level; the fragmentary manner in which they have been applied; the lack of appreciation that has been given to the proper judgement that success or failure needs to be evaluated at the periphery by services delivered and health status improved; the failure to look at health services as a whole; and the absence of a clear understanding that WHO can do some things at the request of ministries of health that no other organization is able to do. WHO should identify and concentrate upon these aspects rather than attempt to give assistance across the board, which it has neither the resources to do nor the need. If it can be stated that the starting point in health service promotion and development in a national administration is a national will, it could be said equally to WHO that there is the need for an international will. (Revised journal abstract.)

0190 WHO, Geneva. *Statistical indicators for the planning and evaluation of public health programmes: fourteenth report of the WHO Expert Committee on Health Statistics.* Geneva, WHO Technical Report Series No. 472, 1971. 40p. Engl.

The committee report focusses attention on information exchange between health planner and statistician, on the types of statistics needed in various circumstances, and on how they could be used to provide meaningful health indicators. Discussion covers health information systems for health planning, education and training considerations for statistical methods in health planning, and research and development in statistical methods.

0191 WHO, Geneva. *Mass health examinations.* Geneva, WHO Public Health Papers No. 45, 1971. 99p. Engl.

Mass health examinations are discussed in the context of a wide variety of health activities, with particular reference to costs, training and manpower, records maintenance and evaluation, health education, epidemiological surveys and disease surveillance, and prescriptive screening. As a public health tool, mass health examinations have considerable value, and can be augmented by moderate planning, evaluation, and research.

0192 WHO, Geneva. *National environmental health programmes: their planning, organization, and administration. Report of a WHO Expert Committee.* Geneva, WHO Technical Report Series No. 439, 1970. 56p. Engl.

This committee report considers aspects of environmental health, such as the impact of science and technology, the backlog of needs, and the scope of environmental health. The planning of national programmes involves definition of major problems (e.g. community water supply, water treatment, air pollution, soil pollution, vector control, etc.), formulation of policies, manpower training, material resources, financing and legislation. Organization and administration of such programmes, international collaboration, public information, and evaluation of programmes are discussed.

0193 WHO, Geneva. *Water pollution control in developing countries: report of a WHO Expert Committee.* Geneva, WHO Technical Report Series No. 404, 1968. 38p. Engl.

It is important to plan water economy, including pollution control measures, early in a country's development. Discharging of sewage and industrial wastes into rivers creates serious water pollution; protection of water resources is essential for public health especially with regard to enteric disease transmitted by water, transmission of virus diseases, and contaminated fish and shellfish. Other health risks arise from chemical pollutants, and of waste water for agricultural and household purposes. In planning water resources, it is necessary to survey existing resources, identify sources of pollution, predict future needs, and coordinate regional planning with environmental health authorities. The water control programme involves different storage techniques, sewerage systems, methods of treatment e.g. irrigation and stabilizing ponds, sludge disposal, and the direct reclamation and reuse of waste water. Fundamental and applied research should be encouraged in developing countries. The training necessary for personnel (managers, university teachers, middle-grade professionals, and auxiliaries) is discussed. Outside assistance may be necessary to meet educational and staffing needs. The public must be informed, using all possible means of communication, about the dangers of water pollution.

0194 WHO, Geneva. *National health planning in developing countries: report of a WHO Expert Committee.* Geneva, WHO Technical Report Series No. 315, 1967. 40p. Engl.

A group of experts attempt to answer fundamental questions about health planning in a developing country. These questions deal with recognizing a country's readiness to plan, determining the resources it needs, and deciding how the plan will be implemented and by whom. The committee's discussion of these questions focusses on socioeconomic development, planning methods, and training for planning.

0195 WHO, Geneva. *Planning of public health services: fourth report of the Expert Committee on Public Health Administration.* Geneva, WHO Technical Report Series No. 215, 1961. 48p. Engl.

An international group of experts expresses views on the following aspects of planning for public health services: planning in relation to economic and social development; surveys as a means of gathering data; establishing priorities and objectives; and implementation and assessment of the plan. With respect to development of health programmes, the committee looks at the programme scope, determination of requirements, and administrative considerations. Illustrations are provided for public health planning as practiced in Sri Lanka, Czechoslovakia, India, the USSR, Egypt, Syria, and the U.K.

0196 WHO, Geneva. *Methodology of planning an integrated health programme for rural areas: second report of the Expert Committee on Public-Health Administration.* Geneva, WHO Technical Report Series No. 83, Jun 1954. 46p. Engl.

A committee report suggests guidelines for planning, organizing, and staffing rural health units. Financial aspects and integration of local health programmes are discussed. Staffing patterns suggested reflect standards possible in developed countries under ideal conditions. However, this report is of interest for the completeness with which ideal goals for rural health services are outlined. The report emphasizes, for instance, that the person in charge of a local health unit should always be a fully qualified and registered physician trained in public health. This early report rejects the idea of using auxiliaries for these posts.

0197 Wilson, J.M. WHO, Geneva. *Mass health examinations: a review of the subject.* In Mass Health Examinations, WHO Public Health Papers No. 45, Geneva, 1971, 9-27. Engl.

The field of mass health examinations is expanding rapidly and embraces a range of health activities, from looking for the scars of smallpox vaccination to the application of a battery of automated biochemical, haematological, and other screening tests. This paper examines the validity of tests used, the importance of establishing a suitable records system, costs in terms of manpower and other resources, staff training, establishment of priorities for any particular form of mass health examination, legal and ethical considerations, health education, epidemiological surveys, and prescriptive screening.

0198 Wolstenholme, G., O'Connor, M., ed(s). Ciba Foundation, London. *Teamwork for world health.* London, J. and A. Churchill, 1971. 242p. Engl.
Individual articles have been abstracted separately under entries 27, 74, 92, 216, 302, and 425..

In a collection of 16 papers delivered at the Symposium on Teamwork for World Health, seven papers deal specifically with health care in developing countries and especially with development and use of auxiliary health workers. A bibliography of over 30 items on rural health care is included.

II.4 Geographic distribution of health services

See also: 0032, 0121, 0130

0199 Bravo, A.L. *Development of medical care services in Latin America.* American Journal of Public Health (New York), 48(4), Apr 1958, 434-447. Engl.

This paper is a review of prevailing patterns for the provision of medical care in Latin American countries, with special reference to Chile, based on the author's personal experience. Developments in Latin America have been conditioned by local standards (political, economic, geographic, etc.). Free or compulsory prepaid medical care has become the answer to the problem created by the high incidence of diseases affecting a population that is largely unable to afford medical care.

All countries of Latin America are covered by some kind of health insurance system. By 1958 medical care services were provided free of charge or through a compulsory sickness insurance scheme for workers and their families and the medically indigent population. Some kind of public health service has existed in all Latin American countries since the colonial period. However, public health units were not widely organized until the 1930's and 40's. The state-financed public health service is responsible for environmental, educational, statistical, and preventive health activities for the whole population. Personal preventive services are provided at the local level by public health units. One hundred and ten references are listed.

0200 de Kadt, E. *Distribution of health in Chile.* Brighton, England, Institute of Development Studies, University of Sussex, Discussion Paper No. 17, May 1973. 43p. Engl.
Originally published by Centro de Estudios de Planificacion National (CEPLAN), Universidad Catolica de Chile, (Doc. S/73 No. 16 - in Spanish) under the title "Distribucion del Ingreso y Desarrollo."

Recent interest in income distribution in developing countries has drawn attention to the complementary question of welfare and its distribution. One aspect of welfare is health: this paper deals with the distribution of health care and the effectiveness of the health services in Chile. It surveys the findings of the more important studies in this field, and engages in a fairly detailed analysis by province of regularly published statistical series on infant mortality and its causes, correlating these data with broad indicators of social and economic development and of availability and use made of health services. The resulting picture is one of considerable inequality in health between main towns and countryside, more developed and "backward" provinces, low and high income groups, educated and uneducated people, well- and ill-housed families, etc. The health services have not managed to reach those most in need, and it is obvious that their organization has not been appropriate to this task. The present government has sought to improve the situation by various measures, including the formulation of schemes to involve the population through community organizations in the health care system; these schemes are discussed and some first impressions of problems and achievements are given, as well as a series of research tasks that will be followed up in the future. Thirty-seven references are listed.

0201 East African Medical Journal, Nairobi. *Rural medicine.* East African Medical Journal (Nairobi), 46(10), Oct 1969, 534-535. Engl.
Editorial.

The problem of providing medical services to the most remote areas of East Africa involves the organization of adequate care for patients, particularly in areas devoid of hospitals or health centres, and the provision of support for doctors working in isolated areas. Working in isolation, without the opportunity of consulting with a colleague can be demoralizing and professionally destructive for a doctor. Provision of an adequate radiocall system, or personal visits by individuals or teams can greatly assist the rural doctor.

0202 **Frenkel, J.K.** *Brief cool summer near the equator: medical interests in Colombia, S.A.* Journal of the Kansas Medical Society (Topeka), 69, Apr 1968, 163-176. Engl.

An American physician reports on medical care delivery in Colombia during an exchange visit. The exchange was part of an ongoing programme of the University of Kansas aimed at raising the level of medical and educational competence in developing countries. Two medical students also participated; one studied pediatric patients, while the other examined the compulsory rural year for medical students. The impact of poverty on both malnutrition and infectious disease was noted, as was the fact that lack of cultural and recreational facilities and an interesting social life, plus the dominance of the conservative Catholic hierarchy in rural towns, discourages interest in rural practice. Only 20% of the medical students had any desire to take up rural practice. Although plans are in progress to unite the social security and general health systems, Colombia has as yet no overall health plan. Nutrition, preventive medicine, and family planning compete for limited funds and manpower. The use of medical assistants is considered a possible solution to the problem of physician disinterest in rural practice. Twenty-eight references are listed.

0203 **Hall, T.L., Diaz, S.** *Social security and health care patterns in Chile.* International Journal of Health Services (Westport, Conn.), 1(4), Nov 1971, 362-377. Engl.

This paper is divided into three parts. The first traces the evolution of health care under social security in Chile from 1918 to the present. The early period saw the establishment of almost 50 different social security funds, each with its own unique characteristics. This was followed by a period of consolidation and reform highlighted by the passage of the Preventive Medicine Law (1938), the creation of the National Health Service (1952), and passage of the Curative Medicine Law for Employees (1968). The significance of these legislative milestones is discussed. The second section examines the degree to which social security coverage affects the utilization of health services. Based on the results of the 1968 health survey it may be concluded that a strong positive correlation exists between social security coverage and the utilization of medical and dental services, along with an inverse correlation between coverage and the unmet demand for care. The paper concludes with a discussion of the tasks facing the new government as it seeks to integrate Chile's different systems of publicly sponsored health care so as to improve efficiency and to make comprehensive service available to all Chileans. (Author abstract.)

0204 **Infante, A.D.** *Regionalizacion como estructura docente. (Regional confinement of the teaching structure).* Revista Medica de Chile (Santiago), 96, May 1968, 348-359. Span.

The division of Chile into health regions closely follows the structure of the National Health Service. The hospitals of Santiago are assigned to broad health zones into which the country has been divided. East hospital is the area base and, as such, acts as regional hospital for other smaller hospitals located in the same zone. The geography of the country presented certain problems to this concept of regionalization, which, at the time of publication of the paper, were referred back for further study. The endemic lack of medical personnel and their inability to meet the demands upon their services were reasons for the establishment of the Postgraduate School of the Faculty of Medicine of the University of Chile. The formative action of the School extends from the University to the zone hospitals to which graduating physicians are deployed. The flow of traffic between zone and regional hospital is two-directional. Patients go to the regional hospital seeking services the zone hospital cannot provide, and doctors from zone hospitals go to regional hospitals to seek advice or supplementary training. Their colleagues from the regional hospitals give consultations in their respective specialities at zone hospitals. This has the advantage of performing the feedback function of transmitting actual field experiences to the Faculty. The National Health Service, although operating on the basis of a national structure, allows zone units to operate with a degree of autonomy to meet regional needs. The paper suggests that the chronic shortage of professional staff could be met by making maximum use of available manpower resources in rural areas in the form of auxiliary health workers. The extent of their training should be proportional to the difficulty of obtaining the services of a physician. Twelve references are listed.

0205 **Journal of the Indian Medical Association, Calcutta.** *Providing work for rural practitioners.* Journal of the Indian Medical Association (Calcutta), 52(4), 16 Feb 1969, 184-185. Engl.

There is a shortage of physicians in rural India primarily because rural conditions are unfavorable to private practice. The majority of people in rural areas cannot afford to pay for services. Required facilities and specialist services are located in the cities. The Indian Medical Association (IMA) has recommended that rural medical practitioners be integrated with India's rural health centres on a part-time basis. Several state branches of the IMA have proposed a cooperative self-help movement. A pilot station could be set up as a basis for investigation, treatment, health education, and family planning. A team of pathologists, technicians, and specialists could make weekly visits to the pilot centre, manned by the doctor to supplement his efforts. The government should, at any rate, play a greater role in helping out the rural practitioner.

II Organization and Planning

0206 Kretchmer, N. *International health - impressions of a medical research team in Nigeria.* American Journal of Diseases of Children (Chicago), 121, Feb 1971, 97-103. Engl.

This article traces the origin and development of the Foundation for International Child Health, which is concerned with training, care, and research projects related to maternal and child health (MCH) in developing countries. To determine the particular MCH needs in Central Africa, a research group visited various parts of East and West Africa; they concluded that Africans must be trained in technology useful to their nation, that these technologists must have modern equipment, that individuals should be trained in their own environment, and that centres of excellence could be established in Central Africa to provide advanced training for these individuals. In response to this initial inquiry, a group of American physicians, research technologists, social workers, and laboratory assistants joined cooperatively with a similar team from Nigeria to study neonatal jaundice and lactose intolerance. The objective of the programme was that the American team would train a Nigerian team in laboratory methodology required for this research project, and leave the Nigerian team in charge of continued investigation and training. The paper summarizes knowledge acquired by the team in Nigeria from an anthropological, social, and medical point of view. Nine references are listed.

0207 McGlashan, N.D. *Distribution of population and medical facilities in Malawi.* Central African Journal of Medicine (Salisbury), 14(11), Nov 1968, 249-252. Engl.

Using a geographical approach, census information of Malawi in 1966 is analyzed to assess distribution of medical facilities and to assess hospital work loads.

0208 Nepal, Ministry of Health. *Health institutions.* Kathmandu, Ministry of Health, n.d. 15p. Engl. Unpublished document.

This document provides maps accompanied by statistical data on Nepal's district health facilities. Numbers of hospitals, health centres, health posts, ayurvedic aushadhalaya, malaria eradication organization, maternal and child health and family planning facilities, smallpox offices, leprosy control project facilities, and tuberculosis control facilities are indicated.

0209 Newkirk, D.D. *Program of rural public health - past, present, and future.* Vanga, Zaire, Vanga Hospital, Department of Public Health, Dec 1972. 12p. Engl. Unpublished document.

This programme report indicates the present (1972) conditions of villagers served by the Vanga Hospital, Zaire. Morbidity and mortality rates are high in all age groups of the population, but particularly so in the 1-5 year olds. In carrying on its preventive medical work the hospital hired auxiliaries. These local young men with 4 months of on-the-job training perform such duties as weighing children, dispensing medicines, and giving injections. Within the hospital, there is a Well Child Clinic every week for children of nearby villages, and a Residential Nutrition Rehabilitation Centre. From this base, auxiliaries, using bicycles or trucks for transportation, carry out the village sanitation project. Rural dispensaries, staffed by a nurse, will be increasing their public health work with the help of the mobile team. The Department of Public Health at the hospital is financed by OXFAM and local village contributions. Rural public health work has concentrated on sanitation, maternal and child health, tuberculosis, nutrition, family planning, and training of village health workers. Phases of the department's preventive medicine programme in all these areas are discussed.

0210 Roemer, M.I. *Social security for medical care: is it justified in developing countries?* International Journal of Health Services (Westport, Conn.), 1(4), Nov 1971, 354-361. Engl.

Social insurance spread from Europe to the developing countries, especially in Latin America, after World War I. In these countries, however, the percentage of persons insured is typically small, so that "inequities" are created relative to the larger noninsured populations. Nevertheless, the social insurance device is justified because of its effects in upgrading the overall health service resources and promoting the general economic development of the predominantly agricultural countries. Moreover, social security programmes are in the long run not obstructive to but promotive of Ministries of Health and their services. Thirteen references are listed. (Author abstract.)

0211 Sharpston, M.J. *Uneven geographical distribution of medical care: a Ghanaian case study.* Journal of Development Studies (London), 8(2), Jan 1972, 205-222. Engl.

Statistical data is presented illustrating the concentration of health services, medical personnel, physicians, hospitals, and health centres in urban areas of Ghana, especially around Accra. As of 1969, popular opinion was against development of broad integrated health services for rural populations. Political and popular forces favoured creation of hospitals for urban areas. Data shows that health services for the country as a whole centred around Accra and that efforts to deploy auxiliary health workers to rural health centres had not been undertaken with determination.

0212 Taba, A.H. *View of the World Health Organization Eastern Mediterranean Region.* Journal of Medical Education (Chicago), 44, Apr 1969, 278-284. Engl.

The WHO Eastern Mediterranean Region comprises 21 member countries of the West Asian and North African subcontinents. The region has an annual population growth rate of more than 2.5%. Considerable progress has been made in certain countries but the health services are still not accessible to a great mass of people, especially those in the rural areas where the majority of the population lives. Intense, sustained effort to increase economic and manpower resources is

II.5 Financial aspects

See also: 0082, 0088, 0120, 0122, 0151, 0165, 0177, 0191, 0196, 0197, 0336, 0337, 0625

0213 Bonnet, P.D., Ruderman, A.P. *Health care systems and financing.* In Reinke, W.A., ed., Health Planning: Qualitative Aspects and Quantitative Techniques, Baltimore, Md., Johns Hopkins University, 1972, 209-218. Engl.

Each country has its own pattern of health care evolved out of its particular political, cultural, and historical tradition. Decision making may be centralized, resulting in a formal, easily recognized system, or diffused, and less formal. Neither the centralized nor the decentralized system guarantees great effectiveness or economy, although the centralized is generally assumed to provide a more equitable system of health care where resources are scarce. Sponsorship may be public or private, but comprehensive care is rarely provided. Advantages and disadvantages of various types of financial sponsorship of health care systems require further research; some of these are discussed and additional readings are listed.

0214 Dunlop, D. *Summary of the ADC workshop on the role of human resource investments in rural development.* Nashville, MCH/FP Training and Research Centre, Meharry Medical College and the Department of Economics, Vanderbilt University, 1973. 24p. Engl. Unpublished document.

At a series of workshops, human resource investments in rural health were discussed. Topics included nutrition, health, nonformal education/communication, and maternal and child health/family planning. Given that nutrition affects the health of mothers and children, mental development, and work performance, research is required to analyze alternative family health delivery systems, through which a package of nutrition, family planning, infectious disease control, and child health services can be delivered. In that health is a basic right and that there are secondary economic benefits from investing in health, further research of the role of health in development is indicated. Since mass communication and interpersonal communication both have their advantages in nonformal education, research should be conducted to evaluate communication costs and benefits. Studies of family planning programmes that were discussed focus on demand, and suggest that research is necessary for development of demand-sensitive family planning programmes.

0215 Fulop, T. *L'educatior sanitaire et l'etat de sante de la population rurale. (Health educator and the state of health of the rural population).* Sante Publique (Bucharest), 1, 1968, 79-84. Fren.

Medical care in the socialist countries, e.g. Hungary, is free of charge and does not raise financial problems for the population. As a consequence the number of consultations is increased. The author stresses the differences in applying medical assistance to patients of different educational levels. Investigations conducted in the rural area disclosed that, in the case of people having 1-4 years of school instruction, fewer appeals are made for medical assistance. This shows that special attention must be paid to persons with a lower educational level, that health education must be strengthened and expanded, and that for optimum results to be obtained from accessibility to medical care there must be an accompanying rise in the level of education. Nine references are listed.

0216 King, M. *New priorities in tropical medicine.* In Wolstenholme, G., O'Connor, M., eds., Teamwork for World Health, London, J. and A. Churchill, 1971, 25-36. Engl.
See also entry 198.

Finding solutions to the problem of providing medical care in developing countries necessitates analyzing the whole epidemiological pattern to ascertain the critical factors involved and to find ways to influence them favourably. The size of a country's economy dictates its capacity to provide basic health services. The problem is aggravated for poor countries by rapid population increase. A comparison of two countries with similar populations: Malawi, with a per capita GNP of U.S. $51 and Zambia with six times that figure, illustrates the superiority of Zambia's achievements in the provision of health care and bears out the argument that countries with a per capita GNP of under U.S. $76 cannot from their own resources provide basic health services on anything but the most unsatisfactory and rudimentary scale, whereas those with GNP's of between U.S. $76 and $150 provide a reasonable level of health care only with great difficulty. International help is needed to enable the poorest nations to develop basic health services, not only for humanitarian reasons, but because of their effect on the economy through increased efficiency of the work force and, in the long term, their influence on population growth through improved maternal and child health.

0217 Medina, E., Kaempffer, A.M. *Planificacion de Salud y presupuestos por programa. (Public health care and budget planning).* Revista Medica de Chile (Santiago), 96, Jun 1968, 434-438. Span.

Separate budgeting of each health programme represents the final monetary expression of the health care planning process. This method has been introduced by the National Public Health Service of Chile with satisfactory results. As this technique is now compulsory in all activities of public administration, the experience gathered over the last 2 years (1966-68) has influenced the training of personnel, definition of action plans, and awareness of operational problems. Given the influence of salaries upon the total cost, it is necessary to define the functions to be performed by each individual; and an exact control on inputs and statistical recording of all actions effected must be maintained. Limitations lie in the difficulty of breaking down some of the expenses of the National Health Services. Generally speaking, the aim behind the new budgeting system is to identify an expense with a definite health care programme. Three references are listed.

0218 Roemer, M.I. *Social insurance as leverage for changing health care systems: international experience.* Bulletin of the New York Academy of Medicine (New York), 48(1), Jan 1972, 93-107. Engl.

International experience shows that the growth of health insurance has had some impact on the patterns of health services. Where the political ideology is more collectivized and where the economic level is somewhat lower, the degree of influence is greater. In some countries, these changes have provided the structural basis for development of national health services. Social insurance provides leverage for health system innovations in disease prevention, medical teamwork, regionalization, and general quality control. Social insurance for medical care has led to the establishment of health centres with innovative staffing patterns. Twenty-nine references are listed.

0219 Stapleton, T. *Prospective in pediatrics.* Journal of Tropical Pediatrics and Environmental Child Health (Kampala), 17, Jun 1971, 71-86. Engl.

Two problems facing developing countries are the rise in population following the introduction of preventive medicine, and the time lag between population increase and production increase. A further difficulty is the narrow distribution of aid, as in the UNICEF milk distribution policy, which helps children reach 18 months of age but does not prevent ensuing years of malnutrition. Postgraduate medical education and research often do not contribute to development of the students' own country. Developed countries (e.g. Australia) can give valuable assistance by sponsoring brief visits to (Australian) university departments by senior Asian lecturers, by arranging reciprocal visits to medical schools in the Asian countries, by consulting on teaching methods, etc. References are listed.

0220 Wolf, A.C., Theberge, J.D. *Las inversiones en salud y el desarrollo en las Americas. (Health investment and development in the Americas).* Boletin de la Oficina Sanitaria Panamericana (Washington, D.C.), 64, Apr 1968, 281-290. Span.

Only in the recent past have expenditures on health, as part of the process of economic growth, begun to be examined on a systematic basis. This is due to the attribution of a key role to technological improvement requiring large amounts of capital or to the difficulty involved in measuring the effects of expenditures that improve the quality and size of the labour force, and that were classified as consumption goods. The combined growth of physical inputs of capital and labour do not explain the historical growth of output achieved; and although there is still considerable uncertainty about the size and components of the economic residual, it appears certain that an improvement in the quality of labour resulting from investments in health and education has accounted for a significant share of the unexplained growth rate. Health is undoubtedly a variable in the economic system. Health investments have an effect on productivity and output of the economy through their influence on the mortality (loss of workers), morbidity (loss of working time), and debility (loss of productivity on the job) of the working population. According to one calculation, the productivity of the labour force of a country may be reduced by as much as 50% as a result of the combined efforts of poor nutrition and bad health conditions. Furthermore, health investments raise the rate of return on other social and economic investments. The interrelations of health with other variables in the economic system point to the crucial importance of a balanced pattern of mutually supporting investments in order to raise the yield. In the Americas there are many low rates of return resulting from a failure to undertake complementary health programmes. Endemic plague in the vicinity of Guayaquil has threatened the potential return from labour development in recent years; the outbreak of yellow fever in Trinidad (1954) produced a sharp decline in tourist arrivals; malaria and malnutrition have resulted in the past in the loss of part of the rice crop in northeastern Brazil. In addition, in 12 Latin American countries preventable losses in output due to inadequate occupational health and safety programmes have been estimated at 15% of the national income of these countries. In the less developed countries it is necessary to concentrate on those categories of eradicable and reducible diseases whose "cost per life saved" is low. Little systematic analysis has been made of the relationship of the economic benefits of health programmes as a fundamental requirement for increasing the efficiency of the services. Health services should be studied from the standpoint of supply and demand: how to develop health services more efficiently and which programmes yield the highest returns in terms of increasing *per capita* income. Economic criteria are not the only ones that should be applied, and health must be viewed as a part of a dynamic economic system composed of interacting elements. The Latin American countries are coming to view health in this light, and it is the duty of economists and planners to ensure that this view is accepted as soon as possible. (Revised journal abstract.)

II.6 Cultural aspects

See also: 0160, 0215, 0356

0221 Kettle, E.S. *Health education at village level.* International Committee of Tropical Medicine Newsletter (England), (8), Mar 1970, 4. Engl.

The author relates useful health education techniques, citing her experiences in Australia and a health exhibit in the Ankole province of Uganda. She recommends the establishment of training schools for health educators in areas similar to those where they will work, supervised field experience for health educators, the inclusion of social anthropology in training courses, and more use of the social anthropologist on the health team.

0222 Messing, S.D., Prince, J.S., Yohannes, T. *Method of health culture research in an African country.* Journal of Health and Human Behavior (Washington, D.C.), 6, Winter 1965, 261-263. Engl.

Research is being conducted in Ethiopia to examine cultural aspects of public health. It was found that paramedical workers trained at the Gondar Public Health College lacked training related to specific problems they would encounter in their assigned regions. The research project discussed here was designed to evaluate specific problems that trainees would encounter in four distinctly different parts of the country. The paper gives examples of field problems that demonstrate the influence of cultural forces on public health work in developing countries. Inclusion of a cultural anthropologist on the health team can be useful in clarifying the cultural factors influencing rural health workers and their work.

0223 Nath, B. *Role of general practitioners in leprosy control.* Journal of the Indian Medical Association (Calcutta), 49(10), 16 Nov 1967, 470-472. Engl.

The general practitioner in India has been disinclined to play a vital role in leprosy control for several reasons. The main reason is fear and ignorance on the part of the general public. Leprosy is believed to be unsightly and highly contagious. Although it is neither in its early stages, doctors are reluctant to see leprosy patients for fear they will frighten away other patients. People tend to hide the disease. There is little appreciation, among doctors and patients, of the fact that early treatment can prevent gross deformities. Physicians could greatly contribute to the National Public Health Programme by opening their doors to these patients and preventing the spread of the disease. They must be educated to do so.

0224 Radoli, O. *Who are the witchdoctors?* Afya: A Journal for Medical and Health Workers, (Nairobi), 7, 1973, 87-89. Engl.

In the Western mind, traditional medicine men in East Africa have often been associated with witchdoctors and their efforts ridiculed. East Africans themselves have always differentiated between spell casters (who are associated here with evil) and Waganga traditional healers. Their function was to treat illnesses with herbs, set broken bones, extract teeth, and in some cases give advice on social and family problems. They have been credited with averting starvation in tetanus epidemics by advising routine extraction of some of the lower teeth to facilitate feeding with liquids, and with the isolation of lepers and yaws victims. When planning medical programmes, the contribution of such indigenous human resources as the Waganga should not be overlooked, since economic factors will continue to limit the influence of modern medicine in developing countries for some time yet.

0225 Twumasi, P.A. *Sick role cycle: a sociological view.* Accra University of Ghana, n.d. 11p. Engl.

The way a society understands and copes with illness, that is the "sick role," is a means of understanding individual and collective reactions to illness. Human behaviour related to the sick role greatly influences the utilization of health care delivery systems. In Ghana, traditional rural behavioural reactions persist after people have moved to urban centres. Disease is understood in behavioural, not biological terms, and a supernatural agency is invoked. Traditional ideas will not change as long as rural health care services remain underdeveloped, poorly distributed, and the emphasis is placed on curative rather than preventive methods. Concrete suggestions to promote a change in attitude include training medical assistants for work in clinics, homes, and rural areas, emphasizing the role of the preventive specialist in health care, and liberalizing medical education toward greater cultural awareness. Five references are listed.

II.7 Epidemiological, family planning, MCH, and nutritional studies

See also: 0100, 0112, 0134, 0140, 0152, 0200, 0291, 0361, 0370, 0439, 0577

0226 Alexander, C.A. *Health problems and economic development.* Participant Journal (New Delhi), 4(6), Dec 1969, 7-10. Engl.

India's principal health programme for the next decade must be family planning. Improvement in health increases the technological productivity of a population. Cost-benefit analysis should be used in establishing health priorities. Efforts must be made to consolidate the gains in communicable disease control and to improve rural and urban health care services. This was begun by establishing 5 000 primary health centres in rural areas.

0227 **American Public Health Association, Washington, D.C.** *Development and evaluation of integrated delivery systems for health, family planning, and nutrition (DEIDS).* Washington, D.C., American Public Health Association, n.d. 3p. Engl.

The American Public Health Association has entered into a contract with the U.S. Agency for International Development to help developing countries extend the delivery of family health services. The contract is to establish family planning pilot projects designed to develop improved low-cost systems for delivering health services, predominantly to rural areas in up to four countries. Emphasis is to be on maternal and child health, nutrition services, and family planning. The primary objective is to extend these services to the majority of mothers and children in the defined project area. It is hoped that the projects will serve to guide national planning and provide prototypes for development of services throughout the country. Details of the projected contractual programme are briefly described.

0228 **Asayesh, K.** *Role of health corp in communicating family planning information in Iran.* Chapel Hill, N.C., University of North Carolina, 20 Apr. 32p. Engl.
Unpublished term paper.

Statistical data reveal that an extensive family planning programme is necessary in Iran. The programme now in operation uses a nationwide information system to achieve its purposes. Services performed in rural areas by health corps members, i.e., young people eligible for military service and given adequate training, include community development, health and nutrition education, and family planning education. Twenty-three references are listed.

0229 **Banerji, D.** *Effect of treatment default on results of treatment in routine practice in India.* Bulletin of the International Union Against Tuberculosis (Paris), 43, Jun 1970, 247-249. Engl.

Owing to the inadequate development of tuberculosis service as an integral part of the general health services in India, more than three-quarters of the patients who seek treatment for tuberculosis are denied opportunities for continuing medical attention. As a result of this lapse, they continue to spread the disease in the community. The major impediments to implementation of tuberculosis programmes in developing countries appear to be organizational, managerial, and technical rather than behavioural factors that lead to inadequate acceptance by patients of the treatment offered because of shortcomings in the patients' motivation. Even with limited resources it is possible to get reasonably satisfactory results, not only in terms of alleviation of suffering, but also in preventing the spread of the disease from them to the community.

0230 **Banerji, D.** *India's national tuberculosis programme in relation to the proposed social and economic development plans.* Indian Journal of Public Health (Calcutta), 9(3), Jul 1965, 103-106. Engl.

Tuberculosis services in India are inadequate. Because of organizational limitations, traditional medical and health services do not reach many tuberculosis patients. Health administrators must be motivated to initiate administrative changes, a community approach should be developed, and the tuberculosis campaign should be extended to include training programmes for medical auxiliaries. Provision of curative services to those already seeking help will motivate others who are not. A rise in the standard of living, progress in education, and mass communication will increase the need for preventive services. Social and economic progress will make available greater resources for health programmes and help control tuberculosis in India.

0231 **Behm, H.** Milbank Memorial Fund Quarterly, New York. *Needed research on Latin American mortality in relation to public health.* Milbank Memorial Fund Quarterly (New York), 43(no. 4, pt. 2), Oct 1965, 338-353. Engl.

This paper deals mainly with research needed on mortality and the relevance of such research to health problems and health programmes in Latin America. Areas for research should be selected according to the outstanding health problems in Latin America, and should be relatively feasible research projects, taking into consideration the methodological aspects as well as the difficulties in obtaining basic data. The following areas for research are suggested, among others: (1) validity of mortality as a health indicator, with consideration of its wise use and the changing relation between the frequency of deaths and the frequency of the disease; (2) socioeconomic determinants of mortality and morbidity as required information for defining the scope of health programmes in underdeveloped communities of Latin America; (3) trends and characteristics of changes in mortality, using the variables provided by available statistics; (4) epidemiological research on specific health problems selected on the basis of excessive and preventable mortality, such as tuberculosis, infantile diarrhea, malnutrition, alcoholism, etc. Mortality under 5 years of age, mainly infant mortality, is a subject of obvious importance; and (5) the extent and implications of deficiencies in mortality statistics, including experimentation in alternative methods of collecting vital statistics. Several conditions favouring current research on mortality in Latin America are discussed, and the rewarding possibilities of analytical studies of the huge mass of basic data available are emphasized.

0232 **Bennett, F.J., Lutwama, J.S.** *Organization of MCH services in developing regions: (I) Health services for school children.* Journal of Tropical Pediatrics and Environmental Child Health (Kampala), 12(1), Jun 1966, 16-21. Engl.
See also entry 357.

The real difficulty of providing a health service for school children is to weld the component aspects of the problem into a whole. This requires good liaison between administrators, teachers, health workers, school-parent committees, and community workers. Only in this way can a service be provided that would deal with the very important environmental factors, provide a personal service for examination, immunization, and treatment, and also ensure that the school child is receiving the correct education in health matters. (Author abstract.)

0233 Black, R.H. *The role of rural health services in disease eradication programmes.* Papua and New Guinea Medical Journal (Boroko, Port Moresby), 13(1), Mar 1970, 7-10. Engl.

Due to the recent trend toward integration of services, successful malaria eradication campaigns are handed over to general health services. These services fail to assure continued malaria control for the following reasons. The eradication process, to be effective and lasting, requires systematic organization and unrelenting follow-up. To ensure total coverage of the population, a programme of active case detection through home visiting by surveillance agents of the malaria service, as compared with passive detection by health centre staff when the sick person comes to the centre for treatment, must be followed by remedial measures of spraying, drug distribution, etc., and a maintenance phase of vigilance against reinfection by visitors or in case of seasonal malaria. As health centre operations reach people only within a small, well-defined radius of the centre itself, health centre records do not reflect epidemic conditions among nonclinic users. Besides, rural health centre staff are not sufficient in number to take on eradication tasks in addition to all the other tasks they are required to perform.

0234 Blankhart, D.M. *Health problems in pre-school children: (5) Central Africa.* Journal of Tropical Pediatrics (Kampala), 14, Dec 1968, 249-252. Engl.

Central Africa consists of Zambia, Malawi, the southeastern part of the Congo (Zaire), and Rhodesia. The sparsely distributed population is concentrated along roads and in mining towns. Zambian children suffer from gastroenteritis, protein calorie malnutrition, respiratory diseases, measles, smallpox, anaemia, and tetanus. Malnutrition is widespread among school children. In 1964 a preventive approach to this problem was adopted, involving the following steps: fact-finding on the incidence and cause of malnutrition; clinics for pre-school children; distribution of protein-rich foods through welfare centres in mining towns; and training of auxiliary health personnel in applied nutrition. Public health education in the home, e.g. through cooking demonstrations and the media, has begun. A weight card called the "Road to Health" is recommended as a useful teaching tool. Two nutrition rehabilitation units are being established. Sixteen references are listed.

0235 Brown, R.E. *Mission to Biafra (January 1969): a study and survey of a population under stress.* Clinical Pediatrics (Philadelphia), 8(6), Jun 1969, 313-321. Engl.

A United States technical mission composed of consultants who had collectively spent about 20 years in Africa and therefore were familiar with general problems of the region was sent to study conditions during the siege of Biafra by federal troops. Hospitals, refugee camps, feeding stations, kwashiorkor centres, government departments, laboratories, farms, yam barns, factories, schools, market places, and research centres were visited. Data and medical records were freely available to the mission for comparison with their own findings. All observations confirmed that famine and infectious diseases as a result of the air and sea blockade, and the resulting overcrowding of refugees, were prevalent and serious. Immediate international relief efforts were called for, and recommendations were made for paramedical teams to be trained on a massive scale to give BCG, tetanus, measles, and smallpox immunization, and to administer antimalarials, antihelminthics, and iron to counteract anemia. The fact that large groups of people were already aggregated for food distribution and other reasons would facilitate these preventive measures.

0236 Brown, R.E. *Editorial: medical assistants and child health.* Journal of Tropical Pediatrics and African Child Health (Kampala), 12(1), Jun 1966, 1-4. Engl.

Developing countries' health problems reflect problems in education and general socioeconomic progress. Some experts consider simple lack of health care to be responsible for underdevelopment; therefore it is easy to conclude that training of health workers must take top priority. Diseases of children are the primary problem. Their control lies in immunization, clean water supply, sanitation, and health education. Prevention of these childhood diseases is much less costly in every respect than cure or rehabilitation. Given sufficient training and supervision medical assistants can perform this work. Nine references are listed.

0237 Carty, C. *Integration of family planning with a public health department.* Journal of the Christian Medical Association on India (Mysore City), 46(10), Oct 1971, 550-551. Engl.

As a first step toward integration of family planning and maternal and child health services in India, children of mothers attending tubectomy camps can be given medical care. Services will concentrate on child care and on health education. Problems involved and possible solutions are presented. Such a programme will help ensure the health of those children living and minimize women's fears about the operation.

0238 Chow, L.P. *Integration of family planning with maternal and child health: experience in Taiwan, Republic of China.* n.p., 27 Jun 1970. 26p. Engl. Unpublished document.

Taiwan's family planning programme is being integrated with a general health programme and in particular with the maternal and child health services. This paper relates Taiwan's approaches to integration. Sixteen references are listed.

0239 Chow, L.P. *Some aspects of the integration of MCH and family planning activities in the general health services.* Baltimore, Md., Johns Hopkins University, n.d. 13p. Engl.
Unpublished document.

Public health goals have been altered by rapid population growth. Although maternal and child health and family planning are legitimate concerns of health departments, the problem of too rapid population growth is not just a health concern. Economic and social viewpoints are involved as well. Pros and cons of integration of family planning into general health activities of maternal and child health activities are discussed. Provocative questions are purposefully raised. More studies have to be done to actually show the health advantages of family planning. Economic incentive is important in motivation for birth control. Integration of family planning with other health services does avoid duplication of effort, but the urgency of the problem and other factors encourage one to consider not integrating the birth control programme with health services. Existing health personnel should support the family planning programme when they contact the population they serve. Fifteen references are listed.

0240 Copping, A.M. *Planning nutrition education in developing countries.* Journal of the American Dietetic Association (Chicago), 53, Aug 1968, 127-129. Engl.

Investigations made in 26 countries indicate that nutrition education is seriously neglected. Before nutrition education can be planned, the background of race, creed, and cultural pattern of the community must be understood. Various approaches to planning are considered. Sixteen references are listed.

0241 Davachi, F. *Medical relief project: Port Harcourt, Nigeria.* In Hughes, J.P., ed., Health Care for Remote Areas: An International Conference, Kaiser Foundation, Oakland, 1972, 126-131. Engl.
See entry 155 for complete proceedings.

In reactivating the services of a war-destroyed hospital in eastern Nigeria, a medical relief team found malnutrition, infectious diseases in children, and problems of the newborn to be primary problems. Education has only begun to correct some poor nutritional habits; children admitted to the hospital with infectious diseases were often terminal cases. Local authorities rejected the idea of a tetanus immunization programme.

0242 David, P. *Need to reconsider, evaluate, and restructure the delivery of family planning medical services in rural India through mobile teams.* n.p., Spring 1969. 29p. Engl.
Unpublished document.

In India, mobile IUCD and vasectomy teams were devised to bring family planning services to rural areas. This paper suggests ways in which delivery of these services can be evaluated and improved upon. Seven references are listed.

0243 Gaur, S.D., Marwah, S.M. *Role of health education in filaria control.* Indian Journal of Public Health (Calcutta), 11(3), Jul 1967, 131-132,137. Engl.

As public participation is essential to filariasis control in India, an educational approach is proposed. General methods for endemic areas involve the following: including basic knowledge about disease transmission in school curricula, in-service training for health centre personnel about personal protection, educating planners about the necessity for sanitary waste disposal, and the elimination of mosquitogenic conditions. Some specific methods, based on the educational approach, as applied in one township are described. Seven references are listed.

0244 Ghosh, S., Bali, P. *Role of health professions in population problems.* New Delhi, Indian Association for the Advancement of Medical Education, 1960, 259-269. Engl.
Preconference paper on the Role of Health Professions in Population Problems.

Staff of the family planning, maternal and child health, and nutrition services must understand that these programmes are complementary. Pediatricians and obstetricians working together are an essential part of the maternal and child health centre. The author questions the right of family planners to stress birth control when there is no assurance for health of children already living. An integrated programme of nutrition, prevention, and treatment of diseases is needed. A second paper discusses planning of demographic education for health personnel.

0245 Guyer, B. *Childhood mobility in Igbo-Ora, Western Nigeria: its relevance to morbidity and the organization of medical care.* West African Medical Journal (Ibadan), 20, Oct 1971, 333-336. Engl.

Life patterns as observed among young children in the town of Igbo-Ora, Nigeria, and the implications of these patterns for morbidity, childhood illness, and health care are discussed. The study was carried out in a town of 30 000 people. Sleeping patterns and mobility of the children were studied, as well as the amount of time spent by children in the local markets. Yoruba children are highly mobile, enabling wide exposure to communicable diseases.

0246 International Confederation of Midwives, London. *International Confederation of Midwives concensus reports I-III.* London, International Confederation of Midwives, Dec 1972. 5p. Engl.

The International Conference of Midwives, held in London in December 1972, defined maternal and child health, family planning, and the functions and responsibilities of the midwife and of the traditional birth attendant. It recommended that midwives be responsible for the inservice education of the traditional birth attendant; that family planning instruction be integrated into each level of midwifery training; and that midwifery be expanded to include family health care in general, through inservice and postgraduate courses in paediatrics, public health nursing, etc. In countries in which family planning is not an accepted part of family health service programmes, it should be included in the training programmes of nurses and midwives. Where family planning services exist, they should be incorporated into maternal and child health services.

0247 Jain, A.M. *Planning and organization of child health services in rural India: II. School health service.* Indian Journal of Pediatrics (Calcutta), 35(242), Mar 1968, 150-155. Engl.
See also entry 248.

Child health care in India could be organized to continue through school health services, especially in rural areas, where children cannot otherwise obtain proper health care. The objectives of such a programme include providing the students and staff with health supervision and maintaining a sanitary environment in the school. Prevention, monitoring, and health education programmes could be maintained through the structure of the school system, if committees of community members were involved on an on-going basis. Community resources, financial and otherwise, could be tapped, and programmes modified to fit the needs of each community.

0248 Jain, A.M. *Planning and organization of child health services in rural India: I. Well child care centre.* Indian Journal of Pediatrics (Calcutta), 35(242), 1968, 146-149. Engl.
See also entry 247.

India has prenatal services but lacks services for children from birth to age 5. Well-child clinics must be organized for the many children living in rural areas. Health centres should monitor the progress of children, provide preventive immunization, instruct parents in health education, etc. Supervision of village health workers is necessary.

0249 Johnson, G.Z. *Health conditions in rural and urban areas of developing countries.* Population Studies (London), 17(3), Mar 1964, 293-310. Engl.

Comparisons of statistical data on infant and child mortality in urban as opposed to rural areas of developing countries show that health service benefits have been felt only in urban areas. Basic advances in preventive medicine should be applied to rural areas through health services and sanitary control. Provision of services should include policy directed at limiting population increase.

0250 Kidane-Miriam, W. Ethiopia, Ministry of Public Health. *Importance of maternal and child health in public health program.* Addis Ababa, Ministry of Public Health, 20 Jun 1970. 9p. Engl. Unpublished document.

Rural Ethiopia lacks medical and health services. The government is emphasizing preventive medical care, and has established health centres and health stations that are the basis of rural health services. A serious lack of health manpower results in continuing reliance on traditional medicine in rural areas. Improvement of the maternal and child health (MCH) services will cover prenatal care, delivery care, postnatal care (including birth control advice), and infant and child care. In all phases of MCH there is the need for health education, environmental hygiene, nutrition, and preventive care. Future planning will depend on careful recording and reporting of vital and health statistics and community data.

0251 Kretchmer, N. *Child health in the developing world.* Pediatrics (Springfield, Ill.), 43(1), Jan 1969, 4-11. Engl.

Nutrition, shelter, sanitation, agricultural productivity and supply, marketing, population, education, and physical environment are the major factors affecting child health in developing countries. Malnutrition is basic to the ills of children in these countries. Nutrition education programmes are often irrelevant since parents are reluctant to prepare more nutritious foods that are often expensive and unfamiliar to them. The author proposes increases in foreign aid and subsidies for health research, especially those research projects that respond to the unique problems of a particular geographic area.

0252 Llinares, V.M. *Higiene y seguridad en el medio rural. (Hygiene and safety in the rural environment).* Reprint; source unknown, 243-266. Span.

Health hazards to the rural dweller are discussed under the broad classifications: (1) the traditional (those resulting from the physical, biological, socioeconomic, and cultural rural environmental setting); and (2) the man-made (those resulting from the applications of modern technology.) Prophylactic measures for dealing with domestic animal-borne diseases, guidelines for the safe use of pesticides and insecticides, prevention and control of forest fires, and elementary safety practices to be followed when using farm machinery are given in some detail.

0253 Lythcott, G.I. *Maternal and child health within a total health system.* In Hughes, J.P., ed., Health Care for Remote Areas: An International Conference, Oakland, Kaiser Foundation, 1972, 145-158. Engl.
See entry 155 for complete proceedings.

In that mothers and children comprise approximately 65% of the population of developing countries and have the highest mortality rate from preventable diseases, and because their health affects the development of the future generation, it is recommended that mothers and children receive highest priority in health services planning. Problems associated with malnutrition, communicable diseases, and child spacing deserve maximum attention. An important beginning is the incorporation of sound epidemiological principles, including reporting, surveillance, and application of the acquired data to the planning and development of categorical programmes of immunization and child health as well as to longer range goals. Categorical programme planning must provide for manpower development of both traditional health personnel and new cadres of workers. Finally, successful integration and coordination of donor activities within recipient nations can go a long way to assist the development and implementation of both short-term and long-term goals.

0254 Martin, J.F. *Family planning courses at African health training institutions: a preliminary contribution to an AID-CPC project.* Chapel Hill, University of North Carolina, School of Public Health, Department of Health Administration, Dec 1970. 15p. Engl.
Unpublished document.

In response to the need existing in sub-Saharan Africa "to assist African institutions which are training health personnel, to increase their capacity for teaching family planning as an integral part of total health services," USAID was presented a project plan with proposals from the Carolina Population Centre (CPC). The intended course of action includes: (1) orientation and motivation of academic leaders; (2) introduction of family planning into selected medical schools; (3) survey of other institutions; and (4) introduction of family planning into other institutions. CPC proposals suggest that consultation and help be offered at the request of the institution, that careful attention be given to the differential needs according to cultural and/or residential groups, that the emphasis be put on timing and spacing of births, and so on. The author identifies areas where action has to be taken and when. These include identifying existing sources of information about family planning in Africa, assessing the situation locally (what is the attitude of the people and the policymakers?), providing accurate, up-to-date information on family planning, organizing research and demonstration projects, and developing faculty and other manpower. The author emphasizes the importance of a low-key approach and the necessity of avoiding paternalistic or authoritarian directives.

0255 Martoy, J. *Tuberculosis campaign in Uruguay.* World Medical Journal (New York), 14, May-Jun 1967, 91-93. Engl.

Uruguay's antituberculosis organization utilizes a network of health centres covering the entire country to administer the following integrated services: economic and social assistance, mass examination, supervision of identified cases, administering of BCG, education programmes, and a national registry of patients.

0256 McDermott, W. *Infection and malnutrition.* In Hughes, J.P., ed., Health Care for Remote Areas: An International Conference, Oakland, Kaiser Foundation, 1972. Engl.
See entry 155 for complete proceedings.

Malnutrition in children does not particularly favour or impede the acquisition of infection but it goes a long way to determining the course of the resulting disease. Demographic transition cannot be achieved using contraceptive technology alone in the presence of high infant and preschool mortality. Present antimicrobial technology will not take care of mortality problems in infants and preschool children; yet the results of experiments quoted in this article support the possibility that nutrition can reduce these mortality problems. The author recommends that in combating microbial disease in technologically underdeveloped areas, all-out efforts be made in the nutrition field and in the development of vaccines.

0257 Mollaret, P. *L'institut de medecine et d'epidemiologie africaines. (The African Institute of Medicine and Epidemiology).* Press Medicale (Paris), 77(12), 8 Mar 1969, 449-452. Fren.

The Institute of African Medicine and Epidemiology in Paris was created by a French-Gabonese agreement in 1967. It is primarily a teaching and research institute specializing in problems of tropical medicine. The following subjects are taught: social medicine, epidemiology, public health, nutrition, and other subjects relevant to African health problems. Projects will be carried out cooperatively between the Institute and African countries.

0258 Moodie, A.D., Wittmann, W., Truswell, A.S., Hansen, J.D. *Socio-economic factors in the aetiology of gastroenteritis and their relationship to the health services.* South African Medical Journal-Supplement: South African Journal of Nutrition (Cape Town), 19 Jun 1965, 498-501. Engl.

Investigations in Cape Town point to an important relationship between gastroenteritis, malnutrition, and infection. Parents of infant patients were interviewed to find out how socioeconomic factors relate to these illnesses and to health service utilization. Overcrowding, lack of hygiene, social disorganization in the family, and other factors were observed. The relationship of these factors to gastroenteritis varied between children 0-9 months old and children 10-21 months old. Poor use of welfare services, weaning from the breast before 3 months of age, and inadequate milk intake were noticeable. Improved standards of health education for mothers and coordination of preventive and curative services are called for. Sixteen references are listed.

0259 Musoke, L.K. *Health problems in pre-school children: (4) East Africa.* Journal of Tropical Pediatrics (Kampala), 14, Dec 1968, 245-248. Engl.

In East Africa, 90% of the population lives in rural areas and an estimated 20% are of preschool age. A recent survey in Uganda determined that up to 25% of these children are undernourished. Birth and infant mortality rates are high. Breast-feeding and early immunization should be encouraged. Nutrition education should be combined with mobile immunization efforts, and health workers should be introduced to modern concepts of health education. Other recommendations include the following: public education through the media; attention to proper mental development among preschool children; and the establishment of more health centres, as it is difficult for rural patients to reach hospitals. There are now three medical schools in East Africa, a malnutrition rehabilitation centre, and several training schools for auxiliary health workers, but the number of qualified is not yet satisfactory.

0260 Narain, B. *Applied nutrition programme.* Indian Journal of Pediatrics (Calcutta), 35(240), Jan 1968, 36-45. Engl.

The government of India reports that the Applied Nutrition Programme has had an impact on food habits, beliefs, and practices. The programme emphasis is on nutrition education, and involves a community development approach to change. The programme focusses on mothers and children and its services extend into village areas. A wide variety of workers from public service disciplines have been trained to promote the programme. Food production personnel and health programme personnel have been involved. The programme is implemented through health centres, women's organizations, schools, youth clubs, farmers' organizations, etc.

0261 Nepal, Family Planning and Maternal Child Health Project. *Family planning and MCH program in Nepal.* n.p., n.d. 11p. Engl.
Unpublished document.

Without accompanying measures to reduce fertility, improvements in maternal and child health care and other health facilities could result in a population growth rate of 3%, which would double Nepal's population by 1995. Although 32% of primary school age population are in school, educational facilities cannot keep pace if the population continues to increase at present rates. An integrated maternal and child health and family planning programme commenced in 1965-66. Organizational charts, goals for the programme, and staff training are outlined.

0262 Ogbeide, M.I. *Relative merits of preventive and curative services in the maintenance of health and nutrition in the rural African child.* Journal of the National Medical Association (New York), 59(4), Jul 1967, 242-250. Engl.

The diseases responsible for high mortality and morbidity rates in African children are largely preventable. A long-term solution to the problem involves balancing investments in preventive and curative services. A temporary solution to the problem of malnutrition and related diseases is the provision of a high-protein food and increased numbers of health personnel. Over the long term it is necessary to raise the economic status of low income groups. Ten references are listed.

0263 Owada, K., Takada, S., Kuzuo, N., Junichi, Y., Fukuoka, M., Matsushita, Y., Iwase, H. *On public health activities in Ceylon and the results of some medical surveys of Ceylonese.* Osaka City Medical Journal (Osaka), 13(2), Feb 1967, 75-101. Engl.

In some respects, the incidence of tropical diseases in Ceylon (Sri Lanka) shows a different pattern from other tropical areas. There have been no outbreaks of cholera, plague, or smallpox for several years. However, there are many vector-borne and parasitic diseases, typhoid fever, and dysentry that can be traced to poor living conditions. Government subsidies to householders for improving toilet facilities have not been entirely successful. Tuberculosis is still an important problem, particularly in the over-15 age groups. Financial assistance is given to patients who continue treatment. Malaria eradication is proving difficult in some areas (e.g., coconut and areca nut plantations) where stagnant water accumulates as this provides breeding grounds for mosquitoes. Some advantage is afforded by the fact that Ceylon is an island and therefore quarantine measures can be effectively enforced. Although there are few doctors, a well-established public health administration and well-developed road system contribute to maintaining good health conditions even in undeveloped districts. Public health nurses give protective inoculations, and medical care at government institutions is free of charge. Increased efforts are needed in environmental, maternal, and child health control. Ten references are listed.

0264 Participant Journal, New Delhi. *Inexpensive family planning and health programme.* Participant Journal (New Delhi), 5(9), May 1971, 33-34. Engl.

The success of a low-cost programme of family planning and maternal and child health care lies in training nurse-midwives to offer professional care. Family planning is effectively taught in conjunction with prenatal and postnatal care. Construction of maternal and child health centres and midwife training schools is essential. The programme's essential elements are: two prenatal visits, provision of a trained birth attendant, three postnatal contacts, accessible obstetric facilities, an accurate records system, and organized village assistance.

0265 Pisharoti, K.A. Central Family Planning Institute, New Delhi. *"Few firsts" in the implementation of family planning programme at the peripheral level.* New Delhi, Central Family Planning Institute, n.d. 16p. Engl.

The national family planning programme of India hopes to lower the birth rate in the country from 40 per thousand to 25 per thousand population by 1973. Success of the programme depends on performance of prerequisite duties by workers at the village, primary health centre, and district levels. The minimum necessary duties of personnel are described. A list of eligible couples should be prepared, a map of each village should be available showing roads, houses, and other information. Contact should be consistently maintained with eligible couples by nurse midwives, family planning workers, health assistants, and other staff. Information on eligible couples and their situation should be kept updated. Community development and publicity techniques should be used to gain group acceptance of family planning. Specific techniques for doing this are discussed. IUD and vasectomy camps can be organized through the primary health centre. A line diagram is used to show the flow of the supply of contraceptives through various channels.

0266 Poulton, E.M. *Organisation of MCH services in developing regions: (III) Records.* Journal of Tropical Pediatric and Environmental Child Health (Kampala), 12, Dec 1966, 80-83. Engl.

The types of records that facilitate the planning, operation, and evaluation of health services are the following: demographic, epidemiological, administrative, patient, and service. For maternal and child health services the family folder is the key record, containing antenatal notes for each pregnancy, progress records for each child attending the child health clinic, etc.

0267 Prasada Rao, D.C., Gupta, S. *Child health in a rural community of south India.* Indian Journal of Pediatrics (Calcutta), 35(246), Jul 1968, 327-330. Engl.

Since the first sociological studies of rural residents in Pondicherry, India, were made, a great deal of social change has taken place. These papers present information from a recent study to reassess socioeconomic status, child health patterns, infant dietary and feeding habits, etc. of this rural community. Children under 12 years of age composed 45% of the population; 50% of the families were pure vegetarians; and 68% of the population was illiterate. Conditions reported can be ameliorated by mass education and higher standards of living. Health education is suggested as a means of dealing with problems within the scope of existing resources.

0268 Raska, K. *Concept of epidemiological surveillance of communicable diseases.* Israel Journal of Medical Sciences (Jerusalem), 4(3), May-Jun 1968, 402-414. Engl.
Fourth Rehovoth Conference on Health Problems in Developing States, Rehovoth, Israel, 15-23 Aug 1967.
See entry 96 for complete proceedings.

Epidemiologic surveillance activities are fundamental to the planning and assessment of communicable disease control measures. Information is collected to a large extent through existing health services and is, to that extent, dependent on the system. Exchange of information between neighbouring countries is extremely important. Distribution of information within the health system is also important. Surveillance should be conducted differently for different diseases. WHO provides technical advice about these processes.

0269 Rosa, F.W. *Impact of new family planning approaches on rural maternal and child health coverage in developing countries: India's example.* American Journal of Public Health (New York), 57(8), Aug 1967, 1327-1332. Engl.

Maternal and child health services now reach only a small portion of people in developing countries. The new emphasis on family planning promises to change this because family planning is best approached from a maternal and child health basis. Implications of this change for India's maternal and child health programme are discussed. Women workers need to be trained to reach rural women. Within a few years it is hoped that each primary health centre will have a female doctor as well as a male doctor. Her function will be to care for mothers and children and do family planning work. Subcentres are now staffed by auxiliary nurse midwives, who are under pressure to fulfill targets for IUD insertions. Most births are attended by village midwives or "dais". Dais need to be better mobilized for family planning work. Maternal and child health services are considered the basis for effective family planning efforts.

0270 Rothert, F.C. *Medical self-help and nutrition courses in Central America.* Journal of the Arkansas Medical Society (Fort Smith), 63(2), Jul 1966, 65-66. Engl.

A training course in nutrition and medical self-help designed for Central America is outlined. The manual used, method of implementing it, type of people trained as course leaders, and follow-up are discussed.

0271 Sai, F.T. *Nutrition in developing countries.* Israel Journal of Medical Sciences (Jerusalem), 4(3), May-Jun 1968, 425-442. Engl.
Fourth Rehovoth Conference on Health Problems in Developing States, Rehovoth, Israel, 15-23 Aug 1967.
See entry 96 for complete proceedings.

It is estimated that half the world's population suffers from lack of sufficient food. Almost all of these people live in developing countries. Low consumption of food is related to low production of it. In developing countries there is a large dependent group relative to production groups. Young rural women who ought to contribute to farm production have their productivity reduced by frequent pregnancies. Tropical conditions may affect calorie intake requirements. Data do not exist to establish accurately adult calorie needs in developing countries; personnel are needed for nutrition work, research, development of inexpensive foods, and population control.

0272 Shelesnyak, M.C. *Population problems: medical and public health.* Israel Journal of Medical Sciences (Jerusalem), 4(3), May-Jun 1968, 517-531. Engl.

Fourth Rehovoth Conference on Health Problems in Developing States, Rehovoth, Israel, 15-23 Aug 1967.
See entry 96 for complete proceedings.

The world population growth rate was 2% in 1966. The burden of this increase can be translated into economic, educational, and environmental terms. To plan approaches and services for developing countries with limited resources, we must assess accurately the influences responsible for this rise in population growth. For developing countries this problem may not be that of devising better contraceptive techniques but of bringing about recognition of the need for reduced family size. The concept of generalized reduction of a percentage of fertility by mass methods should be given careful evaluation, free from prejudice.

0273   Sofoluwe, G.O. *Prevention of communicable disease: the control of communicable diseases in rural workers - the role of university departments.* Journal of Tropical Medicine and Hygiene (London), 73, Nov 1970, 310-317. Engl.
A discussion follows the article.

Nigeria has no government agency specifically responsible for control of communicable diseases among rural workers; disease control is wholly dependent on dispensaries, health centres, and hospitals. The diffuse nature of government control has severely limited success in this field. Although individual members of various university departments have served as consultants to the government, notable achievements by university staff have been irregular and uncoordinated. Several solutions to problems in the field of disease control are presented. The administrative and organizational machinery needs to be improved and it is necessary to establish one multidisciplinary agency to deal with the control of these diseases. Health education needs to be intensified. Technological measures to improve the environment must be intensified. Detailed and accurate preliminary studies on all aspects of the diseases must be conducted, as well as effective assessment. Efforts should be made to increase employment and improve the earning and productivity of rural workers by the control of these diseases. The cooperation of overseas institutes, e.g. the London School of Hygiene, will hasten the solution of these major problems. Fifteen references are listed.

0274   Swallows in India, Madras. *Report on present and planned activities of the health, nutrition and family planning centre at Desia Nagar, New Washermanoet, Madras-81.* Madras, India, The Swallows in India, 1972. 5p. Engl.
Unpublished document.

This report indicates the present health activities of the Swallows in India in Madras State. Antenatal care, postnatal care, family planning, epidemiological care, tuberculosis treatment, general child welfare, etc. are described. A timetable and a system of treatment and advisory work for these activities are included, as well as samples of statistical record forms. This group is increasing its preventive medical work and decreasing expenditures on medicines. A paramedical home visiting programme is being implemented, aiming at intensive educational programmes.

0275   Syme, S.L. *Contributions of social epidemiology to the study of medical care systems: the need for cross-cultural research.* Medical Care (Philadelphia), 9(3), May-Jun 1971, 203-213. Engl.

The nature and magnitude of disease problems in the community have important implications for the priorities that are established for medical care services, for the ways in which such services are organized, and for the urgency with which primary prevention is regarded. The way in which medical care services are organized in the community has implications for understanding disease distributions in that community. The study of medical care systems then inevitably involves study of the magnitude and distribution of disease, and epidemiologic studies of disease distributions must take the medical care system into account. Perhaps most important is that cross-cultural settings provide unique opportunities to explore all of these issues due to the wide variations that exist among the nations of the world in both patterns of disease and in patterns of medical care organizations. Eighteen references are listed.

0276   Taylor, C.E., Hall, M.F. *Health, population and economic development.* Science (Washington, D.C.), 157, 11 Aug 1967, 651-657. Engl.

The relationships between health, population growth, and economic development are complex and vary from one situation to another. Optimum progress occurs when there is simultaneous development in all three areas. Some say family planning should be pursued as a separate programme but evidence presented here challenges this approach. Successful health programmes develop attitudes that encourage change and economic growth. These positive aspects of health work lead to developments that outweigh the much publicized negative influence of population increase. Health programmes are necessary to promote limitation of births. Fifty-five references are listed.

0277   Ten Have, R. *Health services, family planning, and malaria: what about integration?* Nepal, n.p., 14 Oct 1969. 8p. Engl.
Unpublished document.

The term "integration" is often mentioned as a goal of health services. It implies a sharing, among different health programmes, of resources, facilities, and manpower. In Nepal these would be malaria workers, family planning workers, smallpox, leprosy, and tuberculosis control personnel, and hospital and health centre staff. Before integration can take place it is necessary to consider which supplies, buildings, transportation, equipment, and finances exist in sufficient quantity to allow it. A study should be conducted in a limited area where integration of malaria control, family planning, and maternal and child care could be tried. Such a study would provide essential information on the practical problems of integrated health care.

II Organization and Planning

0278 **Thailand, Ministry of Public Health.** *For consideration family health project.* Thailand, Ministry of Public Health, 1969. 4p. Engl.
Unpublished document.

The Government of Thailand's health plans include family planning. Targets for the number of family planning acceptors are being established. Some acceptors are given service at provincial hospitals and health departments. If paramedical personnel are allowed to distribute contraceptives, the numbers of contraceptive acceptors at provincial and municipal levels might be greater than expected. Projects need to be started to test a variety of innovative approaches. New types of family planning workers, leaders, and personnel for health and development projects in rural areas must be trained. Use of incentives for recruiting acceptors should be considered. Training and utilization of family health educators are discussed.

0279 **Ukeje, M.A.** *Integration of maternal and child health activities.* Tropical Doctor (London), 3(4), Oct 1973, 182-184. Engl.

Maternal and child health activities have been separate in Africa in the past. At present, there are twice as many under-five clinics as maternal clinics in Zambia; service offered in maternal clinics is often inadequate. An integrated maternal and child health clinic would save time for the mother who needs both services, facilitate record keeping, and provide clinical staff with a more complete understanding of the family health situation. One drawback is the need for privacy in maternal health care; this could be overcome through the use of portable screens, and the employment of unskilled assistants as babysitters.

0280 **WHO, Geneva.** *Organization and administration of maternal and child health services: fifth report of the WHO Expert Committee on Maternal and Child Health.* Geneva, WHO Technical Report Series No. 428, 1969. 34p. Engl.

An international group of experts express their views on the organization and administration of maternal and child health (MCH) services. Particular areas of discussion are: aims and problems of concern in MCH services, planning, administrative functions, outreach, relation of family planning to other MCH activities, school health programmes, adoption, day care, handicapped children, training, evaluation, and legislation.

0281 **Wurapa, F.K., Neumann, A.K.** *Project summary of the Danfa Rural Health and Family Planning Project.* n.p., 17 Jul 1970. 5p. Engl.
Unpublished document.

The Danfa Rural Health and Family Planning Project in Ghana is a comprehensive teaching, research, and service project. It was initiated by the Department of Prevention and Social Medicine of the Ghana Medical School. It involves other university departments as well as governmental departments, and receives technical or financial support from international organizations such as WHO, UNICEF, IPPF, and USAID. The University of California provides specialists in epidemiology, operational research, family planning, and health education, and will help to build up a biometric data processing centre. The health centre offers family planning as a normal part of its comprehensive services. The project will research questions of vital importance to the development of health programmes in Ghana.

0282 **Ziai, L.** *Iran: family planning model in the context of the existing health services.* Chapel Hill, N.C., n.p., 1970. 20p. Engl.
Unpublished document.

The need for population control in Iran and integration of family planning and maternal and child health services are discussed. Iran's family planning programme provides oral contraceptives and inserts intrauterine devices through a network of centres and mobile teams. Training and education for family planning involve medical personnel, auxiliary health workers, and military personnel. Thirteen references are listed.

III Primary Health Care — Implementation

III.1 Rural inpatient care

See also: 0085, 0299, 0319, 0350, 0616, 0688

0283 Courtejoie, J., de Hertaing, I.R. *Country hospital in the tropics.* Kinshasa, n.p., n.d. 12p. Engl.
Hospitals in Zaire should not limit themselves to treating emergencies and avoidable diseases, but should develop aspects of preventive medicine. Hospital and medical personnel could contribute to the development of the entire region by, e.g., distributing antimalaria tablets in schools and prenatal clinics, and impressing upon people the need to take worm medicine, be vaccinated, eat a balanced diet, etc.

0284 Institute of Rural Health and Family Planning, Gandhigram. *Avvai rural medical service, Gandhigram: Kasturba Hospital.* Gandhigram, Institute of Rural Health and Family Planning, 1966. 4p. Engl.
Unpublished document.
The Kasturba Hospital at Gandhigram, India, provides local villages with the following services: an Auxiliary Nurse Midwife Training Centre, regular weekly antenatal and postnatal services, a family welfare planning programme including sterilization facilities, and an IUD programme.

0285 Joubert, C. *Ghana: the Valco medical service.* In Hughes, J.P., ed., Health Care for Remote Areas: An International Conference, Oakland, Kaiser Foundation, 1972, 73-79. Engl.
See entry 155 for complete proceedings.
The VALCO medical service at Tema, Ghana, was established by the Kaiser Foundation in 1964, during construction of an aluminium smelter. The emphasis in this health service is on preventive medicine. Occupational and nonoccupational health care, as well as care for workers' dependents are aspects of the medical services discussed here.

0286 McPhail, J.E., Wilson, E.E., Eckersley, L.W. WHO, Geneva. *Study on the working of primary health centres in Uttar Pradesh, India.* Geneva, WHO, 1963. 31p. WHO/SEA/RH/14. Engl.
Unpublished document.
Observations and recommendations of a WHO study team in Uttar Pradesh, India, are presented. The study embraced four primary health centres, and examined these aspects of health care: outpatient and inpatient care; referral services; communicable disease control; public health nursing; environmental control; health education; the (pharmaceutical) compounder; school health services; district-level supervision; cooperation with block administration; medical education in relation to rural health service; and future prospects of a primary health centre medical officer. Two annexes provide special reports on the functioning of health visitors and midwives in four selected primary health centres.

0287 Turner, J., Abramson, A.S. *Paraplegic management in rural India.* Rehabilitation Record (Washington, D.C.), 12, Nov-Dec 1971, 10-12. Engl.
Twenty-five rehabilitation research and demonstration projects are being supported by SRS in India. At Vellore, associated with the Christian Medical College, a paraplegic project is being conducted. Its chief investigator, Dr M. Berghese, is attempting to modify Western rehabilitation methods to suit local cultures and economic conditions. A study of patients' homes was conducted to develop architectural modifications and aids and to determine vocational and transportational problems. The requirements for such items as specialized shoe material, devices for indoor mobility, toilet facilities, etc. were noted in the study. Procedures to prevent patients' discomfort are being studied. At the institute, training is given in many trades such as tailoring, brush making, and radio repair. The project also incorporates medical research at the hospital, utilization of local materials, and development of adaptions for braces and crutches.

0288 WHO, New Delhi. *Short study of primary health centres: inpatients, bed strength, staffing and allied matters.* New Delhi, WHO, 1966. 14p. WHO/SEA/PHA/56. Engl.
Unpublished document.
A short study of 139 primary health centres in India presents statistics on the number of beds and yearly admissions, the distribution of doctors, nurses, and auxiliary personnel, average length of stay, distance of referral hospitals from health centres, number of laboratory tests performed, etc. The 99 doctors involved in the study expressed the need for consulting services,

improved communications, better referral hospitals, etc.

0289 Zaire, Department of Public Health. *Programme de sante publique en zone rurale: bilan et projets du departement de sante publique, Hopital de Vanga (Zaire). (Public health programme for the rural sector: evaluation of projects of the Department of Public Health, Vanga Hospital).* Kinshasa, Department of Public Health, May 1973. 22p. Fren.

Village public health activities of the Vanga Hospital, Zaire, include health education and motivation, health inspections, distribution of medicine, and an annual follow-up visit. In this paper procedures dealing with the following are analyzed: mother and child health, tuberculosis, nutrition, and family planning. Village health workers assist in the villages by promoting health, coordinating visits of the mobile health team, keeping records of health statistics, etc. These health workers are usually married, 25-35 years old with fewer than five children, and have at least 6 years of primary education.

III.2 Rural outpatient care

See also: 0029, 0048, 0074, 0104, 0146, 0174, 0226, 0284, 0285, 0350, 0365, 0366, 0460, 0616, 0642, 0689

0290 American Friends Service Committee, Philadelphia. *Pilot project in rural health and rural economy: Guatemala.* Philadelphia, American Friends Service Committee, May 1973. 2p. Engl. Unpublished document.

Pilot health programmes using auxiliary health workers were started in five Guatemalan villages. Support came from students, village committees, university faculties, etc. The villages chosen were rural resettlement cooperatives of people from several language groups. Local people assisted in building health centres. Villagers were trained as health promoters, with a view to their providing preventive and curative care for the village after 2-3 years of supervision, experience, and training. The project was expanded to include developments in rural economy.

0291 Arole, R.S. *Comprehensive rural health project, Jamkhed: leprosy control and treatment integrated with comprehensive rural health programme.* n.p., Apr 1973. 4p. Engl. Unpublished document.

Modern methods of treatment make it unnecessary to isolate lepers. Domiciliary treatment is safe for most patients. Traditional social attitudes, however, discourage patients from taking advantage of advanced medical care. In the rural area of India chosen for a comprehensive health programme, 11-15 persons per 1 000 have leprosy. The main centre of work is in Jamkhed, although there are plans to expand the geographical distribution of services. Leprosy patients are encouraged to attend general outpatient services at the clinic. They are assured their condition will be kept confidential. During routine home and school visiting sessions, new cases are identified, and without the public knowing it leprosy patients are brought under treatment. Objectives of the programme are complete integration of leprosy care with other aspects of comprehensive health care and continued outpatient care of cases.

0292 Arole, R.S. *Comprehensive rural health project, Jamkhed, India.* Contact (Geneva), 10, Aug 1972, 1-9. Engl., Fren.

Address given to the Christian Medical Commission, Geneva at its annual meeting in June 1972.

A phased health programme for rural India is described. A health centre based in Jamkhed, India, with 10 subcentres in neighbouring villages provides diagnostic, emergency surgery, and medical care facilities. Initially funded by the Christian Medical Commission, the centre is intended to be self-sustaining after 6 years of operation and will serve up to 80 000 people in 55 villages. The programme, which will be coordinated with other government programmes, aims at reducing population growth rates and infant and child mortality, and treating lepers and the chronically ill. To achieve these goals, the support of the entire community is sought. In participating villages a consultative committee including representatives from all strata of society is formed. This committee decides on priorities, appoints reliable nonprofessionals, and activates the community to cooperate in various aspects of the programme. Prerequisites for starting work in a village include provision of a place to work and housing for visiting nurses, and village cooperation in child care and immunization. Under-five clinics, a family welfare and nutrition programme, mobile clinics, and school health projects have been started. The cooperation of indigenous practitioners is enlisted in feeding programmes, antenatal care, treatment of leprosy and tuberculosis, etc.

0293 Attia, S.E. WHO, Alexandria. *Report on a visit to the Syrian Arab Republic, 24 June to 8 July 1969.* Alexandria, WHO, Sept 1969. 32p. WHO/EMRO /69/948. EM/RH/16 Syria General. Engl.

This report is related to the development of the Five Year Plan for Basic Health Services and Training for 1971-75, for the Ministry of Health of the Syrian Arab Republic. Prior to the plan there were over 140 rural health centres in the country. Different centres have been developed to cover independent aspects of health service without much coordination and without meeting the real needs of the population. Services are unevenly distributed and understaffed. Subcentres must be developed as one means of systematically reaching all of the population. The plan is an integral part of the socioeconomic plan for the country for the same period.

0294 Baxter, A.J. *Long journey to Kasama on foot.* Zambia Nurse (Kitwe, Zambia), 2(1), Jan 1966, 14-18. Engl.

The author joined the Northern Rhodesian Nursing Service in 1919. In 1924 she volunteered to serve in a health outpost in Kasama, Zambia where a new hospital was to be built. Early services included midwifery, treatment of malaria cases, and emergency surgery.

0295 Beghin, I.D. *Nutritional rehabilitation centers in Latin America: a critical assessment.* American Journal of Clinical Nutrition (Bethesda, Md.), 23(11), Nov 1970, 1412-1417. Engl.

Although Nutrition Rehabilitation Centres (NRC) are not the universal solution to preschool child malnutrition, and cannot be a substitute for economic development, increased education, or strengthened health services, in six Latin American countries they make an important contribution to the solution of nutritional problems. An effective operation must include low costs, broad coverage, effective education of the mother, and adherence to a set of rules governing operation of the centre. The NRC should be integrated within the health centre as a service whenever possible, but can also be located wherever malnutrition exists. The number of rehabilitation centres should be higher than the number of health centres and provide wider coverage. They can serve as starting points for community development programmes or for applied nutrition programmes in communities deprived of health services. Because of the demonstrated flexibility of this effective and inexpensive formula, the author recommends its general application. Seventeen references are listed.

0296 Bolton, J.M. *Medical services to the aborigines in West Malaysia.* British Medical Journal (London), 2, 29 Jun 1968, 818-823. Engl.

The aboriginal people of West Malaysia were first provided with medical care in 1955. The original reasons for this aid were military, but after Malaysian independence the service became part of the Malaysian government's rural development programme. Aborigines are of many language and ethnic groups. During the war for independence they had been forced to leave the jungle and settle in camps at the edge of the jungle. A high mortality rate was the result. Later they were allowed to return to the jungle and were treated with Western medicine only when they presented themselves at police posts. Their acceptance of Western medicine was superficial and a matter of convenience. With the Malaysian government's second 5-year development plan, funds were allocated to expand services to the aborigines. Gradually there has been an improvement in the relationship between the aborigines and the government's various development programmes. Maternal and child health services, leprosy, tuberculosis, and malaria control services, flying doctor and emergency services have been set up. Jungle medical posts have been set up, manned by aborigines trained as auxiliary health workers. Midwifery services are also available.

0297 Bruce, S. *Busoga eye project.* Nursing Times (London), 63(38), 22 Sep 1967, 1281-1282. Engl.

In 1963, a survey conducted in the Lake Victoria area of Uganda indicated the seriousness of the trachoma problem there. The African Medical and Research Foundation decided to attempt a project to eradicate the disease from the area. The Royal Commonwealth Society for the Blind supported the project. Eighty schools were visited and 2 719 children were found to have active trachoma. The programme was then extended into the homes of the people. A mobile vehicle was equipped and a nurse, a health educator, and a driver were recruited. It was difficult to get the children to cooperate fully with treatment through the schools alone. Home and school efforts were then coordinated. The organization of treatment, education, and the administration of achromycin are described. Records show that people were cured following 6 months of treatment. However, many thousands more remain in need of this service.

0298 Bull, G.M. *Impressions of a medical tour of eastern and western regions of Nigeria.* West African Medical Journal, (Ibadan), 9(4), Aug 1960, 139-144. Engl.

This report presents observations of Nigerian government hospitals, health and maternity centres, dispensaries, mission hospitals, and other health institutions. One problem in Nigeria is providing health services to a large population on a very small budget. Expenditures for public health would provide health services for more people at less cost, but public pressure is for development of curative services. Physician education encourages graduates to take urban posts, leaving the field of public health neglected. Demand for outpatient services in hospitals has increased greatly. Many patients seeking help from outpatient departments were government employees and scholars looking for an excuse for time off. In Umuahia Mission Hospital special hours were designated for care of civil servants and for school children. As a result, total outpatient attendance fell dramatically. A first step in outpatient care should be filtration of patients by some system based on the kind of care they need. Patients saw a physician at the rate of one patient every 30 seconds. This is unrealistic in terms of proper diagnosis. The improvement of outpatient care is a research subject deserving high priority.

0299 Byer, M.A., Dyer, H., Gourlay, R.J., Standard, K.L. *Role of the health centre in an integrated health programme in a developing country.* Medical Care (Philadelphia), 3, 1966, 26-29. Engl.

The advantages of an integrated and comprehensive curative and preventive medical service are described. The role of the health centre in such a service is emphasized, and a broad plan for the regionalization of health centres providing community care in Jamaica is described. (Author abstract.)

III Primary Health Care — Implementation

Abstracts 0300-0307

0300 Central Treaty Organization, Ankara. *Teaching health centres.* Ankara, Central Treaty Organization, 1962. 45p. Engl.
Conference on teaching health centres, Ankara, Turkey, May 1962.

The conference was attended by public health experts from Turkey, Iran, Pakistan, USA, and U.K. Their purpose was to explore the benefits of health centre training for medical students, to consider the organization and duration of said health centre training, and to suggest administration and staffing requirements for such a health centre training institution. Summary discussions of the three areas are reported. It is recommended that such meetings be held on an annual basis, that representatives of appropriate international agencies be invited to participate in future health conferences, and that a health representative be added to the CENTO staff to serve as liaison and coordinating officer.

0301 Chablani, T.D. *Einfuhrung der ganzheitsmedizin durch haupt-gesundheitszentren auf dem lande. (Promotion of comprehensive medical care through the main health centre in rural areas).* Zeitschrift Fur Die Gesamte Hygiene Und Ihre Grenzgebiete (Berlin), 13, Nov 1967, 877-880. German.

The author maintains that the urgent demand for health protection in rural India can only be met by promoting the main health centre, the backbone of medical services in rural areas, and by providing it with a well-equipped and complete team of health workers. (Revised journal abstract.)

0302 Dadgar, M., Saroukhanian, G. *Health corps in Iran: an approach to the better distribution of health resources in remote areas.* In Wolstenholm, G., O'Connor, M., eds., Teamwork for World Health, London, J. and A. Churchill, 1971, 37-55. Engl.
See also entry 198.

Iran's unique use of military personnel in health services is examined, particularly in terms of the Health Corps' potential for training future manpower. Although Iran's Ministry of Health provides 810 clinics in addition to some 400 clinics run by the Health Corps, health manpower is still not satisfactorily distributed. Most physicians live in urban areas. Women are accepted into the Health Corps and represent 10-15% of all medical school graduates. The programme has been supported enthusiastically by rural communities.

0303 de Glanville, H., ed(s). *Administration: health centres/small hospitals.* Afya: A Journal for Medical and Health Workers (Nairobi), 7, Apr 1973, 60-62. Engl.

One of the problems of running small health units is that their staff are rarely trained as administrators. Scientific principles need to be applied in administering these centres. Poor administration may result in poor public relations, high staff turnover, low patient load, and a totally unhappy atmosphere. Duties of health centre administrators that increase staff effectiveness and job satisfaction are outlined.

0304 Dimataga, A.L. *Rural needs and problems.* Newsette (Makati-Rizal, Philippines), 8(2), Apr-Jun 1968, 13-14. Engl.

Two billion of the world's population live in rural areas. In the Philippines the needs of people in the rural area have become quite clear. The Philippine Government alone cannot provide the massive funding required to meet growing requirements of rural areas. Civic and religious groups play an important role in supplementing government services. The activities of the Opon Puericulture Centre and Maternity House include maternal and child health services. Family planning services have been recently added. Each month an average of 1 000 patients attends the clinic.

0305 Du Toit, A.E., Johnson, S., Coster, M.E. *Functions of a health centre.* South African Medical Journal (Capetown), 45, 20 Mar 1971, 307-319. Engl.

The first health centre in South Africa was opened in Johannesburg in 1969 to serve a predominantly white section of the community. Due to an inadequate concept of the functions of such a centre a survey was undertaken by the health personnel of the local authority to determine how far the needs of the community were being met by existing services and how improvements could be made within the limits of enabling legislation and finances. The ideal functions of such a health centre are defined. In the meantime only interim measures can be introduced prior to lifting of legislative and financial barriers wherever possible. Forty-seven references are listed. (Journal abstract.)

0306 Fendall, N.R. *Health centres: a basis for a rural health service.* Journal of Tropical Medicine and Hygiene (London), 66, Sep 1963, 219-232. Engl.

This article discusses comprehensive rural health services, widespread distribution of health centres, and the use of auxiliary health workers. Health centres are the local level unit through which national health care reaches all the people. At health centres, integration of curative and preventive medicine is necessary. Examples are taken from Kenya. Seven architectural plans show various designs of health centres. Eighteen references are listed.

0307 Fendall, N.R., Killen, O.H., Southgate, B.A. *National reference health centre for Kenya.* East African Medical Journal (Nairobi), 40(4), Apr 1963, 118-123. Engl.

The health centre is an institution where curative, preventive, and promotive health services are coordinated and from which services radiate to the community. The National Reference Health Centre in Kenya has three main functions: (1) providing medical care for a rural African community and functioning as a model for other centres; (2) training all categories of rural health workers; and (3) providing research facilities. Two types of training are undertaken: (1) short courses for medical officers, public health inspectors, and public health nurses who supervise health centres; and (2) longer practical courses for the auxiliary health centre staff. Research activities are directed mainly toward local field research on mortality and morbidity statistics, epidemiology of local diseases, the sociological impact of the rural health service, etc. Six references are listed.

0308 Fendall, N.R. *Health centres in Kenya.* East African Medical Journal (Nairobi), 37(3), Mar 1960, 171-185. Engl.

The health centre concept is the only realistic approach, both economically and for the future health of the population of underprivileged countries, where the population is essentially rural. However, certain fundamental working principles must be followed to achieve success: (1) the health centre is the institution where all three arms of the service — curative, preventive, and promotive — are coordinated; (2) it exists at the periphery and is the direct link with the family in its home and community environment; (3) it must be supported by a planned hospital and health service but these exist to support and reinforce the health centre, not vice versa; (4) staff must be infused with a sense of vocation and provided with practical in-training at a health centre; (5) the building and staffing of health centres must not precede the training of staff, or the whole project is likely to fall into disrepute; (6) although in its final state the health centre will encompass much more than a pure health programme, it should not attempt to reach this stage at the beginning: it should be designed and staffed to keep just a little ahead of the people it is serving in both education and service; (7) the unit should be capable of being reduplicated in sufficient numbers throughout the country so that the national economy is not overburdened; (8) once a health centre is established in an area it must be the paramount institution: the public must be educated to turn to it always and all other health activities should be channelled through the centre; (9) staff should be recruited from the indigenous population; (10) an adequate transport system is essential; (11) comprehensive records are very desirable and in due course are essential for future policy planning; (12) the distinction between a general practitioner health centre and a consultant or chief health centre must be drawn clearly; and (13) the provision of beds in a centre should be sufficient for emergency cases (patients being transferred to home or hospital) and normal maternity cases where home conditions are unsatisfactory, etc. In addition to the above recommendations the author discusses staff training, health education, and the mobile health unit. Thirteen references are listed.

0309 Fisek, N.H. Hacettepe University, School of Medicine, Institute of Community Medicine, Ankara. *Account of the activities of the Etimesgut Rural Health District, 1967, 1968 and 1969.* Ankara, Hacettepe Press, 1970. 40p. Engl.

The Etimesgut Rural Health District was established by the Ministry of Health of Turkey in 1965. Medical staff and hospital services were provided by the Hacettepe University; paramedical staff and financial resources were provided by the Ministry of Health. The objectives of the project are to provide health care for persons living in the district, to provide training facilities for medical and paramedical personnel in rural health practice, and to carry out research in rural health administration and epidemiology of health and disease. This report provides a detailed description and evaluation of the project.

0310 Flavier, J.M. *Rural public health: a search for an answer.* Philippine Journal of Nursing (Manila), 37(1), Jan-Mar 1968, 24-31. Engl.

Of the Philippine population, 75% live in rural areas and about 75% of deaths amongst these rural people are due to communicable and preventable diseases. These deaths represent a great loss in manpower and productivity, costing the nation a staggering amount annually. Only about 26% of the cases resulting in death are seen by a physician and only about 32% of the births are delivered by a licensed midwife or a physician in rural areas. The rural health unit concept is well accepted, although implementation has been difficult. There is a great need for continuous training of new medical personnel, since those stationed in rural areas seem to migrate to the towns and cities. A corps of dedicated workers is called for.

0311 Forbes, C. *Interim report on the Gatundu comprehensive child health clinic (C.C.H.C.).* Nairobi, University of Nairobi, Department of Pediatrics, n.d. 4p. Engl.
Unpublished document.

Since 1972 a comprehensive child health clinic has been operating out of the Gatundu Self-Help Hospital. This project developed after experts concurred that under-five clinics proved the best way to deliver health care services to children. The project is built from analysis of health needs of children in a community. Resources to meet needs are brought together. The clinic is actually a maternal and child health clinic. Procedures and patient records are described. Dramatic reduction in the death rate between 1972 and 1973 is credited to the establishment of the Comprehensive Child Health Clinic. Problems of clinic operations are listed. Real community involvement and participation has not yet been accomplished. Overcrowding still hinders optimal functioning.

0312 Iran, Ministry of Health. *Health corps: a new approach to the better distribution of the health resources, on the occasion of the tenth anniversary of the White Revolution in Iran.* Iran, Health Corps Organization, Jan 1973. 33p. Engl.

A new programme for delivery of health care to the rural communities of Iran is outlined. The Health Corps consists of physicians, dentists, pharmacists, health educators, etc., along with a supporting group of high school graduates i.e. auxiliary health workers.

During a training period of 6 months (which includes military training), Corps members receive instruction in rural health education and public health. Mobile teams led by a physician and supported by medical aides are the most dynamic section of the Corps. Statistical data on activities in family planning, public health, waste disposal, water supply and treatment, and health education are presented.

0313 Jackson, P. *Egbe hospital: past, present and future.* Saving Health (London), 11(3), Sep 1972, 41-43. Engl.

The experience of a doctor who is the sole physician in a 120-bed hospital in Kwara State, Nigeria is reported. The history of early medical service to the area is described. Present work in a newly built maternity ward calls for educating women to seek antenatal care and delivery. Clinics for antenatal, postnatal, and family planning have been established. An average of 200 outpatient patients are seen a day. The author feels he should be doing direct spiritual missionary work but is limited by not speaking Yoruba. Mission work therefore is done by deed rather than by word of mouth. The future of this kind of work looks bleak because it is difficult to get non-Nigerians to come and work in the area, and Nigerian physicians work in urban areas. Efforts to "Nigerianize" the staff is part of the hospital's policy but Nigerian physicians demand salaries roughly on par with those paid in the United Kingdom.

0314 Maar, S.A. *Follow-up survey of outpatients in a medical clinic for Africans at Harare Hospital in Rhodesia.* Central African Journal of Medicine (Salisbury), 19(7), Jul 1973, 151-154. Engl.

In a prospective study of 233 medical patients discharged from a medical unit of Harare Hospital in Rhodesia, only 115 (49%) attended their follow-up appointments. Reasons for this are discussed in relation to social factors, discharge diagnosis, and readmission 18 months later. Twelve references are listed. (Revised journal abstract.)

0315 Matovu, H.L., Bennett, F.J., Namboze, J.N. *Kasangati health centre - a community approach.* East African Medical Journal (Nairobi), 48(1), Jan 1971, 33-39. Engl.

A description of the Kasangati Health Centre (Uganda) is presented and records for the 4 years have been reviewed to evaluate the services' effects on the community, concentrating mainly on trends in maternal and child health. Patterns of morbidity, mortality, and some vital rates are given. Also reviewed are immunization and prophylaxis as bases for mass prevention and treatment. Progress in local acceptance of the centre's services is attributed to its strong emphasis on health education and a community approach. Ten references are listed.

0316 Moles, G. *Medical mission work in Africa: the present and the prospect.* Saving Health (London), 10(4), Dec 1971, 76-81. Engl.

Many persons ask how long Christian medical work in Africa will continue. The author believes it will be recognized as needed and will be sought after in the future. Part of the role the mission plays reflects the massive need for medical work to be done in Africa. The medical mission centre at Vom, Nigeria, is in a rural area and serves many persons. A private clinic held several times weekly serves the needs of senior service Nigerians and expatriates. Vom is also a training school for nurses, midwives, and laboratory assistants. The author maintains the purpose of being in Nigeria is to get the Gospel across. Problems include financial ones, since government hospitals charge no fees whereas mission hospitals have to charge fees. The government provides a grant but this does not cover all costs.

0317 Rao, P.S., Benjamin, V., Richard, J. *Methods of evaluating health centres.* British Journal of Preventive and Social Medicine (London), 26, 1972, 46-52. Engl.

Scientific evaluation of health centres leads to more effective planning. An evaluative study of health centres in Tamil Nadu, India, produced a statistical breakdown of the following evaluative indices: effort expended by health centres per person-unit and per activity-unit per week; percent of population served by a primary health centre in relation to distance from centre; percent of persons utilizing outpatient services from subcentre and nonsubcentre areas per year; percent of mothers and children who made use of maternal and child health services in subcentres and nonsubcentres; and community response to health centre services, etc. These indices were created from the most readily available data and do not relate achievement to need or compare input with output. Further study would require more sophisticated techniques. Evaluation can be hindered by weak statements of programme objectives and by lack of resources. However, given time restraints, etc., available data can provide insight into programmes. Nine references are listed.

0318 Rao, P.S., Richard, J. *Measuring community responses to health centre programmes.* Indian Journal of Medical Research (New Delhi), 58, 7 Jul 1970, 938-946. Engl.

The interest, enthusiasm, and initiative of the local citizens figures significantly in effective community health service. Although those who need the services most fail to take advantage of them due to ignorance, tradition, etc., the more educated and well-to-do tend to make maximum use of available health services on their own without too much effort on the part of the health centre. In evaluating programme effectiveness, we therefore need to identify those factors that have been hindering the full utilization of the health centre services by the total community, and measure the response of the community in terms of their knowledge, attitudes, and utilization of the health services. In this paper, the design and conduct of such a study is described and discussed, using the rural area served by the teaching health centre of Christian Medical College and Hospital, Vellore, and that of six primary health centres in the adjoining districts of North Arcot and Chingleput. The structure of the questionnaire used is described. As an alternate to sampling from general public, three suitable types of respondents were identified, viz., the patient, the community worker, and the community leader. Based on the distance from the health centre or subcentre, the area served was divided into three segments. Representative samples of general public, patients, workers, and leaders from each segment were chosen and interviewed. The responses from these four groups were compared. The community workers gave the least valid estimates of the true response in the community. The patients also were not found suitable for representing correctly the community response, and the interview had to be rather brief. Valid and reliable estimates of community response were obtained from community leaders, when selected on the basis of the length of their stay in the area and intensity of contact with the public. Five references are listed. (Journal abstract.)

0319 **Roberts, J.M.** *Rural health centre projects in North Nyanza.* East African Medical Journal (Nairobi), 37(3), Mar 1960, 186-203. Engl.

In North Nyanza, Kenya, health services developed from hospital work in urban areas to curative work in rural dispensaries and later to preventive work in rural health centres. Health centres are now the basic unit providing comprehensive care. The centres are operated and financed by the local authority. Mobile health units, which are also run by the local authority, provide a service to remote areas and in immediate environs around the district hospital. This paper describes aspects of health centre operation such as financing, water supplies, transport, equipment, and staff. Experience in North Nyanza indicates that training of health centre staff should be carried out in the practical atmosphere of a health centre as opposed to a provincial hospital; training centres should be developed where health centre practice is already well established.

0320 **Roemer, M.I.** WHO, Geneva. *Evaluation of community health centres.* Geneva, WHO Public Health Papers No. 48, 1972. 42p. Engl.

This report clarifies the various meanings of "health centre," reviews the literature on evaluation of their activities, and proposes research studies for developing countries. Eighty-six references are listed.

0321 **Schulman, D.P., Schulman, S.** *Nurse as catalyst.* American Journal of Nursing (New York), 68(9), Sep 1968, 1890-1894. Engl.

The nurse can initiate continuing action in the community. In Colombia a North American nurse served as a catalyst in initiating services in a small clinic in a slum area of Bogota. The nurse began as a volunteer, introduced into the community by a priest who had helped the people build the clinic. The nurse was able gradually to enlist the participation of several private physicians, social workers, and religious workers. Three years after leaving the area the involvement of these Colombians in the clinic continues. A part-time Colombian nurse works in the clinic and a physician holds regular weekend clinics there.

0322 **Segall, M.** *Medical care in North Vietnam.* Lancet (London), 6 Jun 1970, 1224. Engl.
Letter to the editor.

Health service efforts in North Vietnam before 1964 concentrated on providing services to people in the countryside. Nearly all the villages in the plains and two-thirds in the hills had health centres. Staff consisted of nurses, midwives, assistant doctors (trained for 3 years), and health instructors, drawn from the countryside and going back to their own villages to work. The clinics were responsible for health education, immunization, maternity care, birth control advice, and treatment of minor illnesses. Before bombing began in 1965, the village clinics were supported by 50-bed district hospitals, and above these were the larger provincial and specialist hospitals. Although 265 hospitals had been destroyed by 1970, the decentralized character of the health system permitted continuous medical care.

0323 **Seoul National University, School of Public Health, Seoul.** *Chunseong Gun community health service: Report 1. Summer training program of 1972; Report 2. Field training of students, Shindong Myon Health Sub-station activities.* Seoul, Seoul National University, School of Public Health, Apr 1973 and Apr 1974. 108p. and 79p. Engl., Korean.

Since 1959, when the Seoul National University School of Public Health was set up, it has been recognized that field experience is an important part of the medical student's training, and consequently several health centres in Seoul were selected for the purpose. Problems arose, however, because health centre staff were ill-equipped to lead students in their field work and most were too busy with their own activities to devote time to supervision and training. To correct this unsatisfactory state of affairs, in 1972 the School set up its own training and demonstration centre, supervised and operated in conjunction with the local health authority of Chunseong Gun Community. The results of the experimental training programme for 1972 and 1973 are evaluated. Maps, curriculum, and demographic and other data are included.

0324 **Shepherd, P.** *Crossroads of the tribes.* Saving Health (London), 12(2), Jun 1973, 33-35. Engl.

Haicota is the town representing the crossroads for three tribes (Baria, Ilit, and Cunama) in Ethiopia. The historical and cultural background for the groups is sketched. The Haicota hospital is thus strategically placed. This is a mission hospital and medical work is considered part of the church-building efforts in the tribal area. At one point village clinic work was interrupted when Liberation Front activities were in force and the government restricted movement of foreigners outside the main towns. Otherwise the mission of the hospital and its dispensaries continues.

0325 Soumah, A. *Health centres to serve rural Africa.* World Hospitals (Oxford), 1968, 63-64. Engl.

In Africa only the most specialized medical services should be developed in urban centres. The real overall need is for the development of rural health centres providing outpatient and inpatient care through combined curative and preventive medical work. Centres with 50 to 200 beds are recommended. Building costs depend on costs of materials in each local area. An attempt is made to estimate appropriate percentages of funds for various elements in the health centre building.

0326 Stanley, A. *Back door clinic.* Reprint; source unknown. 1p. Engl.

Health care for African employees on Europeans' farms in Rhodesia depends largely on the farmer's wife's knowledge of medicine. Transportation of the sick and injured to hospitals is a problem, since ambulance service is expensive and distances are great. African children often suffer from burns and scabies, and medicines are given out when available by the farmer's wife without much knowledge of diagnosis or cure.

0327 Vogel, L.C. *Kenya-Netherlands-Israel Project for Operational Research in Outpatient Services: report on second quarter of 1973.* Nairobi, n.p., 30 Jun 1973. 7p. Engl.

Unpublished document. This report should be read in conjunction with the Annual Report for 1972 and with the First Quarterly Report for 1973 (see entry 328). See also entry 329.

As of 1973, the Kenya-Netherlands-Israel Project for Operational Research in Outpatient Services (KNIPOROS) was continuing and construction of the clinic building was in progress. Plans for the preliminary experiment were complete. This report covers agreements and decisions for the second quarter of 1973. Appended to the report is a pamphlet describing the project, which will provide general outpatient care, antenatal care, infant and preschool care, and family planning. A second appendix describes criteria for evaluating the project, i.e. efficiency, cost-effectiveness, quality of care, and acceptability of care to the people.

0328 Vogel, L.C. *Kenya-Netherlands-Israel Project for Operational Research in Outpatient Services: report on the first quarter of 1973.* Nairobi, n.p., 6 Apr 1973. 5p. Engl.

Unpublished document. This report should be read in conjunction with the Annual Report for 1972 (see entry 327). See also entry 329.

This is a detailed report on the decisions taken and the agreements reached, during the first quarter of 1973, by the Kenya-Netherlands-Israel Project for Operational Research in Outpatient Services (KNIPOROS). The report includes comments on the current state of the construction of the KNIPOROS clinic building and the rate of social and operational research.

0329 Vogel, L.C. *Early history of KNIPOROS (Kenya-Netherlands-Israel Project for Operational Research Outpatient Services) covering the period up to ultimo 1972.* Nairobi, Medical Research Centre, 30 Dec 1972. 22p. Engl.

See also entries 327 and 328.

This document is intended for those interested in the early history of the Kenya-Netherlands-Israel Project for Operational Research in Outpatient Services. Appendices include ground plans for the building that will serve as the study cum service area. Experiments are described that will develop improved techniques for handling outpatient care. Aspects of management to be evaluated include prescription by "code," prepackaging of drugs in the pharmacy, a new supply system, and new layout of injection rooms.

0330 Wells, M. *Planning of health buildings.* Tropical Doctor (London), 3(4), Oct 1973, 177-181. Engl.

Health centres are replacing hospitals as the nucleus of nation-wide health delivery in underdeveloped countries. A limited number of large hospitals, often teaching institutions, supported by a large number of smaller hospitals, supported by still larger numbers of health centres and clinics, is generally considered the most desirable system of health delivery in underdeveloped countries. Ideally, the local clinic or centre relies on the hospital for visits by supporting staff and referrals. This paper discusses the shortcomings of this system in serving rural areas, i.e., poor communication between clinics and hospital, inadequate staffing, and the fact that the clinic is forced to be a more self-contained unit than it was originally designed to be. The author suggests that clinics in remote areas be made more self-sufficient by staffing them with locally trained medical assistants, and later community-trained doctors, and by expanding their facilities to include more beds and hostels for housing the families of patients. At the same time, effective communication with the local hospital should be maintained.

0331 WHO, Brazzaville. *Health services as a factor in regional integrated rural development.* Brazzaville, WHO, 6 Nov 1969. 11p. WHO/AFR/PHA/55. Engl., Fren.

A rural health care delivery system based on a study of rural development problems is outlined in general terms. The establishment of health centres and satellite subcentres for rural populations is recommended. Objectives, activities, staffing patterns, resource allocation, etc. will differ from country to country, and from situation to situation. The system should be established and then developed gradually over years. The importance of mother and child care is emphasized. Staff training relevant to local needs is a high priority. Health centres should be integrated with community development, agricultural extension, and adult literacy programmes. Five references are listed.

0332 Woolman, A. *Mountain nurse.* Saving Health (London), 10(4), Dec 1971, 65-69. Engl.

A description of difficult work in a rural hospital in Lesotho is given. The hospital is the nearest help for hundreds of villages and is staffed by 11 people. As a newly independent nation, the people are not yet used to independent action. Part of the work is to encourage all staff to attain as much independence of thought and action as possible. Local personnel, even the trained, are reluctant to take on responsibility for work if a European is near at hand. This pattern by local personnel is logical within the context of their upbringing and culture. The centre is growing both in bed space and clinics for children. The antenatal clinic is being extended. A series of outstation clinics are visited monthly and these must be visited by horse. Disease conditions present are aggravated by malnutrition. Venereal disease is epidemic. Head wounds are common as a result of local fights. Working in South Africa takes the men away from the villages and presents problems for those left behind as well as for the men who leave.

0333 Yen, Y.T. *Use of medical students in studying health center operations in Taiwan.* Journal of Medical Education (Chicago), 46, May 1971, 466-469. Engl.

In Taiwan, students of preventive medicine and public health studied the activities of 13 health stations. They recorded such health centre activities as prenatal care, treatment of venereal disease and tuberculosis, family planning, general medical care, and immunization, as well as home visits for antenatal and postnatal care, family planning, etc. Comparison of student observations indicates that interobserver differences are increased in recording the working pattern of multiphasic staff, including public nurses, inspectors, and health workers. In the health stations, where an extensive variety of functions are performed and integrated approaches are adopted for each staff member, the researcher should be an experienced and well-trained public health worker in order to record comprehensive information about activities. Students should have a more advanced knowledge of public health practice before their assignments to health centre settings can provide a really effective educational experience.

0334 Zaghloul, A.Z. WHO, Alexandria. *Assignment report: basic public health and medical care services (model community health centre, Safwa) 20 November 1965-21 April 1967.* Alexandria, WHO, Aug 1967. 21p. WHO/EM/PHA/119. Saudi Arabia 0029/FIT. Engl.

Statistical data on health care in Saudi Arabia show that services are urban, centralized, and curative. A community health centre established in 1964 in the growing town of Safwa attends 250 patients per day. Careful family records are kept and a weekly report of communicable diseases is made. Maternal and child health services, health education, school health, and health surveys have been activities of the community health centre. Objectives of the health centre were largely fulfilled with the exception of sanitation objectives. One recommendation is that training of Saudis take place on a level adequate to fill the nation's needs so that the country will not have to rely on expatriates. Midwives and auxiliaries need to be trained. Statistical data on the social background of Safwa residents is presented.

III.3 Mobile units and services

See also: 0062, 0071, 0242, 0289, 0423, 0481

0335 African Medical and Research Foundation, Nairobi. *Flying doctor services training centre.* Nairobi, African Medical and Research Foundation, Feb 1973. 9p. Engl.

The African Medical and Research Foundation's flying doctor service is responsible for emergency ambulance flights and routine surgical, medical, and health education visits to outlying East African hospitals and clinics in rural districts. The Foundation also has mobile land units comprised of a medical assistant, two nurses, and other auxiliaries. These units spend 2 weeks each month in remote areas bringing curative and preventive medicine to static and nomadic population groups. The training centre programme trains doctors, nurses, medical assistants, radio operators, pilots, health educators, and administrators. Curricula are given for each type of course. Subjects covered at the centre include "bush" medical practice; radio control operation; radio repair and maintenance; "bush" flying; aircraft maintenance; flying doctor service administration; flying doctor service accounting; health education; motor vehicle maintenance; camping; hospital workshop, woodwork, and metal work; and survival techniques.

0336 African Medical and Research Foundation, Nairobi. *Medical development: Southern Sudan.* Nairobi, African Medical and Research Foundation, May 1972. 43p. Engl.

The African Medical and Research Foundation presents its recommendations for medical development in southern Sudan. The proposals include creation of a flying doctor service and other mobile services, development of rural dispensaries, and establishment of training centres for paramedical personnel. Several appendices present estimates of projected capital expenditure and personnel requirements.

0337 African Medical and Research Foundation, Nairobi. *A flying doctor service: (and) a radio-communications network.* Nairobi, African Medical and Research Foundation, n.d. 6p. Engl. Unpublished document.

The African Medical and Research Foundation now has about 70 radios in use in support of its flying doctor service. This radio communications network allows emergency and nonemergency medical traffic to be handled, to the benefit of patients and administrators of the programme. PYE SSB 130 radios costing U.S.

$1 140 (Shs. 8000/-) each are used. Details concerning the use of these are provided and may be of interest to persons considering establishing this kind of service. The cost and type of aircraft used are also given. This service is as cheap as road travel, and time saved in reaching rural patients is considerable. The use of aircraft allows specialists to reach more sections of the population, permits supervision of rural auxiliary staff, etc.

0338 **Bodenheimer, T.S.** *Mobile units: a solution to the rural health problem?* Medical Care (Philadelphia), 7(2), Mar-Apr 1969, 144-154. Engl.

The fundamental problem of rural health is the extremely low density of health professionals per unit of surface area resulting in large distances between patient and services. To deliver services in rural areas, either stationary facilities or mobile units can be used. The underdeveloped world has had considerable experience with different varieties of mobile units. From this experience, certain principles can be derived that are useful in choosing between stationary and mobile facilities for specific situations. The first consideration is the geographic-demographic layout. Second is the type of health service desired, with mobile units most applicable to periodic health services employing simple facilities, but not desirable for comprehensive care. The third factor in deciding between stationary and mobile systems is the determination of which provides more benefits per cost. Although mobile units are an attractive method for rural health service delivery, stationary facilities are often preferable. Forty-one references are listed.

0339 **Burkitt W.R.** *Rural mobile medicine in Kenya.* East African Medical Journal (Nairobi), 46(10), Oct 1969, 541-547. Engl.

This article describes one line of approach that has been used in Kenya whereby the centrally based specialist can actively supervise "eye-trained" medical assistants in various parts of the country. The emphasis is on the administrative and economic aspects of an ophthalmic programme, but it is thought that the general approach could have a wider application to other spheres of rural medicine. A brief account of the development of the work is given; the problems encountered and the lessons learnt are discussed, and certain general principles for its success are outlined. Finally, the expenditure involved is detailed. (Author abstract.)

0340 **Burkitt, W.R.** *Work of the Kenya mobile eye unit with clinical observations on some common eye diseases.* British Opthalmology (London), 52, Apr 1968, 329-334. Engl.
Unpublished document.

Medical assistants with opthalmic training carry out preventive and curative work in three districts of Kenya by means of a Mobile Eye Unit. Since the publication of this article, the assistant has taken charge of the Unit, although he has no recognized medical qualifications. The Unit staff visits health centres in a Land Rover carrying camping equipment, operating equipment, and drugs. Preparation of the community greatly contributes to the success of the visit. The unit performs cataract operations, distributes eye glasses, does trachoma surveys, treats trachoma and eyestrain, and generally attempts to educate the community in the prevention of blindness.

0341 **Christian Medical Association of India, Bangalore.** *Summary report: CMAI Family Planning Project, All India Conference of Mobile Teams, June 2-6, 1970.* India, CMAI Family Planning Project, 1970. 23p. Engl.
Unpublished document.

The Christian Medical Association of India (CMAI) conducts various programmes in health through Christian mission hospitals in India. The summary report of this conference sponsored by the CMAI outlines the themes of discussion at the conference. The objective of the mobile teams was to motivate hospital staff toward family planning work by conducting visits for training and follow-up purposes. Eight teams from various parts of India presented reports. Hospital senior staff did not show much interest in family planning and the size of the vans proved cumbersome for India's roads. A total of 3 880 persons attended training programmes conducted by the mobile teams over a 5-month period. Some of the teams felt that hospital staff did not understand the objectives of the family planning project and considered the visits inspection tours. Comments of participants are recorded. Better health education through training is recommended for nurse educators.

0342 **Cox, P.S.** *Value of mobile medicine.* East African Medical Journal (Nairobi), 46(10), Oct 1969, 548-552. Engl.

Mobile medicine has an important place in the medical services in East Africa. Full and "scientific" evaluation is impossible owing to the number of variable and subjective factors, but for both patients and medical personnel, visits by expert teams are welcome and necessary. A plan for the development of these services is needed. This should include a budget for the establishment of medical centres and arrangements for visits on all levels. An air ambulance service should be set up. (Author abstract.)

0343 **de Glanville, H.** *East African flying doctor service.* Kenya Nursing Journal, (Nairobi), 1(1), Jun 1972, 41-42. Engl.

The flying doctor service of East Africa is intended to send out surgeons, to assist isolated hospitals and dispensaries, and to evacuate emergency cases. Aircraft operation costs compare favourably with a Land-Rover. During 14 years the African Medical and Research Foundation has also operated a mobile clinic and a health education service that publishes *The Defender*, a health education magazine for the public, and *Afya*, a monthly medical journal for paramedical personnel. The Foundation is financed by charitable organizations, individuals, local governments, churches, and some Western governments.

0344 Duraiswami, P.K. *Multipurpose role of mobile hospitals in rural India.* Journal of the Royal College of Surgeons of Edinburgh (Edinburgh), 16(2), Jul 1971, 185-187. Engl.

Only one in five of India's primary health centres has more than one doctor. Rural areas do not attract physicians and competition amongst doctors in urban areas results in emigration to Western countries. Thus a new approach to physician education has been devised by the government health services directorate: this entails training medical personnel in total community medicine, enabling them to provide comprehensive health care and win the confidence of villagers. The new scheme proposes that each state select a medical college and provide it with a 50-bed mobile training/service hospital. Each unit is to cover an entire district with a rural population of about 1 million. Involvement of medical postgraduates in this work will prepare them for work in district hospitals and eventually in primary health centres as funds become available.

0345 Graver, V. *You have to be ready for anything.* Zambia Nurse (Kitwe, Zambia), 2(5), Jun 1967, 16,19. Engl.

The East Africa Leprosy Research Centre at Alupe, near the Kenya/Uganda border, conducts village surveys through a mobile visit programme. Camps for the survey are about 2 miles apart, making it possible for women and children to walk to them. The mobile van visits villages, schools, and health centres, setting up two tents: one for examination of males and one for females. In addition to patients, those suffering from polio and other diseases are treated.

0346 Holz, P. *Mobile clinic to combat trachoma.* Eye Ear Nose Monthly (Chicago), 45, Oct 1966, 85-86. Engl.

Eye disease among South Africans follows a distinct geographical pattern. The incidence of trachoma is highest in the northern parts of the Republic. A vaccine is being tested in field trials in an effort to immunize the African population. A mobile unit, staffed by a surgeon, nurses, and social workers distributed antibiotic ointment and performed operations for entropion, a condition resulting from trachoma. Operations are performed in the mobile unit only if all available hospitals in the area are full. All children attending school for the first time were treated for trachoma. Other tours by mobile units treated cataracts. The mobile unit of the Bureau for the Prevention of Blindness had performed 3 100 operations between 1952 and 1966.

0347 Laha, N.M. *Transport organisation: an important component in comprehensive health care - its nationalisation.* Indian Journal of Public Health (Calcutta), 15(4), Oct 1971, 150-151. Engl.

Efficient transportation is one of the key elements in providing health services. It ensures mobility to health personnel and ensures transport of materials and patients when necessary. It was recommended that the state be responsible for the maintenance of mobile transportation fleets in India. By establishing regional workshops (on mobile unit maintenance) and establishing mobile units in Varanasi and Gorakpur (in Uttar Pradesh), the number of inoperable vehicles was reduced. The maintenance of vehicles through such an organization can assist the government by speeding up repair and minimizing expenditure.

0348 Rehabilitation Record, Washington, D.C. *Eye camps in rural India.* Rehabilitation Record (Washington, D.C.), 9, Sep-Oct 1968, 28. Engl.

It is estimated that 2 million of the 3 million blind people in India can have their sight restored; they are the people needing surgery, treatment, or simply spectacles or instruction in proper eye care. A mobile eye hospital was operated as part of a demonstration project designed as a prototype for rehabilitation of the blind in rural areas.

0349 Sharma, B.N. *Surgery in camps.* Journal of the Indian Medical Association (Calcutta), 53, 16 Oct 1969, 408-410. Engl.

Providing medical aid to 300 million Indians living in rural villages is a problem. Health centres, medical aid centres, and dispensaries are few and far between. Ideally, centres should be staffed by a surgeon, a physician, a gynecologist, an ophthalmologist, and an anaesthetist, but it will take a few decades before such service can be provided. Surgical camps are a practical way of providing necessary surgical service to villagers. Young physicians practicing in these camps can often gain more experience in a variety of surgical problems than they can in hospitals. These camps are held in Rajasthan 10 months a year. The 2-month rainy season serves as a planning period. People are notified that the camp will be held in their area, provided local people raise funds to feed the patients. The camps are strategically located within easy access of several communities. Camp equipment and costs are described. In India 50-60 units would probably serve the national need.

0350 Vintinner, F.J. *Mobile rural health services program in Central America and Panama.* American Journal of Public Health (New York), 58(5), May 1968, 907-914. Engl.

A mobile rural health service program known as PUMAR (Programma de Unidades Moviles para Areas Rurales), initiated in 1963, provides basic medical care and preventive medicine services for 2 million people living in the rural areas of Costa Rica, El Salvador, Guatemala, Honduras, Nicaragua, and Panama. As a programme of the Alliance for Progress, the Ministries of Public Health assisted by the U.S. Agency for International Development (USAID) and other public and private organizations are now bringing essential services for better health and greater hope for the people previously isolated from centres of population. Self-help is a cardinal factor and through cooperative community actions basic health facilities have been constructed, health programmes implemented, environmental sanitation improved, and roads, bridges, schools, athletic fields, and other community facilities built or established. Foundations have been laid for

III Primary Health Care — Implementation

permanent responsible local groups who can take leadership in community health and development activities and there is a growing change of attitude toward civic responsibility and pride in local organizations and achievements. With improved health and a feeling of new hope for a better life in the spirit of the Alliance for Progress, the people in the rural areas of the five countries in Central America and Panama will become an important component in the total economic and social progress of the region. (Author abstract.)

0351 Westwater, K. *Dentistry with the Zambia flying doctor service.* Dental Practitioner and Dental Record (Bristol), 20(2), Oct 1969, 60-62. Engl.

In Zambia the population is sparse; the greatest concentrations are near the copper mines and the capital city. This complicates efforts to deliver care to rural people. A flying doctor service has provided fully qualified medical and nursing care since 1967. Dental care was added to the service as it became apparent that a great demand for this service existed. Dental care is very acceptable and particularly desirable for children. By 1969, school dental programmes had treated approximately 1 600 children. By constructing dental chairs locally and building up emergency supplies at each airstrip, the equipment airlifted daily was reduced to a box of instruments, a general anaesthetic apparatus, a prosthetic box, and a foot engine.

0352 Wilkinson, J.L., Smith, H., Smith, O.I. *Organization and economics of a mobile child welfare team in Sierra Leone.* Journal of Tropical Medicine and Hygiene (London), Jan 1967, 14-18. Engl.

In Sierra Leone malnutrition was recognized as widespread after a survey was conducted in 1956. The initial solution, the distribution of food supplements, accomplished little in obtaining the cooperation of village mothers or in improving the welfare of the children. It became clear that prevention and treatment of malnutrition was more effective when linked to the prevention and treatment of infective diseases. Now a mobile child welfare team is responsible for visiting villages within an area of 200 square miles. This paper details the organization, time utilization, and cost distribution of the service. Immunization is supplemented by skim milk distribution and nutrition education. Very ill children are transported to the hospital. Infant mortality has been reduced from 332 to 156 per thousand live births. Five references are listed.

0353 Wood, A.M. *Communication with rural areas by radio, light aircraft and mobile land units.* Journal of the Royal College of Surgeons of Edinburgh (Edinburgh), 16(1), Jan 1971, 202-205. Engl.

Two factors influence communications in rural areas of East Africa: (1) there is one doctor per 30 000 people, and the majority of doctors serve in urban centres; and (2) government spending per person for health is only 10 shillings. The author discusses work of the African Medical Research Foundation (AMRF). A radio network was installed, linking rural hospitals first to Nairobi and later to aircraft and mobile units, to serve for medical consultations, discussion of hospital matters, arrangement of specialists' visits, and for boosting morale. Seven light aircraft evacuate emergency cases, assist doctor visits, transport supplies, and assist supervision of field projects. Operational costs of the donated planes are not considered expensive under the conditions prevailing in Africa. An advantage of this programme is that rural areas get more medical and surgical coverage. A disadvantage is the inadequate follow-up, e.g., the doctor must leave the patient 2 or 3 days after an operation. An important educational benefit of the system is the presence of consultants in the field, where 85% of the population is situated. For East Africa, a combination of the radio network and aircraft with mobile units on the ground is the best method of health care delivery.

0354 Wood, A.M. *Problem of communications in medical practice in East Africa.* East African Medical Journal (Nairobi), 46(10), Oct 1969, 536-540. Engl.

Two-thirds of Kenya is sparsely populated and relatively inaccessible by road or telephone. Peripheral hospitals in these areas are poorly equipped and understaffed. Improved communication between these outlying hospitals and major centres in Nairobi can be accomplished through radio communication and the flying doctor service. Light aircraft can evacuate a patient needing treatment at a larger centre, fly in medical staff for specialist cases, and transport supplies such as drugs, blood, etc. Aircraft operate at a similar cost per mile as a Land Rover with the advantage of being much faster. Problems encountered by the flying doctor service involve returning the patient after treatment, weather conditions, clearing an airstrip, etc. An unplanned benefit is rural development around the airstrip.

III.4 Community health education

See also: 0056, 0059, 0062, 0187, 0221, 0237, 0258, 0283, 0564, 0591

0355 Anderson, J.K. *Health education in Africa.* Journal of the National Medical Association (New York), 59(4), Jul 1967, 251-253. Engl.

The overwhelming need for health education in Africa is apparent even after the most cursory consideration of some of Africa's health problems. Eighty-five percent of Africans live in small rural villages far from health services. Tradition shapes their views on health matters. At most some are exposed periodically to a mobile health team. Health behaviour known to be of importance in breaking the chain of infectious disease is difficult to introduce where traditional views dominate and services are lacking or infrequent. A number of inspiring health education projects have been carried out, however, in Africa. Ethiopia, Ghana, Liberia, Upper Volta, and Chad are among the countries that have lead in the development of professionally trained health educators at the national level. Most health educators now in developing countries were trained in the United States, where the profession was first established. Health education is, however, beginning to be taken seriously in African countries and included in their national plans.

0356 Arole, R.S. *Community participation in a community health programme.* Journal of the Christian Medical Association of India (Mysore), 48(4), Apr 1973, 168-169. Engl.

Community health programmes succeed best when health personnel work not only for the community, but with the community. In a programme in Jamkhed, India, health personnel sought to involve the community from decision-making stages on up to the building of health centres. During 2 years, with community cooperation, the project immunized 12 000 children in 30 villages. The health project responded to famine in the project area by organizing volunteers to provide care and food supplements for children under five. Another need was for the provision of emergency care and simple medical treatment in the village. Interested persons from villages were given training to meet this need and were supplied with drugs. Through formation of youth clubs, school children were encouraged to participate in health education. Promotion of the programme depends on the ability to utilize existing community structures.

0357 Bennett, F.J., Letlhaku, L. *Organization of MCH services in developing regions: (II) Health education.* Journal of Tropical Pediatrics (Kampala), 12, Sep 1966, 32-36. Engl.
See also entry 232.

Health education is part of the everyday work of every maternal and child health service worker. Education is used in prenatal clinics to allay fears, improve maternal nutrition and general health, and prepare mothers for child care. However, education is often difficult, requiring skilled personnel with proper training. This paper stresses a flexible, innovative approach to education, requiring continuous evaluation of present programmes to provide constant feedback for use in future programmes. The educator must reassess the situation at every session. Maternal education activities involving husbands, group discussions, and demonstrations in hospital wards and outpatient clinics, and the employment of a local woman to give health instruction, are examples of various approaches. It is most important that health education be communicated in a form acceptable to village people, rather than in a form that seems simple to a Western-educated person.

0358 Bennett, F.J. *Development of health education in Uganda, 1946-1966.* International Journal of Health Education (Geneva), 9(1), 1966, 39-46. Engl.

The demobilization of Ugandan men who had served in World War II was probably the greatest impetus to health education in Uganda, since a large number of men had been trained in hygienic practices. The Uganda Medical Service sponsored health days, health weeks, and demonstration films. Uganda is now one of 15 African countries with a Health Education Division in its Ministry of Health. In all training schools, there are now individuals who have had some theoretical training in health education. Among the problems that have arisen are a lack of continuity in the direction of the Health Education Division and lack of any long sustained coordinated programme at the community level. The ground work for acceptance of health education has been established, but the country has yet to launch an ongoing sustained programme. Twenty references are listed.

0359 Courtejoie, J. *Health education in the primary and secondary school: an account of a practical experiment in health education undertaken by the Centre for Health Education, Kangu-Mayumbe, Congo Kinshasa.* Kinshasa, n.p., n.d. 14p. Engl.
Unpublished document.

Health education could be integrated with school curricula in many ways. The author explains how existing subjects, class projects, and outings could be oriented towards greater health awareness. Health technicians could influence the health activities of their patients by explaining procedures as they perform them. Students could be responsible for disinfecting and spraying school premises, and school medical inspection could be accompanied by explanations.

0360 Galli, E.A. *Development of nutrition education among some urban non-white communities in the Republic of South Africa.* South African Medical Journal-Supplement: South African Journal of Nutrition (Cape Town), 23 Dec 1967, 1223-1226. Engl.

This is a report of the development of a nutrition education programme to alleviate poor nutrition among nonwhite workers in a South African transportation company. Poor nutrition accounted for prolonged illnesses, absenteeism, low productivity, and increased accidents. Diets were evaluated and showed deficiencies in use of milk and vegetables and frequent use of refined cereals. In liaison with the health clinic, a health education programme was begun based on data about the causes of poor nutrition among the workers. This programme and its successful results were later extended to the community. The work included a child feeding scheme, nutrition education through the Alexandra University Clinic and Health Centre and through the Entokozweni Welfare Centre and the Maize and Egg Control Board of Alexandra Township. Successful results after 3 years included reduced worker absenteeism, improved child health, and increased community demand for and use of nutrition information. Five references are listed.

III Primary Health Care – Implementation

0361 Garcia, A.L. *Educacao Sanitaria e Esquistossomose. (Health education and schistosomiasis).* Revista Brasileira de Malariologia e Doencas Tropicais (Rio de Janeiro), 18, Jan-Mar 1966, 175-188. Portuguese.

In the 10 years since the last schistosomiasis symposium, living conditions in much of Brazil have not improved. Incidence of schistosomiasis and areas affected have even increased. In certain areas the physician to inhabitant ratio is 1:28 000. Low educational standards, isolation, and malnutrition in such underprivileged communities do not favour the establishment of health care as a concept. The largely experimental health education programmes run by the National Department for Rural Endemic Diseases are characterized by their flexibility. They have been invaluable in the training of auxiliary health workers. But the most urgent need now is for the preparation of educational programmes, based on preventive rather than curative principles, to reach the people. Work done in other countries employing theories from the behavioural sciences, such as group dynamics, is extensively cited to illustrate how changes in attitude can be brought about. Twenty-four references are listed.

0362 Gereda, R. *Educadores rurales en salud oral. (Rural educators in dental health).* Guatemala, Universidad de San Carlos de Guatemala, Facultad de Odontologia, n.d. 8p. Span. Unpublished document.

In view of the lack of oral education among the inhabitants of Guatemala's rural communities, a programme has been instituted whereby dentistry students spend 1 year in field practice selecting and training community leaders in basic oral care. The leaders then pass this knowledge on to the inhabitants of their respective communities. The oral health educators are the link between the rural community and government health services. This document lists manpower and material resources available for the programme and subjects to be covered. It emphasizes the important role of the community leader in achieving the broadest possible social participation.

0363 Kassel, M.B. *Community organization for allied health manpower: manpower for the human services.* Chicago, Illinois State Department of Labour, Human Services Manpower Career Centre, Jun 1971. 132p. Engl.

This monograph is the fourth in a series summarizing the progress of the Human Services Manpower Career Center, a special research and development project funded by the U.S. Department of Labour. It presents a developmental model and guidelines for organizing a working coalition of concerned community groups, for identifying major tasks, and for proceeding to problem-solving joint actions. Suggestions for the composition, objectives, and organizational structure of a force can begin to attack the major problems involved in allied health manpower planning and development. A set of proposed Illinois guidelines for programmes for physicians' assistants and a description of 25 barriers that restrict effective recruitment, training, and utilization of allied health manpower are appended. (Author abstract.)

0364 Mgobozi, P. *My experience as a health educator in a Bantu tuberculosis hospital.* South African Medical Journal (Cape Town), 43, 19 Jul 1969, 908-910. Engl.

As a result of health education the percentage of patients not attending regularly for outpatient treatment at a Bantu tuberculosis centre after discharge from hospital fell from 59 to 21% after 9 months, and to 12.5% after a further period of 15 months. The number of patients absconding from hospital at Christmas time fell dramatically after 2 1/2 years of health education. The general absconding rate has fallen less. Some difficulties encountered in health education are discussed. (Revised author abstract.)

0365 Morley, D. *Nutrition education in rural societies.* Proceedings of the Nutrition Society (London), 29(2), Dec 1970, 230-236. Engl.

Efforts to communicate more effectively with rural populations include the establishment of nutrition rehabilitation centres where mothers see their children's health improving with changes in diet. In East Africa one centre is an effective combination of an under-fives' clinic, a nutrition rehabilitation centre, and a demonstration farm. In Malawi, a positive approach to child nutrition has been encouraged through a system of "road to health" cards. Using the card, the child's progress is documented and observed for improvement. This card indicates to mothers how their children are progressing in relation to health crises and diet. The health worker has the positive objective of promoting adequate growth and not just preventing malnutrition. If this educational programme can be linked with an effective immunization programme against measles, whooping cough, and tuberculosis, rapid improvement in child nutrition can be expected. Eight references are listed.

0366 Patel, T.B., Ambwani, G.J., Shah, M.H., Panchal, R.M. *Knowledge, attitude and practices of community concerning primary health centre.* Indian Journal of Public Health (Calcutta), 15(1), Jan 1971, 3-13. Engl.

Application of a knowledge, attitude, and practices (KAP) type study was used in several Indian villages to estimate health care recipients' responses to a rural health centre. Results show that awareness of the centre is directly proportional to the ease with which it is reached. Although a wide range of services were offered, most respondents thought medical treatment was the main function of the primary health centre. Villagers considered the sanitary inspector as a vaccinator against smallpox, and the health visitor as an attending midwife. Most respondents did not know the health centre vehicle could be used to transport the very ill. Where maternity beds were provided, only 20% of total deliveries were institutional; women preferred the services of an untrained village dai (midwife). Only

5.8% of respondents attended well-baby clinics for regular health checkups of their children. The need of villagers was felt to be for medical aid whereas planner's goals were for preventive measures supplemented by curative services. Results of this study point out the necessity of introducing a health centre to the community through mass communication media and of bridging the gap between what is expected of a primary health centre and what impact it actually makes.

0367 Rao, G.K. *What was the highest success in health education in the Media Division of the Health Education Bureau, Madras, and how it was achieved.* Madras, Health Education Bureau, Media Division, n.d. 1v.(various pagings). Engl. Unpublished document.

In 1954 a Health Propaganda section was formed by the government of Madras. After 1957 it became part of the Central Health Education Bureau. With external advice and aid from the Government of India the programme was upgraded and expanded after 1960, and the Media Division took over the activities of the propaganda section. The activities of this section are reviewed in this report. Included in the programme is a Radio Rural Forum. Local units of government were supplied with community listening sets, and, with the help of the Community Development Department and All India Radio, programmes designed to encourage group discussion among the village listeners were set up. These include a wide variety of health subjects. The Division also previews and pretests films for training programmes and for village adult health education.

0368 Rao, N.M. *Nurse and the community.* Nursing Journal of India (New Delhi), 60(1), Jan 1969, 27-30. Engl.

The role of the nurse has changed from treatment to preventive work. Health education has become part of the nurse's functions in malaria, tuberculosis, smallpox, venereal disease, trachoma, maternal and child health, family planning, and nutritional work. Today a community approach calls for the cooperative interaction of all members of the health team. By nature of their professional training, responsibilities, and placement in the community, public health nurses, health visitors, midwives, auxiliary nurse midwives, and trained dais shoulder the major responsibility for community health services in India. Principles of extension education must be understood by nurses and understanding of educational methods and teaching aids and their place in programme development is called for. Appropriate uses of media in education are discussed.

0369 Samarasinghe, C.E. *Health education in Ghana.* Ghanaian Nurse (Accra), 5(1), Feb 1969, 13-18. Engl.

Public health education is successful to the extent that the people assume responsibility for the betterment of their own health. With this aim in mind, the Ministry of Health in Ghana set up the Health Education Unit as a source of knowledge of the principles, techniques, and methods of health education, for the use of the Ministry staff and other agencies. Local health education committees have been formed throughout the country and health education in the schools is in the planning stage. Community education in Ghana has been proven a most effective approach, especially in areas where health centres already exist and where staff take an interest in preventive as well as curative medicine.

0370 Saxena, K.N., Saxena, M.N. *Health education in dermatology.* Indian Practitioner (Bombay), Aug 1966, 589-592. Engl.

The morbidity rate of skin diseases in India is quite high. An education programme about skin care will begin by establishing what people know, feel, and do about skin diseases. Mothers should be told about skin care in antenatal clinics. During infancy, attention should be paid to cleanliness, and any infections treated by a dermatologist. Care should be taken to protect toddlers from contact with animals. Education in personal hygiene is needed for school teachers, industrial workers, military personnel, and old people. Six references are listed.

0371 Sengupta, A. *Programme building operation for promotion of family planning: the Indian Statistical Institute clinic experiment.* Journal of the Indian Medical Association (Calcutta), 49(1), 1 Jul 1967, 19-28. Engl.

A family planning programme was begun at the Indian Statistical Institute in Calcutta. Two clinics (male and female) were operated using an extension approach. A community level extension education programme was built up in which clinic personnel, community leaders, and supporting organizations worked together in a coordinated way. Volunteer group leaders promoted family planning among their fellow employees and clinic personnel spent considerable time contacting employees in the Institute. This pilot project was set up in an organized way in order to systematically study the factors influencing acceptance of family planning. These factors were analyzed for future evaluation of the educational and organizational aspects of family planning programmes. Statistical data were kept and are included in the article. Group meetings, conducted after personal contact with potential clients, turned out to be most useful in motivating employees to accept family planning methods. It appears from this programme to be possible to set up a family planning programme in an institute such as this at a minimal cost, with workers themselves acting as volunteer promoters and distributers. Five references are listed.

0372 Sugiono, M. *Village social development organization in Indonesia.* Paediatrica Indonesiana (Djakarta), 8, Mar-Apr 1968, 76-81. Engl.

The Village Social Development Organization (VSDO) is a social organization that coordinates community activities in Indonesia. Its objectives are to develop social responsibility in rural communities and to lessen the suffering of rural people. Practical work is done in cooperation with rural governments and involves strengthening weak and handicapped community members, prevention of socially detrimental habits (opium use, alcoholism, gambling), and promotion of a good environment. Participation in education is extensive. It is suggested that future activities encourage economic development. Funds for the VSDO come from the mutual cooperation of villagers and the government. Some tangible results have been the building of rice mills, the provision of accommodation for the poor, the transformation of jungle into rice fields, etc. Five references are listed.

0373   Sundram, C.J. *Influences of public health education.* Medical Journal of Malaya (Singapore), 20(3), Mar 1966, 182-185. Engl.

Phases of health education have focussed on law enforcement, health information, "fear appeals," "unadorned truth," and "attention-getting." Today health education programmes are behaviour-focussed, i.e. they aim for effective changes in individual behaviour to attain community or national health. The emphasis is on constant evaluation of educational programme results. Ten references are listed.

0374   Tsai, J.F., Wang, W., Niu, L.C. *Survey on the health status of the less privileged people in Cheng-Chung district, Taipei City.* Journal - Formosan Medical Association (Taipei), 65(7), 28 Jul 1966, 354-360. Engl.

A health survey conducted in the slum areas of Taipei City, Taiwan, revealed that people with greater need for medical care are less informed about services available at a public health centre. Awareness increases with educational level. The public health nurse is the primary communication agent between the centre and the public and should be trained in health education methods and techniques. Nine references are listed.

0375   Valenzuela, V.C. *Training for health development.* Journal of the Philippine Medical Association (Quezon City), 41(9), Sep 1965, 652-656. Engl.

There is a need to reexamine efforts aimed at raising the level of health of the Philippine population. Major problems are provision of adequate food, better housing, improved sanitation, communicable disease control, medical care facility expansion, extension of medical care to rural areas, efficient use of available manpower and facilities, health personnel training, health education for the public, and improved collection and research of health statistics on local problems. In meeting these problems planning on a national scale is obviously necessary. Management is difficult since modern management practices conflict with traditional systems, which rely on loyalty to kinship groups. At the community level, health development must be made part of total community development. The training of health personnel can be shared by several departments and institutions. Training of personnel must be hierarchical, from the national level to the regional, provincial, and municipal levels. Training for health development is part of training for community development.

IV Primary Health Manpower — Training and Utilization

IV.1 Primary medical care

IV.1.1 Professional

See also: *0031, 0036, 0041, 0087, 0094, 0095, 0257, 0467, 0482, 0496*

0376 Aguirre, A. *Community medicine at the University of Valle.* In Lathem, W., Newbery, A., eds., Community Medicine: Teaching, Research, and Health Care, New York, Appleton-Century-Crofts, 1970, 51-64. Engl.
A discussion follows the paper. See also entry 162.
The community medicine programme at the Universidad del Valle, Colombia, first emphasized the individual and disease, gradually focussed on the family, and finally evolved into a Department of Preventive Medicine and Public Health striving for comprehensive medical care. The present programme involves rural and urban community health care, and provides medical students with community experience. The university's extension into the community is through a hospital and its system of satellite health posts. Young physicians are trained through lectures and field work. They participate in training auxiliary health workers.

0377 Akinkugbe, O.O. *Role of teaching hospitals in a developing country.* British Medical Journal (London), 1, 24 Feb 1973, 474-476. Engl.
If one were to consider concentration of physicians in urban areas as itself reflective of the health situation in a country, one would be overlooking the concept of the health team as the most crucial unit of medical manpower. With the new emphasis on planning and the team approach to health service organization, the urban teaching hospital takes on the new function of relating itself to this overall effort. The measure of their success is the degree of their identifying their objectives with overall national health priorities. Teaching in hospitals must change from that emphasizing the sophistication of the hospital environment to that emphasizing practical work and learning. In Nigeria the teaching load is tremendous. With state ministries of health seeking doctors as teachers, and rural communities needing doctors as practitioners, it is necessary for universities to collaborate with government in physician and auxiliary training. Manpower training, research, popularization of preventive measures, etc., all require coordinated university and government effort.

0378 Ali, D.S., Backett, E.M., Dowling, M.A., El Borolossy, A.W. WHO, Geneva. *Aspects of medical education in developing countries: selected papers presented at the second WHO conference on medical education in the Eastern Mediterranean Region.* Geneva, WHO Public Health Papers No. 47, 1972. 116p. Engl.
Selected papers presented at a conference on medical manpower and physician education in the Eastern Mediterranean region deal with the following topics: objectives of medical education in developing countries; medical curricula; student evaluation of medical education; the integrated teaching of medical sciences; audiovisual media; teaching of social medicine and epidemiology; the establishment of new medical schools; and the particular problems of medical education in Iran.

0379 Allen, L.R. *Community medicine at the All India Institute of Medical Sciences.* In Lathem, W., Newbery, A., eds., Community Medicine: Teaching, Research and Health Care, New York, Appleton-Century-Crofts, 1970, 79-90. Engl.
See also entry 162.
In 1965 the All India Institute of Medical Sciences set up, in cooperation with Haryana State Health Service, a research and training project on comprehensive rural health care at Ballabgharh. The project's objectives are: to evolve an adequate pattern of health services that could be extended on a national scale to all community development blocks (each community development block consists of roughly 100 villages and about 80 000 people) and to develop an extramural organization that would provide medical students, nurses, and other health workers with practical experience in comprehensive rural community medicine delivery. Staff of the departments of Medicine, Surgery, Pediatrics, Obstetrics-Gynecology, and Social and Preventive Medicine of the Institute are responsible for developing and implementing the programme, assisted by basic health workers, auxiliary nurse-midwives, and sanitarians. The main problem is shortage of trained manpower: the brain drain of physicians from India and the disinclination of those remaining to work in rural areas are reasons cited. The motivation of parents and students,

and the attitudes of students, faculty, and the community to innovation and change contribute. It was felt that a pioneering spirit was lacking, although a growing number of faculty were undertaking research programmes in nutritional disorders, diarrhoea, and heart diseases, etc.

0380 Argentina, Department of Social Welfare. *Programa de cursos de capacitacion de personal para el sector salud. (Programme of personnel training courses in the health field).* Buenos Aires, Ministry of Social Welfare, 1974. 45p. Span.

This document lists all courses in the health field offered by the Department of Social Welfare, Argentina, in 1974. Twenty-two courses are offered at the professional level, 13 courses at the technical, and six courses at the auxiliary level. Several courses on sanitation of the environment and related activities are offered at the professional and technical levels. Course number 32 deals with construction techniques applied to the sanitary improvement of the rural dwelling. One page is devoted to each course, outlining its purpose, organization, starting date, qualification requirements, and the number of students to be admitted.

0381 Banerji, S.C., Siddhu, C.M. *Study of the factors and attitudes of medical officers, working at primary health centres in Uttar Pradesh.* Indian Journal of Medical Sciences (Bombay), 19(10), Oct 1965, 789-794. Engl.

A study of factors influencing the attitudes of medical officers in primary health centres of Uttar Pradesh, India, reveals reasons for dissatisfaction with rural postings. Doctors in the study were generally dissatisfied with their remuneration and hours of work. Many centre doctors did not receive enough training in social and preventive medicine to appreciate opportunities in rural areas. They also lacked administrative training necessary for effective utilization of their staff. Nine references are listed.

0382 Bennett, F.J. *Medical manpower for occupational health in the tropics - professional staff: needs and training.* Journal of Tropical Medicine and Hygiene (London), 73, Dec 1970, 324-335. Engl.

Symposium on the Health Problems of Industrial Progress in Developing Countries.

Statistics of medical manpower for East African countries and Nigeria indicate that there will be difficulty in reducing the doctor-population ratio below 1:10 000 before the end of the century. Rapid expansion of training at the auxiliary level will be essential, and the basic health organization will have to include the rural health centre run by auxiliaries but supervised by professional staff. Most occupational health work will be in relation to agricultural jobs, and will require occupational health specialists, occupational hygienists, health inspectors, public health nurses, industrial health nurses, etc. Local training courses for these workers must be established at universities, and teachers will have to be recruited initially from institutes abroad. Curricula must include communicable diseases, nutrition, health education, and socio-medical problems related to inadequate housing, poverty, migration, and urbanization. Field work in people's homes and their places of work is an important part of training. Institutes in industrialized countries can be most helpful by containing their specialized courses for occupational hygienists and medical graduates, by seconding teachers for short periods to universities in developing countries, and by providing funds and workers for combined research projects. Forty-four references are listed.

0383 Bevan, P.G., Manson-Bahr, P.E., Pinkerton, J.H. *Medical education in Burma, 1969.* British Journal of Medical Education (London), 4, 1970, 67-75. Engl.

A report on medical practice in Burma focusses on medical education. The article outlines the historical development of medical education since 1924. Increased life expectancy and decreased infant and maternal mortality rates have placed an overburdening weight on existing health facilities. This has created the need for an increase of medical staff in teaching hospitals and improved postgraduate training. Aspects of medical education surveyed in this report include medical research, the undergraduate curriculum in medicine and surgery, traditional teaching techniques, postgraduate training, obstetrics, and gynecology.

0384 Buri, P. *Medical education: responsibility and objectives.* In Lathem, W., Newbery A., eds., Community Medicine: Teaching, Research, and Health Care, New York, Appleton-Century-Crofts, 1970, 17-32. Engl.

See also entry 162.

Physician education must be oriented toward the needs of the individual, the community, and the nation. Medical educators must confront the problem of relating education to local needs while maintaining a level of hospital medicine that meets international standards; the entire faculty of the medical school must become involved in developing a community health programme. The institutional objectives should also include involvement in national health planning, and integration of programmes of medical education with related programmes aimed at improving the social, economic, cultural, and educational conditions of the nation. A discussion is included.

0385 Buri, P. *Community medicine at the Ramathibodi Hospital Faculty of Medicine.* In Lathem, W., Newbery, A., eds., Community Medicine: Teaching, Research and Health Care, New York, Appleton-Century-Crofts, 1970, 105-120. Engl.

See also entry 162.

Thailand's vital statistics and disease patterns, health budget, health manpower, and facilities are reviewed against the background of the development of medical education at the country's leading medical schools. In the field of rural health care, the uneven distribution of physicians and general lack of trained health personnel, plus the fact that provincial hospitals follow the traditional system of university hospital care, result in delivery of care to rural communities not being effective. Furthermore, there is little communication between the hospitals and the rural health centres. Medical students are not positively motivated to serve in rural settings as their traditional training does not equip them to work through a health team and with community resources. The Ramathibodi Hospital Faculty of Medicine, a constituent of Mahidol University, has undertaken to train a strong cadre of graduates who could be deployed as district health officers and teachers in provincial medical schools. A joint Faculty-Ministry of Health programme, using a rural district as a teaching and research laboratory, will train the complete spectrum of health personnel. The curriculum of the medical school is given. Discussion centres on the organization of the programme and the level of participation of faculty staff. The experience of Puerto Rico is quoted as an example of successful application of the principle of university, students, and government integrating efforts to achieve appropriate training in community health care delivery, proving that it is not impossible to attract physicians to rural areas given the right motivation and training.

0386 Campos, P.C. *Community medicine at the University of the Philippines.* In Lathem, W., Newbery, A., eds., Community Medicine: Teaching, Research, and Health Care, New York, Appleton-Century-Crofts, 1970, 33-50. Engl.
See also entry 162.

A programme in community medicine began at the University of the Philippines with short-term assignment of interns to different barrios, or rural communities, in the province of Laguna. This was followed by the establishment of a teaching and research centre in Bay, Laguna. The programme (training, research, service) and facilities are described, and the following suggestions are put forward on the basis of this experience: the programme should be truly community-oriented; the training programme should include all aspects of health care; the programme should have relevance to problems of the community; there must be continuity so students can follow through from problem to remedy to bigger but related problems; the programme must be acceptable to everyone directly involved and adaptable to change; and it should be geared to the resources of the community. A discussion follows the paper.

0387 Cebrian U.J. *Aprendizaje a traves de la discusion de casos en la escuela de salud publica del Peru. (Learning through case discussions at the School of Public Health in Peru).* Boletin de la Oficina Sanitaria Panamericana (Washington, D.C.), 61(8), Aug 1966, 152-158. Span.

The author describes an experiment carried out at the School of Public Health of Peru during the discussion of the topic "Role of Human Relations in Health Institutions," which formed part of the instruction in public health administration given to a group of physicians. The teaching method was the presentation of a series of practical problems, followed by the study and discussion of the same problems by the students, organized as a working group. In this way the participants identified a number of factors that were not conducive to good relations among the staff of a health institution, as well as others that could create more harmonious relationships. The method used enabled the members of the group to take an active and direct part in the discussion. What is learned in this way tends to remain longer with the individual and has a greater possibility of influencing his conduct than what is acquired through the traditional lecture-type class. (Journal abstract.)

0388 Chablani, T.D. *Rural training programme for rotating housemen (1963-65) and its impact on the trends in morbidity patterns.* Indian Journal of Public Health (Calcutta), 12(4), Oct 1968, 201-207. Engl.

A rural training programme was used in Kurali, India, to train physicians in preventive and social medicine. The programme gave interns a chance to practice their skills and to treat health problems in terms of the community as a whole. The rural health centre sought to provide early diagnosis and treatment, to provide maternal and child care, to control communicable diseases, and to collect vital statistics. Interns stayed in the village and practiced there for 3 months. Their basic activities are listed. Statistical data for a period of 3 years show a decline in morbidity rates, particularly for infants and preschool children. This decline is attributed to the introduction of preventive medicine. Six references are listed.

0389 Chablani, T.D. *Praxis der gesellschaftsmedizin, der gesellshaftsdiagnose und der gesellschaftstherapie. (Practice of social medicine, diagnosis, and therapy).* Zeitschrift Fur Die Gesamte Hygiene Und Ihre Grenzgebiete (Berlin), 12, Apr 1966, 264-271. German.

Success in the community laboratory depends on cooperation on the part of the community physician, his assistants, the public, and the social scientists. The physician's role is rapidly becoming preventive in nature and social in function. The community relies on him to determine the course of disease and encourage prevention through essentially educational measures. He is also to be the promoter of positive conditions that make for physical, mental, and social well-being. The family and the community gain from this approach because they play an active part in it. The country in question, in this instance, is India. (Revised journal abstract.)

0390 Christian Medical College Hospital, Vellore, India. *Account of Christian Medical College and Hospital, Vellore, South India.* Vellore, Tamil Nadu, Christian Medical College, n.d. 15p. Engl. Unpublished document.

The history and current (1970) activities of the Christian Medical College of India are outlined. A series of tables covers the undergraduate medical curriculum, postgraduate courses, nursing education, paramedical courses in radiology, physiotherapy, pharmacy, laboratory technology, etc., and hospital activities.

0391 Davidson, L. *Training doctors for Africa.* Lancet (London), 1, 14 Mar 1964, 599-601. Engl.

The great majority of Africa's doctors are civil servants or medical missionaries. The number of doctors ranges from one per 6 000 to one per 100 000 population, depending on the area. The major load of medical care is in the hands of the general duty medical officer. He handles impossibly diverse and demanding tasks. There is no universal solution to problems of health care in Africa; problems are too varied. Transportation is a decisive factor in provision of care. Since teamwork is essential, physicians need leadership training. Preclinical teachers must be trained if African countries are to expand their physician education facilities.

0392 Doege, T.C., Bangxang, H.N. *Laboratory in community medicine: examples from northern Thailand.* Journal of Medical Education (Chicago), 46, Nov 1971, 989-994. Engl.

Medical education at Chiang Mai University, Thailand, includes health-related projects such as a village immunization study, an investigation of BCG vaccination in school children, and a survey of health problems in a pottery factory. These projects are more successful in training future physicians to solve health problems and determine health policies than are didactic lectures and hospital-oriented experiences. Projects relating the basic and clinical sciences to the principles of epidemiology and community health could benefit all medical curricula and contribute valuable health data. Thirteen references are listed.

0393 Dowling, M.A. *Aspects of planning, conduct and evaluation of training for medical and other health staff.* Transactions of the Royal Society of Tropical Medicine and Hygiene (London), 63(2), 1969, 171-186. Engl.

A discussion follows the paper.

In most tropical countries there is a shortage of teachers and training facilities. To use existing facilities to the full, attention must be paid to three aspects of teaching: training courses with shorter programmes, teaching methods adapted to staff shortages, and improved evaluation of student and teacher performance to ensure that teaching remains dynamic and open to modification. To carry out these aspects of teaching, a programme of teacher training must be developed. References are listed.

0394 Gilles, H.M. *L'enseignement de la sante publique a l'Universite d'Ibadan, Nigeria. (Teaching of public health at the University of Ibadan, Nigeria).* Annales des Societes Belges de Medecine Tropicale, de Parasitologie et de Mycologie Humaine et Animale (Anvers), 45(5), 1965, 603-604. Fren.

Since most medical students are not interested in public health, a separate programme was set up in 1962 at the University of Ibadan in Nigeria, to integrate public health and other disciplines with internal medicine and pediatrics. The first-year curriculum concentrated on social and cultural aspects of life in Nigeria. Interdisciplinary instruction related nutrition, infectious and noninfectious diseases, climate, genetics, and community life. In the second year, sanitation is taught through study of a family in Ibadan. In the third year, students follow the health of a family assigned to them. Urban and rural differences are studies in terms of health problems presented by various ways of life. In the final year, study centres on case work, observation, and clinical and laboratory work in the hospital.

0395 Gonzalez, C.L., Vidal, E.L., Sierra, C.A., Colmenares, A., Rojas, F.A. *Ensenanza de la medicina preventiva y social en la Escuela de Medicina "Jose Vargas", Universidad Central de Venezuela. (Teaching of social and preventive medicine at the Jose Vargas School of Medicine, Central University of Venezuela).* Boletin de la Oficina Sanitaria Panamericana (Washington, D.C.), 58, Mar 1965, 209-215. Span.

The authors describe the origin, development, and future plans of the Department of Preventive and Social Medicine recently established at the Jose Vargas School of Medicine of the Central University of Venezuela in Caracas. The Department began to function in January 1962 with a training programme for the first and second years of the medical career. In the following academic year (1962-63) the programme extended into the third year, and in 1963-64 into the fourth year. The Department hopes to cover a 6-year training programme. Its method of work is based on a greater coordination with the other departments of the School of Medicine, and on the continuous teaching of preventive and social medicine throughout the entire medical curriculum. Theoretical training is reduced to a minimum and greater emphasis is placed on objective teaching and on practice, which is offered at the preventive, medical, and social institutions of Caracas and surrounding areas. The present curriculum includes: first year, statistical methods in medicine; second year, social and anthropological aspects of medicine, microbiology, and epidemiology; third year, specialized microbiology and epidemiology, and applied preventive and social medicine, i.e., basic notions of environmental sanitation, health promotion, and social problems; and fourth year, clinical aspects of preventive medicine. The proposed plan for the fifth year includes the study of the country's most important health problems and of the administrative and technical methods used to solve them. For the sixth and last year, a rotating internship will give the medical student an opportunity to practice integrated medicine under supervision at urban and rural health centres. The Department hopes to contribute toward the School's objective of training physicians in such a way that they will develop the attitudes and knowledge required to meet the country's existing needs in the medical, health, and social fields.

0396 Grzegorzewski, E. *Worldwide needs in medical education and their fulfillment.* Journal of the American Medical Association (Chicago), 180(11), 16 Jun 1962, 940-943. Engl.

The most acute medical education needs in developing countries are related to insufficient numbers of doctors. Comparison of the ratios of doctors to population shows extreme differences between developing and developed countries; the distribution of medical schools presents a similar picture. Another problem is the poor quality of graduates from many of these schools. The problem of a common basis for training medical students all over the world is receiving much attention. All medical schools should instill in their students the desire to constantly revise the content of technical knowledge and methods of its application in a continuing process of self-education, and should provide students with the philosophical and methodological basis to do it. Modern trends in medical education and principles of its organization and administration at the various levels of socioeconomic development should become more widely known among medical and general educators, public health administrators, and other responsible groups not only in the developing countries but also in the countries giving assistance. A thoroughly prepared "inventory of needs" is a natural start for education planning.

0397 Haile Selassie I University, Faculty of Medicine, Addis Ababa. *Medical and public health training facilities in Ethiopia.* Addis Ababa, Haile Selassie I University, Faculty of Medicine, Department of Preventive Medicine and Public Health, May 1970. Engl.
Unpublished document.

Tables are used to show facilities in Ethiopia for medical and public health training, nurse training, and dresser training.

0398 Hobson, W. *Training programme of the World Health Organization.* Journal of the Royal Institute of Public Health and Hygiene (London), 28(12), Dec 1965, 336-339. Engl.

The solving of many health problems requires a sufficient number of well-trained personnel. Many parts of the world suffer from a lack of trained medical staff, and where they do exist, distribution is uneven, with rural areas suffering most from the deficiency. By arranging international conferences, interregional travelling seminars, and exchange programmes; providing teachers and educational advisers with fellowships, teaching equipment, and books; publishing Technical Report Series, directories, and the results of special studies and surveys, etc., WHO supports the efforts of all countries, and particularly those of the developing nations, to overcome their difficulties in the training of health manpower to meet the demand.

0399 Janssens, P.G. *Tropical health care system in transition: teaching tropical medicine in a developing country.* Bulletin of the New York Academy of Medicine (New York), 48(10), Nov 1972, 1276-1289. Engl.

The objectives of medical education must be formulated according to the actual jobs to be carried out. Thus, no single pattern of medical education can be selected. Western curricula and its equivalent have been established at universities in many emerging countries, where the pattern of curricula is poorly adapted to local needs and there is resistance to change. The general duty tropical medical officer (M.O.) or tropical doctor must be a jack-of-all-trades; he should be trained to make the greatest impact on health, in the quickest, least expensive way possible. Training should emphasize preventive medicine and community outreach. Community-oriented activities prepare the physician for teamwork. Reappraisal of medical schools and faculties should be done by local personnel and the educational arrangements tailored to their needs. Institutes engaged in postgraduate education for medical activities in the tropics should train students to operate in tropical conditions a primary health service or a peripheral hospital, participate in teamwork, understand the community health problems, and train and encourage national professional and auxiliary personnel to take over at all levels of responsibility. The teaching of public health overseas must be an integrated part of the medical curriculum. The tropical doctor is thus a combination of medical practitioner and public health expert.

0400 Lange, W.G. *Deployment of surgical manpower in South America.* Journal of the Royal College of Surgeons of Edinburgh (Edinburgh), 16(1), Jan 1971, 205-209. Engl.

The efficiency of surgery in developing countries depends on the technical capacity of their surgeons and the equipment of their hospitals. Rural surgeons in Argentina lack access to professional contacts. Although the building of rural hospitals is alleviating this situation somewhat, few surgeons stay in rural practice. If surgeons are to be attracted to rural areas, conferences must be held for people from developing countries. Financial assistance is required if hospitals are to be organized and equipped in a reasonable period of time.

0401 Lucas, A.O. *Community medicine at the University of Ibadan.* In Lathem, W., Newbery, A., eds., Community Medicine: Teaching, Research, and Health Care, New York, Appleton-Century-Crofts, 1970, 91-104. Engl.
See also entry 162.

The historical background to medical education in Nigeria and a brief description of the medical care situation in the country are given. The activities of the various departments of the University of Ibadan Medical School in community medicine, in particular the Ibarapa Project, are outlined. This project, organized on an interdepartmental basis under the direction of the Department of Medicine, is operated by a team of two doctors, a public health engineer, health visitors, and clinical workers, augmented by visiting staff from the Liverpool School of Tropical Medicine, and lecturers from other faculties of Ibadan University, such as the Department of Sociology. Assignment to the project is an integral part of the training of 4th-year students from both Ibadan and Lagos medical schools, following training in the departments of medicine, surgery, pediatrics, and, sometimes, obstetrics and gynecology. Difficulties arise in setting up such a programme: the experimental area soon becomes atypical, the size of the area can present problems of interviewing, and distance from the teaching hospital can determine whether the unit functions as part of the hospital or as a separate entity. The project's main objective was to show medical students the other side of medical care: care within the community, in both rural and urban settings, which is complementary to that given in the hospital.

0402 Lutwama, J.S. *Community medicine at Makerere University College.* In Lathem, W., Newbery, A., eds., Community Medicine: Teaching, Research and Health Care, New York, Appleton-Century-Crofts, 1970, 65-78. Engl.
See also entry 162.

The effective teaching of social and preventive medicine in developing countries requires a full specimen of public health services in which medical students can participate. In response to this requirement, the community medicine programmes conducted by the Makerere Medical School at Kasangati, Kampala, and Ankole districts, East Africa, enable students to meet health visitors, advisers and inspectors, nurses, midwives, etc. in working situations where they can gain insight into the background, skills, and duties of these cadres. Students also acquire experience in such community-oriented activities as health education, environmental sanitation, and compilation and interpretation of vital statistics. The increase in the number of undergraduates, and changes in the disease patterns and character of the society as it becomes less rural and more urbanized, require adjustments to be made in approach, e.g. greater involvement of the school in the training of other members of the health team, in cooperation with government agencies, and the development of suitable curricula. Four references are listed.

0403 Mann, K.J. *Israel physician: his training, responsibilities and rights.* Israel Journal of Medical Sciences (Jerusalem), 6(1), Jan-Feb 1970, 145-153. Engl.

An analysis of undergraduate, graduate, and postgraduate medical education in Israel reveals the following: there are enough physicians to meet medical needs, admission policies are up-to-date, the students' backgrounds involve physical, social, and behavioural sciences, etc. Fourteen references are listed.

0404 Mann, K.J. New York Academy of Medicine, New York. *Role of the family and community health center.* Bulletin of the New York Academy of Medicine (New York), 42(9), Sep 1966, 742-755. Engl.

Israel's Family and Community Health Centre at Kiryat Hayovel, a suburb of Jerusalem, was established in 1953. It provided comprehensive medical care for the community and gave the medical and nursing schools some control over community health facilities for teaching and research. This paper evaluates the Centre's contribution to the training of family physicians, family nurses, and public health nurses, and discusses the part it played in training undergraduate medical and nursing students. It is concluded that the Centre has demonstrated an effective pattern for the provision of medical care to a community in an emerging society. Family physicians and nurses trained in the Centre have since filled key positions in community health services. Training in the Centre is also seen to be instrumental in changing the physician's image of himself as a "scientist" to that of a "healer."

0405 Manuwa, S. *Training of senior administrators for higher responsibilities in the national health services of developing countries.* West African Medical Journal (Ibadan), 16, Dec 1967, 213-221. Engl.

Training of medical personnel for top administrative posts in developing countries is important for two reasons. First, shortage of such persons makes it important that the health administrator be knowledgeable in all aspects of public health. Secondly, training can help the administrator establish priorities within which to use the limited resources that characterize developing countries. Training of physicians without formal qualifications in public health will differ from that of physicians with public health training and from senior administrators without medical qualifications. Curriculum suggestions for training are outlined. Universities in developing countries should take steps to establish community-oriented schools of public health and tropical medicine. Ten references are listed.

0406 Molina, G., Jimeno, C. *Teaching social science concepts in a clinical setting in preventive medicine.* Milbank Memorial Fund Quarterly (New York), 44, Apr 1966, Suppl., 211-225. Engl.

The initial contribution made by the behavioural sciences to the teaching of preventive medicine, integrated into the clinical period in one of the government hospitals used by the University of Chile Medical School is discussed. Integration of social scientists into medical education programmes has been facilitated by adapting social science content to the needs of clinicians, and contributions of the social scientist have been well accepted. Social science and administrative principles are valuable additions to statistical, epidemiological, and educational services offered by a preventive medicine group. Social scientists have fully participated in the whole planning process, and have assumed major responsibilities for study and teaching of sociocultural factors influencing disease, patient care, and educational processes. Twenty references are listed.

0407 Neumann, A.K., Prince, J.S., Gilbert, F.F., Lourie, I.M. *Danfa/Ghana comprehensive rural health and family planning project: preliminary report.* Ghana Medical Journal (Accra), 11(1), Mar 1972, 18-24. Engl.
See also entry 413.

In 1965 a comprehensive rural health demonstration, teaching, and research project began in Ghana as a teaching activity of the Department of Social and Preventive Medicine of the Ghana Medical School. The project arose in response to the Ghanaian government's desire to accelerate development in the rural sector, including training of physicians for rural service. Goals of the Danfa project include investigation of the conditions of rural life, research into effective uses of health manpower, training of a variety of types of rural health workers, and provision of a model comprehensive rural health care programme through the Danfa Health Centre. Future work includes studies on family structure and stability in rural areas of Ghana, the role of village registration in updating census data, the role of local midwives in rural maternal and child health and family planning programmes, the relationship between traditional medical practitioners and government health services, etc.

0408 Odeku, E.L., Williams, G.A., Esan, G.J., Otitoju, E.O., Oduntan, S.A., Banjo, B. *Medical education and training.* In Akinkugbe, O.O., Olatunbosun, D., Esan, G.J., eds., Priorities in National Health Planning: Proceedings of an International Symposium, Ibadan, Caxton Press (West Africa) Ltd., 1973, 183-234. Engl.
See entry 123 for full report of symposium.

The chapter covers six papers on medical education and training. The first paper emphasizes the need for education and research to identify exact areas of need in the health care system. It likens the health problem of developing countries to a health project in Ghana, in which the community leaders stated their needs, in order of priority, as "hospital, water, good roads, latrines, improved farming, schools, and transport." He stresses the necessity for functional definitions of health manpower and for their periodic evaluation. The second paper makes specific suggestions for training physicians, nurses, midwives, and sanitary workers in Nigeria. Paper three calls for admission into Nigerian medical schools of candidates with strong personality and high motivation even if their scientific background is not of the highest level. Logic and medical ethics must be included in preclinical courses and the quality of clinical instruction improved. Problems relating to the education of medical ethics must be included in preclinical courses and the quality of clinical instruction improved. Problems relating to the education of medical teachers and to research are also discussed. The fourth paper calls for the establishment in Nigeria of a training programme in hospital administration that would consider local needs. Paper five emphasizes the importance of the medical anaesthetists and medical assistants in anaesthesia. The final paper observes that excessive support is given to specialists and teaching hospitals to the disadvantage of rural health care programmes. It suggests that Nigeria should adopt suitable elements of the Chinese public health system. Subsequent discussion centered on the training of hospital administrators, reducing the training period of doctors, criteria for admissions into medical schools, medical assistants and rural health delivery, and the need for doctors to improve their image and live by example rather than precept.

0409 Prywes, M. *International aspects of governmental and academic health center relationships.* Journal of Medical Education (Chicago), 46, Dec 1971, 1019-1034. Engl.

The influence of government on medical personnel training and deployment is discussed. Financial and licencing controls exercised by government can be vital to consumer interests. Beneficial effects of state influence can be seen in licencing control and deployment of medical personnel to rural areas of Mexico, Chile, Tanzania, and Bolivia. Government support for medical education is important and academics need to distinguish between benefits of control and the fear of losing academic freedom, in relation to government's influence in the health field. Thirteen references are listed.

0410 Prywes, M. *Principles and methods for undergraduate medical education in developing countries.* Israel Journal of Medical Sciences (Jerusalem), 4(3), May-Jun 1968, 638-655. Engl.
Fourth Rehovoth Conference on Health Problems in Developing States, Rehovoth, Israel, 15-23 Aug 1967.
See entry 96 for complete proceedings.

A great deal of published material now exists on experiences, needs, and perspectives for medical education in the developing world. Medical schools must be developed within developing countries themselves, to meet national needs. Certain principles and methods for implementing programmes need to be stressed. An evaluation of the applicability of medical courses is required. Coordination between the medical institutions of a country is necessary. Anxiety about standards and international recognition in developing countries impedes innovative pragmatic clinical approaches.

0411 Ramos, R. *O Treinamento de Planejadores do Setor Saude. (Training courses for health planners).* Revista de Saude Publica (Sao Paulo), 2(2), Dec 1968, 207-215. Portuguese.

The World Health Organization attaches the same importance to the training of key personnel in the field of health planning as it has in the last few years to the utilization of human resources in the implementation of health programmes. Objectives and content of current health planning courses, and a comparative study of such courses given in the USA, Trinidad and Tobago, Chile, and Brazil are included. WHO's role, through its regional offices, in establishing and consolidating these courses throughout Latin America is analyzed.

0412 Rundle, F.F. *Community distribution of doctors as a challenge to medical education and training.* Medical Journal of Australia (Sydney), 1, 23 May 1970, 1064-1065. Engl.

The problem of making medical education more relevant to community needs is discussed in relation to physician distribution figures for several Asian countries. Consideration for people in rural areas rarely enters undergraduate medical programmes in developing countries. New programmes like the one in Bangkok, Thailand, should introduce students to both community and clinical medicine toward the end of their preclinical studies. Field work, surveys, and analyses of medical care programmes are of immense educational value. In addition to the physician's traditional abilities, graduates will have skills in cooperative leadership and management. Five references are listed.

0413 Sai, F.T., Wurapa, F.K., Quartey-Papafio, E.K. *Danfa/Ghana comprehensive rural health and family planning project: a community approach.* Ghana Medical Journal (Accra), 11(1), Mar 1972, 9-17. Engl.
See also entry 407.

The Ghana Medical School opened in February 1964. The objective of the School was primarily to produce physicians who were generalists rather than specialists. A rural community health project was set up to help train doctors in community health problems. In 1967 a group of seven villages outside Accra were chosen as an experimentation area for training health workers to meet needs of rural people. Local leaders were interviewed and their priorities were recorded. These included a hospital, roads, latrines, improved farming, schools, and transportation. These leaders offered land for a clinic and, with community participation, a centre was built. The project made careful note of the cost and the benefit of various activities, for future use in physician training. Twelve references are listed.

0414 Standard, K.L. *Education for community health practice.* In Hughes, J.P., ed., Health Care for Remote Areas: An International Conference, Oakland, Kaiser Foundation, 1972, 66-69. Engl.
See entry 155 for complete proceedings.

Jamaica has established national goals for family doctor services, which it hopes to make available to everyone. Curricula must be adapted to educate physicians for community practice. A Department of Social and Preventive Medicine has been created to provide physicians with community experience. In this department students help establish their own objectives. A community health aide training programme has also been developed.

0415 Tiwari, I.C., Marwah, S.M. *Approach to interns' training in rural areas.* Indian Journal of Public Health (Calcutta), 14(1), Jan 1970, 6-10. Engl.

All of India's medical colleges have an internship of 1 year including 3 months of rural residential training under a department of preventive and social medicine. No guidelines exist for rural training and each training centre is evolving its own approach. The rural internship training provided by Banaras Hindu University is described. The programme includes seeking villagers' participation in health activities, maintaining family health and health records (family folder), preparing village exhibitions, etc. Since evaluation is considered an important part of health care delivery, interns evaluate some aspect of services. Interns participate with all departmental staff in weekly seminars to discuss village programmes and short-term evaluative studies. Internship has the dual purpose of interesting young doctors in rural work and developing a research approach to rural health problems. Experience in this programme indicates the necessity for operational studies of all aspects of rural interns' training, frequent seminars to discuss topics picked up from field investigations, and visits by medical faculty members to the village health centres.

0416 Velasquez, G. *General practitioner and the evolution toward "community medicine".* Israel Journal of Medical Sciences (Jerusalem), 4(3), May-Jun 1968, 656-664. Engl.
Fourth Rehovoth Conference on Health Problems in Developing States, Rehovoth, Israel, 15-23 Aug 1967.
See entry 96 for complete proceedings.

Over the past 15 years, many countries have tried to improve medical education. Emphasis has been on training more specialized professionals who know the social and engineering sciences. Specialization has become a subject of controversy. The Universidad del Valle in Colombia is attempting to become a basic vital force in the community. Medical education relates to overall regional development. The university participates in national and regional health planning and is training physicians and others to contribute within the needs of the nation as a whole. Various current views of community physician practice are discussed. The objectives and curriculum of the Universidad del Valle's community physician training programme are given.

0417 West African Medical Journal, Ibadan. *WHO assistance to meet critical shortage of health personnel training for doctors, nurses, and health workers.* West African Medical Journal (Ibadan), 15(2), Apr 1966, 53. Engl.

WHO aids Africa by providing assistance to university schools of medicine, departments of nursing, and midwife training institutions for teaching and training all categories of health workers.

0418 WHO, Alexandria. *Medical education in the Eastern Mediterranean Region: the need for teacher training.* Alexandria, WHO, Jul 1970.

10p. WHO/EM/RC20/5. EMRO/70/978. Engl. Unpublished document.

There has been a great increase in the number of faculties of medicine in member countries of WHO's Eastern Mediterranean Region during this century. Additional trained medical teachers are urgently required to fill teaching positions in these schools. The present study analyzes a sample of regional medical schools to evaluate the adequacy of the teaching staff. Information from schools of medicine in Afghanistan, Ethiopia, Iran, Iraq, Israel, Lebanon, Pakistan, Sudan, Syria, Tunisia, and Egypt were analyzed. Considering various factors it is estimated that the task for institutions of medical education in the region in the next 5-10 years is to train about 5 000 new teachers. The responsibility of medical schools and health authorities in providing these teachers is discussed.

0419 WHO, Geneva. *Internationally acceptable minimum standards of medical education: report of a study group.* Geneva, WHO Technical Report Series No. 239, 1962. 59p. Engl.

In establishing a basis for comparison of international medical education, the following problems are considered: selection of students, curriculum, methods of teaching, and adequacy of standards. Existing arrangements for the above are reviewed. Although premedical education is fairly uniform in content, secondary education varies greatly, exposing people of different educational levels to medical training. Admissions are regulated in different ways. Examples of curricula show that all medical schools include human anatomy, biochemistry, etc. but differences occur in time assigned to these subjects. Some countries have government-controlled curricula, whereas others have private systems. The following are a few of the recommendations put forward: that the general education of prospective medical students extend over 12 years; that medical faculties review curricula constantly; that the minimum length of medical study be 4 years, with a fundamental content for all countries; that medical schools exist as part of a university; that teaching staff control academic policy; and that medical schools in developing countries be assessed by outsiders, e.g. WHO.

0420 WHO, Geneva. *Teaching of the basic medical sciences in the light of modern medicine: eighth report of the Expert Committee on Professional and Technical Education of Medical and Auxiliary Personnel.* Geneva, WHO Technical Report Series No. 209, 1961. 31p. Engl.

The preventive concept of medicine can be promoted in preclinical medical courses through the training of teachers and selection of students, textbooks, and curricula, and must be continued during the clinical years of study.

0421 WHO, Geneva. *Expert committee on professional and technical education of medical and auxiliary personnel: second report.* Geneva, WHO Technical Report Series No. 69, Jun 1953. 26p. Engl.

Each country should have adequate medical education facilities. Medical schools should be leaders in the community, demonstrating and teaching for the benefit of individuals within the community. The general practitioner must be trained in comprehensive medicine and must work with allied health professionals. Medical schools should not accept more students than they can educate well. Students should have a broad educational background to augment their influence in the community. The medical school should establish and maintain a department of preventive and social medicine with faculty members of high personal and academic merit.

0422 Yankauer, A., Villarreal, R. *Community health service area as a pediatric teaching facility in Latin America.* Journal of Medical Education (Chicago), 42, Nov 1967, 1015-1022. Engl.

It has been recognized for a number of years that the teaching hospital is inadequate as a facility to promote learning of community medicine and comprehensive patient care. This paper indicates how in Latin America the scope and quality of undergraduate medical training can be improved by using the community and community health services as a facility. This pedagogic concept is particularly relevant to Latin America where regionalization of services, with health service areas extending out peripherally from a base hospital, is accepted as a planning principle. Such decentralization of authority plus a national concern for future manpower needs provides a link between health authorities and medical educators. The pedagogic approach described is especially relevant to pediatric practice, since half of all deaths in Latin America occur in children. Basic pediatric skills such as the assessment of child growth, development, and nutritional status, the techniques of a pediatric physical examination, and the establishment of parental rapport in history-taking are acquired more readily in a community health area than in a teaching hospital. Internship and residency programmes already established are either a compulsory period of service in a rural area or a small hospital, or a hospital pediatric residency. If the community health area facility is to be utilized, the university is obligated to prepare the student for a role within the national health services, and to plan and execute operational research designed to serve the administrative needs of the national health services.

IV.1.2 Lower- and middle-level health workers

See also: 0028, 0029, 0040, 0045, 0054, 0055, 0067, 0198, 0222, 0302, 0323, 0335, 0363, 0380, 0382, 0390, 0572

0423 African Medical and Research Foundation, Nairobi. *Medical development: Botswana.* Nairobi, African Medical and Research Foundation, Jul 1972. 33p. Engl.

African Medical and Research Foundation investigators report to the Government of Botswana on the health development plan and give advice concerning the possibility of setting up a flying doctor service and radio communications network for Botswana. Entrenchment of the old medical system based on Western models has been a barrier to change and further innovative development. The report suggests a training programme for auxiliary workers, a low-cost building programme, a flying doctor service, and a radio communications network to link up rural units. It is suggested that auxiliaries play a greater role in hospitals and participate in the training of other personnel. Recommendations for recruitment and training of various categories of auxiliary health workers are presented.

0424 Arole, M. *Comprehensive rural health project, Jamkhed: the village level worker.* n.p., Jan 1973. 2p. Engl.
Unpublished document.

A comprehensive health project serving 30 villages is in operation in Jamkhed, India. As the rural economy cannot support the services of qualified physicians, a three-tier system of health care delivery was devised in which a physician (first-tier) delegates responsibility for primary health care to a nurse and paramedical worker (second-tier), and women recruited from the villages are trained as village-level workers (third-tier) to provide liaison between the team and the community. An advantage of the system is the closeness of the village-level workers to the people they serve. They can, by their example, convince their peers to use the services where the more educated nurse/paramedical worker fails. For instance, a nurse who stayed in a village for 6 months was unable to persuade a single woman to undergo tubectomy. An illiterate village woman, after herself being convinced to undergo the operation, persuaded 75 others to follow suit. Village-level workers are instructed on various health topics 2 days a week, with the aid of flash cards and charts, which they are taught to use in their promotional work in the villages. Eight workers have been trained so far and results are encouraging.

0425 Baker, T.D. *Paramedical paradoxes: challenges and opportunity.* In Wolstenholme, G., O'Connor, M., eds., Teamwork for World Health, London, J. and A. Churchill, 1971, 129-141. Engl.
See also entry 198.

General agreement on the importance of the paramedical worker makes it difficult to explain the low priority given their recruitment, training, and supervision. These workers are less expensive to train and utilize than are professional workers. Training in paramedical schools is often more traditional than relevant. Four-year anatomy courses reduced to 4-week courses do not have content relevant to auxiliary health workers destined to remote areas. The paramedical problem should become the interest of a foundation, in that teaching techniques need to be updated, the art of supervision needs to be taught, and greater attention needs to be focussed on problems of career development for these workers.

0426 Balasegaram, M. *Malaysia and its problems.* Journal of the Royal College of Surgeons of Edinburgh (Edinburgh), 16(1), Jan 1971, 192-196. Engl.

The Malaysian population is diverse both racially and linguistically. Physicians are faced with a complexity of attitudes, as each racial group has distinct health care preferences and beliefs that influence their acceptance of Western methods of treatment. Since most physicians practice on the populous west coast, auxiliary surgical workers (who reflect the racial composition of the country) need to be trained. Health centres are being built by the government at an encouraging rate in all rural areas.

0427 Boohene, A.G. *Physician assistants in a developing country.* World Medical Journal (New York), 9(2), Mar-Apr 1972, 35-37. Engl.

In Ghana two types of medical auxiliaries are being trained and utilized: health centre superintendents and nurse anaesthetists. Candidates are selected from among experienced male and female nurses. After 1 year of training under the supervision of a medical officer, the health centre superintendent is posted to a rural or urban health centre. In the rural health centre, he is leader of the health team, undertaking preventive and curative health work. The nurse anaesthetist, trained for 6 months by an accredited anaesthetist, works mainly in hospitals and, like the health centre superintendent, is not allowed private practice and is relatively poorly paid in relation to his work and responsibilities.

0428 Brooke, D.E. *Role of the medical assistant.* Tropical Doctor (London), 3(4), Oct 1973, 174-176. Engl.

Too often developing countries attempt to build technically advanced health services that only serve an elite segment of the population. Medical assistant training makes less expensive care for more people possible. These workers undergo training and are selected for their willingness to work in remote areas. Supervision of medical assistants by physicians is necessary, but is often a weak point in programme implementation. Too often medical assistants are left on their own for extended periods of time. Medical assistants are likely to provide the backbone of medical care for years to come. Their function can be improved through experimentation and research.

0429 Brown, R.E. *Augmenting medical care in the remote areas of developing nations.* Clinical Pediatrics (Philadelphia), 5(10), Oct 1966, 582-584. Engl.

To achieve lasting progress the developing countries need to experience balanced growth. Socioeconomic growth and progress in the areas of health and education are equally vital. Many experts see the shortage of health manpower as a factor limiting progress, and to meet the need all available human resources must be utilized. Programmes for new types of auxiliary health workers should include refresher courses and adequate supervision, and should emphasize preventive medicine. Clinic organization and group dynamics training would also prove useful to auxiliary health trainees. Well-trained medical assistants in a well-organized programme can offer care to remote areas that would otherwise not be reached by modern services. Since these workers receive lower salaries than physicians, they can be deployed at lower cost. Western medical educators should consider it an obligation to devise a simplified system of medicine for workers in auxiliary health programmes. Eleven references are listed.

0430 Browne, S.G. *Training of medical auxiliaries in the former Belgian Congo.* Lancet (London), 1(7812), 19 May 1973, 1103-1105. Engl.
A training programme for medical auxiliaries in the former Belgian Congo (Zaire) is discussed with respect to admission requirements, curriculum, teaching staff, examinations (leading to the official title of *infirmier*), and continuing activities. Nine references are listed.

0431 Browne, S.G. *Role of the medical auxiliary in field surveys in tropical Africa.* Transactions of the Royal Society of Tropical Medicine and Hygiene (London), 58(5), Sep 1964, 370-376. Engl.
The valuable contribution made by teams of medical auxiliaries in the course of mass surveys in tropical Africa is illustrated by examples drawn from a circumscribed medical control area in the ex-Belgian Congo (Zaire). It is shown that the training of these auxiliaries can with advantage be orientated toward the investigation of various endemic diseases, and that both during training and afterwards they are able, when suitably directed and supervised, to collect essential clinical, pathological, and entomological data. When such mass surveys are followed by the provision of treatment through a system of village dispensaries, manned by qualified auxiliaries whose training has had a bias toward preventive medicine, the cooperation of the rural inhabitants is assured. Nineteen references are listed. (Revised author abstract.)

0432 Canada, Department of National Health and Welfare. *Community health worker in Indian and Eskimo communities.* Ottawa, Department of National Health and Welfare, n.d. 9p. Engl.
The functions of the community health worker in Indian and Eskimo communities of Canada are outlined. Details are given on the selection procedure, the training programme, and the relationship between the community health worker and public health nurse. Also discussed are their job descriptions and the role of each office in the health programme. The paper concludes that the health worker should be given in-service training and included in professional group discussions to raise his confidence in the performance of his duties.

0433 Chang, W.P. *Health manpower development in an African country: the case of Ethiopia.* Journal of Medical Education (Chicago), 45, Jan 1970, 29-39. Engl.
This paper reviews Ethiopia's manpower programmes designed to provide basic health services. Haile Selassie I Public Health College and Training Centre at Gondar trains teams of health workers for rural health centres. The health officer, community nurse, and sanitarian are key members of the team. Their training emphasizes preventive medicine with a team approach. The Gondar College is not a second-rate medical school, nor a stepping stone to a university course in medicine; but rather it is a first-rate institution for training rural health workers. Recent changes in the health officer's curriculum to meet the requirements of the University resulted in the programme becoming more academic and less service oriented. The training programme should avoid the "near doctor" concept: curriculum of the Gondar College should clearly emphasize preventive medicine and public health. A definite career structure, with future professional advancement and respectable status has to be developed for the health officers. Selection of limited numbers of health officers for a tailored medical course is based on the critical need for public health oriented physicians. The Gondar training scheme could serve as a model, with appropriate modifications, for other developing countries. Five references are listed.

0434 Daynes, J.A. *Health education personnel.* South African Medical Journal (Cape Town), 47, 24 Feb 1973, 295-296. Engl.
This paper outlines health education work to be done in the Bantu areas of South Africa. This includes general health instruction for hospital patients and for those attending clinics attached to hospitals and clinics in the community, and special instruction in cultivating vegetable gardens, the care of food animals, and the preventive aspects of certain deseases such as kwashiorkor, tuberculosis, and bilharzia. It is suggested that health education personnel be trained and given the titles *Bantu health educator* (responsible for health education policy in the district as well as for the training, supervision, and transportation of the health instructors) and *Bantu health instructor* (general health instructors to assist the health educator, and special health instructors for such areas as care of gardens, backyard farming, and food preparation). Three or more of each type of health instructor are recommended for each district. The *Bantu health educator* would be selected from graduates of the diploma course in public health nursing; *Bantu health instructors* should have a junior certificate and special interest or experience in their chosen field of work. Methods of transportation for these personnel in the district are suggested.

0435 Deuschle, K.W. *Training and use of medical auxiliaries in a Navajo community.* Public Health Reports (Washington, D.C.), 78(6), Jun 1963, 461-469. Engl.

The Cornell-Navajo Field Health Project involved the training and employment of Navajo medical auxiliaries. Trainees from various educational levels were selected for their interest in health work and willingness to undergo training. Trainees were drilled in bilingual transmission of medical concepts. Curriculum included personal health, growth and development, epidemiology, immunology, dental care, nutrition, family life, and special disease conditions such as infant diarrhea and tuberculosis. Instruction in nursing procedures and supervised field work were essential aspects of training. Evaluation of the Navajo medical auxiliaries was based on expert analysis of their medical interpretations and on assessment of their value by the professional staff, the community, the trainees, and Public Health Service physicians and nurses. It was unanimously agreed that Navajos with restricted or limited education could be trained individually or in small groups to carry out clinic and field work under supervision. Thirteen references are listed.

0436 Elliott, K. *Doctor substitutes.* Health and Social Service Journal (London), 7 Jul 1973. 1p. Engl.

Redistribution of medical manpower is a worldwide necessity, but an overwhelmingly difficult task. Many countries are now providing substitutes for physicians, i.e. medexes, feldshers, barefoot doctors. Seven such auxiliary health workers can be trained for the same amount of money as one medical doctor, and much more quickly. China has been the forerunner, with barefoot doctors providing primary care, prevention, health education, etc. Western countries are becoming active in this field: America has training schemes for medical care auxiliaries. Although it is true that in communities that lack good sanitation, clean water, and adequate food their contribution is limited, they do provide practical help where none previously existed.

0437 Ennever, O., Marsh, M.C., Standard, K.L. *Community health aide training programme.* West Indian Medical Journal (Kingston), 18, 1969, 193-201. Engl.

Fourteenth Meeting of the Standing Advisory Committee for Medical Research in the British Caribbean, Trinidad, Apr 1969.

See also entries 484 and 614.

An experimental programme to train Jamaican village residents as auxiliary health aides has improved community care. Health aides assist trained nurses. Under professional supervision they recognize the important signs of illness, refer patients to appropriate sources of care, carry out clinic duties, and provide health education for the community. Aides began working as volunteers but are now paid for their services.

0438 Fendall, N.R. *Auxiliaries and primary medical care.* Bulletin of the New York Academy of Medicine (New York), 48(10), Nov 1972, 1291-1300. Engl.

Persons of minimal educational background must be selected, appropriately trained, and utilized to provide medical and health care with the financial and manpower resources of developing countries. The great quantitative demand in these countries is for care of the ambulant sick; the major demand is at a basic level, and comes from the rural areas. In delivery of medical care the emphasis will shift from professional to auxiliary health workers and from urban to rural areas. A medical organization with adequate referral and supervision systems can utilize auxiliaries to advantage, not as replacements for physicians but as "assistants" and "substitutes." Supervision must be properly performed by physicians so that auxiliaries function satisfactorily. Auxiliary training should stress practice and should emphasize the human element. Duties must be defined and functional details studied. Audiovisual methods of learning are important at this stage. Teachers must be aware of field conditions, be adept in their vocation and involved in continuous evaluation and research in the field.

0439 Fendall, N.R. *Auxiliary personnel in specialized programmes with special reference to tuberculosis.* In Proceedings of the Twentieth International Tuberculosis Conference, New York, 2-6 Sep 1969, Amsterdam, Excerpta Medica International Congress Series No. 205, 170-173. Engl.

Twentieth International Tuberculosis Conference, New York, Sep 1969.

Health care in developing countries must cope with slender financial resources, lack of trained manpower, an excessive fertility pattern, a predominantly rural population, and the prevalence of communicable diseases and malnutrition. Efforts to reduce the number of communicable diseases are inhibited by maldistribution of professionally trained personnel, and the education of such personnel. Auxiliary personnel can increase medical outreach at a realistic cost. Auxiliaries have a minimum of learning and although they retain contact with traditional cultures, they are also acquainted with the modern. Informed supervision is essential. Training should be pragmatic and didactic, and should include such core subjects as body structure and functions, basic sciences and biology, mass information techniques, etc. Auxiliaries, given adequate supervision, can be deployed in both general and specific health programmes to advantage. Seven references are listed.

0440 Fendall, N.R. *Auxiliary in medicine.* Israel Journal of Medical Sciences (Jerusalem), 4(3), May-Jun 1968, 614-636. Engl.

Fourth Rehovoth Conference on Health Problems in Developing States, Rehovoth, Israel, 15-23 Aug 1967.

See entry 96 for complete proceedings.

It is often argued that conditions in emerging countries vary, yet characteristics of these countries are sufficiently similar to warrant advocating the use of auxiliary personnel in medical and health care delivery. Types of auxiliaries used so far include the medical assistant, the dental auxiliary, the auxiliary midwife-pediatrician, the junior health worker or auxiliary sanitarian, the laboratory auxiliary, the compounder or pharmaceutical auxiliary, and the nursing, physiotherapy, and radiography auxiliary. Selection, supervision, training, and status of these personnel are discussed. Their roles must be precisely defined by job and market analysis. Training should be of an empirical practical nature.

0441 Fendall, N.R. *Medical assistant in Africa.* Journal of Tropical Medicine and Hygiene (London), 71, Apr 1968, 83-95. Engl.

Developing countries cannot afford to deliver health care via trained physicians. However, as the prevention, recognition, and diagnosis of most illnesses found in these countries are known, the task could be taken over by trained auxiliary health workers. A work force, including nurses, pharmacist-auxiliaries, and midwives, of which at least 40% were career-oriented, would be trained in relation to the actual tasks required of them. The empirical approach would be emphasized. In Thailand, traditional physicians are retrained in simplified home remedies. Examples of auxiliaries at work in various settings are given in case studies from the Sudan, Uganda, Kenya, Tanzania, and Malawi. Functions of physicians' assistants, medical assistants in general outpatient and casualty services, and workers in rural health centres are outlined. Five references are listed.

0442 Fendall, N.R. *History of the Yaba school of medicine, Nigeria.* West African Medical Journal (Ibadan), 16, Aug 1967, 118-124. Engl.

The Yaba School of Medicine in Nigeria began training auxiliary health workers in 1930. The School was designed to train auxiliaries capable of practicing medicine independently in such a way that their practices would be maximally accessible to the African population. The School's objectives took into consideration the experiences of programmes in Singapore, Madras, and other areas of the British administrative control, as well as assessments of the availability and potential of trainees. A 4-year programme was proposed emphasizing pharmacy skills, minor surgery, bandaging, sterilization, and hygiene. Training was long and intensive; the number of graduates was low because of the rigid standards imposed. A brief history of training and results is given. Lessons from this study are relevant to current issues concerning auxiliaries in health work.

0443 Fendall, N.R. *Auxiliary health personnel: training and use.* Public Health Reports (Washington, D.C.), 82(6), Jun 1967, 471-479. Engl.

Comprehensive medicine is beyond the present reach of developing countries, but integrated medicine, i.e. a balanced programme of curative, preventive, and promotional medicine, is not. The use of auxiliary health workers offers a means of achieving integrated medicine. This paper reviews the main types of auxiliary health workers (single-purpose, multipurpose, and all-purpose), their selection, training, and function.

0444 Fendall, N.R. *Utilization and training of auxiliary health personnel for developing areas.* Industry and Tropical Health (Boston), 6, 1967, 153-162. Engl.

Physicians placed in remote health posts are prone to dissatisfaction. Since the costs of training and supporting physicians are high, it is preferable for a few dedicated physicians to work through auxiliary health workers. If medical care can be broken down into its component parts, less-trained individuals can perform many of these jobs. Many diseases, for instance are easy to diagnose and cure. Various types of auxiliary health workers are described, with examples from Thailand, Ghana, East Africa, and Fiji. Given proper support and training, auxiliary personnel can function effectively in the outreach efforts of health delivery systems.

0445 Fendall, N.R. *Medical planning and the training of personnel in Kenya.* Journal of Tropical Medicine and Hygiene (London), 68, Jan 1965, 12-20. Engl.

Kenya's long-term health development plan gives priority to rural health centres. While central government retains control of regional hospitals and training, regional government maintains district hospitals, and local authorities maintain control of personal and environmental services. Regrouping of professional personnel means that the experienced are withdrawn to regional centres and auxiliary medical staff accept more responsibility. Two aspects of training require urgent attention, namely the training of doctors in administrative work and public health, and the training of medical assistants as physician substitutes. Proposals for training multipurpose auxiliaries, nursing staff, laboratory workers, public health personnel, etc. are presented. Twelve references are listed.

0446 Flahault, D. *Training of front line health personnel: a crucial factor in development.* WHO Chronicle (Geneva), 27(6), Jun 1973, 236-241. Engl.

Primary care health personnel can play an important part in development of health services and in community development. The workers must have sound technical training and be firmly motivated toward development. Determining the type of personnel needed, establishing adequate training programmes, and utilizing these personnel are problems that must be overcome in each developing country. Some basic solutions to these problems and the role of WHO are considered.

0447 Flahault, D. *Training of rural health personnel.* WHO Chronicle (Geneva), 26(6), Jun 1972, 243-249. Engl.

The world's rural population is characterized by its vast and growing size, its isolation, and its low standard of living. By training large numbers of auxiliary personnel, ensuring their constant supervision, and giving them mobility to reach remote populations, a basic minimum service can be provided to people who have hitherto been completely without health care.

0448 Freyvogel, T.A. *Work at the Rural Aid Centre (RAC), Ifakara, Tanganyika.* Acta Tropica (Basel), 21(1), 1964, 91-95. Engl.

The Rural Aid Centre (RAC), Ifakara, Tanzania, provided 3-month training courses for persons referred from other government work to become auxiliary health workers in rural areas. Planning for 3-and 4-year training courses is mentioned. Students were reportedly pleased with RAC training, and with its proximity to a modern hospital and well-equipped laboratories. Field experience in nearby villages interested students intensely, many of whom had not been to rural areas before. These rural visits gave students valuable insights for their future work. Subjects taught included clinical medicine, pathology, rural hygiene, epidemiology and medical entomology, laboratory techniques, identification of venomous animals, and control of ecto-parasites. Course contents were coordinated with teaching at the Medical Training Centre in Dar-es-Salaam. Seven references are listed.

0449 Fry, J. *Primary medical care in Africa: M.D., or M.A.?* Journal of the Royal College of General Practitioners (Dartmouth, England), 21, Jun 1971, 356-361. Engl.

The inequality of medical care between the developing nations and the developed ones is quite evident. Poverty, which dominates problems in developing nations, is related to lack of educational progress, poor housing, urban-rural migration, etc. In Africa, common diseases are preventable ones, for the most part. Health centres in East Africa are manned by medical assistants who, with 2-3 years training, diagnose and treat common diseases. Although these workers are to be supervised, supervisory visits are rare. Physician-medical assistant relations are good, but medical assistants usually work in isolation.

0450 Geigy, R. *Rural medical training at Ifakara: Swiss help to Tanzania.* Lancet (London), 26 Jun 1965, 1385-1387. Engl.
See also entry 485.

Tanzania is greatly in need of qualified health personnel. At present, the medical auxiliaries are the key personnel entrusted with health care in remote areas. The Swiss-supported Rural Aid Centre at Ifakara, guided by the Swiss Tropical Institute, trains auxiliaries for rural work. The Centre's location facilitates practical learning under conditions typical of most of the country. The alienation of urban or university-trained personnel in the face of rural practice is thus avoided. Objectives, duration, and syllabus for courses in medical auxiliary training are described.

0451 Giulani, C. *Ecoles de la sante publique en Tunisie. (Public health schools in Tunisia.)* Revue de l'infirmiere et de Assistante Sociale (Paris), 16(4), Apr 1966, 345-347. Fren.

The institutions for auxiliary health workers in Tunisia teach over 1400 students. The female students, coming away from their protective family and local environments as they do, require that this be taken into account in their training and placement. Four schools train auxiliaries. Scholarships for female students and improved employment possibilities increase respect for the training. Girls trained are mostly from well-to-do families. In general this limits the career and these workers and their work are not well known to the general public. Auxiliaries are underutilized.

0452 Harrison, T.J. *Training for village health aides in the Kotzebue area of Alaska.* Public Health Reports (Washington, D.C.), 80(7), Jul 1965, 1-8. Engl.

The State of Alaska is unique in the management of its health problems. Rigorous weather and lack of communication and transportation across great expanses of land prevent the distribution of adequate medical care, especially among the Eskimo (and Indian) populations. A programme of training permanent village residents in the rudiments of medical care has been developed by the Public Health Service to spread the effectiveness of the limited medical personnel and facilities. Two 5-day training sessions for groups of 8-10 health aides were conducted at Kotzebue in February and May 1964. The training was designed to improve the aides' ability to fulfill basic medical needs in a simple effective manner with the materials at hand. Scores on a test given the aides on the first and last days of the course revealed that intial medical knowledge and degree of improvement was similar for both groups. (Revised journal abstract.)

0453 Institute of Rural Health and Family Planning, Gandhigram. *Development of an aptitude test for selection of trainees for health educator's course.* Gandhigram, Institute of Rural Health and Family Planning, 1969. 2p. Engl.
Unpublished document. See also entry 477.

An aptitude test measuring admissability to a health educator's course examines personal data, attitudes toward public health, family planning, and community work, knowledge of disease, personality, and reactions to specified practical and real situations. Test scores plus interview scores determine admission of candidates.

0454 Institute of Rural Health and Family Planning, Gandhigram. *Narrative report on the working of the Institute of Rural Health and Family Planning, Gandhigram, presented to the Governing Council of the Institute at its third meeting on 21/5/1966.* Gandhigram, Institute of Rural Health and Family Planning, 1966. 1v.(various pagings). Engl.

Unpublished document. See also entries 82 and 542.

Narrative reports of the Institute of Rural Health and Family Planning, Gandhigram, India, outline the organization and objectives of the project begun in 1959. Its main objectives were related to the evolution of a model pattern of rural health services to be duplicated in other parts of the country. The work programme consisted of a survey phase and an action phase. The Family Planning Communication Action Research Centre was added in 1962. Despite problems such as building shortages and a lack of qualified staff, the programme is progressing due to staff enthusiasm and international backing. The Institution seeks solutions to the problems of auxiliary manpower training, health education and other issues relevant to rural health care delivery. A summary of the decisions taken in 1966 is included.

0455 Jensen, R.T. *Primary medical care worker in developing countries.* Medical Care (Philadelphia), 5(6), Nov-Dec 1967, 382-400. Engl.

The need for nonphysician delivery of health care in developing countries is reviewed in terms of economics, training, and preventive-care realities. Programmes to train auxiliary workers are described, using as examples the programmes in Kenya, Tanzania, Uganda, Nigeria, Congo (Zaire), Ethiopia, India, and Sudan. Selection and training of workers in each case reflects the availability of educated employable persons for rural work as well as the readiness of administrators and policy-makers to accept auxiliary health worker programmes. Ethiopia's programme is praised for its long-term planning approach to training and use of rural workers. A review of these programmes reveals such problems as status, career security, and advancement possibilities of trained auxiliaries. The common objections to auxiliaries are analyzed. Higher level training is proposed, as well as career advancement through continued training of successful auxiliaries. Physicians should not feel threatened by advancement of subordinates through structured career training, but rather should enjoy their leadership role in developing such programmes. Eighteen references are listed.

0456 Kerr, C.B. *Regional use and training of paramedical personnel.* In Clinical Proceedings of International Planned Parenthood Federation, London, IPPF, Aug 1972, 29-37. Engl.

South East Asia and Oceanic Regional Medical and Scientific Congress, Sydney, Australia, 14-18 Aug 1972.

The overall medical manpower situation in South East Asia and Oceania is summarized in relation to population growth parameters. The necessity of using paramedicals in an effective family planning delivery system is stated, noting that in this region the use of paramedical personnel has not been completely accepted. Indonesia, the Philippines, and Thailand demonstrate increased training and utilization of nurses, midwives, and other paramedical workers. Problems are discussed such as the quality of contraceptive care provided by auxiliaries in outlying areas; provision of supplies by paramedicals in the field; the relationship between doctors and auxiliaries; the incorporation of traditional practitioners; and the training of paramedicals.

0457 Kesic, B. *Adiestramiento y empleo de personal auxiliar de salud publica en America Latina. (Training and utilization of auxiliary health workers in Latin America).* Boletin de la Oficina Sanitaria Panamericana (Washington, D.C.), 60(6), Jun 1966, 469-485. Span.

The training and utilization of auxiliary health workers cannot be tackled on the basis of a universal formula applicable to all Latin American countries. Different geographic, economic, social, educational, and health conditions require specific approaches adjusted to the needs and possibilities of each country. The auxiliary health workers represent a special category of permanent health workers with precisely defined tasks and responsibilities. As substitutes for individual categories of professional and technical health workers they should be considered as a transitory measure to meet exceptional needs. The problem of training and utilizing auxiliary health workers should be dealt with as an integral part of the national health plan. The training programmes for auxiliary health workers should be: (1) drawn up on the principle of teamwork and of integrated medicine, which approaches each health problem from the social, preventive, and curative aspects; and (2) adjusted to the specific nature and actual conditions of their future work. The teaching programmes should also instill a sense of responsibility, a sense of correct human relations, and a proper ethical attitude. One year should be the minimum and 2 years the maximum length of training, and trainees should be recruited locally. Practical field work in health institutions, under the permanent guidance and supervision of competent teachers, should be applied. Primary school should be considered as the minimum, and primary school plus 2-3 years of secondary school as the maximum of general education. The recruitment age for auxiliary health workers should be between 18 and 30 years. Through a continuous system of inservice training and through refresher courses, learning should become a life-long task of auxiliary health workers.

0458 League of Red Cross Societies, Geneva. *Report on the first regional Red Cross seminar for the training of auxiliary health workers in the rural community: Niamey, Niger, 29 Nov-8 Dec 1971.* Geneva, League of Red Cross Societies, 1971. 1v.(various pagings). Engl., Fren.

A regional seminar for the training of auxiliary health workers in rural communities was held in Niamey, Niger, in 1971. Seven French-speaking African Red Cross Societies attended. The report of Niger's Red Cross Society on training *hygiénistes-secouristes de village* (auxiliary health workers in rural communities) was used as a basic reference for group discussion. Included in the agenda were discussions of health problems particular to West Africa, planning of health programmes, training procedures, teaching aids, programme implementation in rural settings, and evaluation and readaptation of programmes. A village close to Niamey was chosen for demonstration purposes. It was agreed by participants that to meet the health needs of the countries they serve, auxiliary health workers must be trained for health education, accident prevention, first aid, and basic health care work.

0459 Loefler, I.J. *Teaching and training for surgical practice in Zambia and the neighbouring countries.* Journal of the Royal College of Surgeons of Edinburgh (Edinburgh), 16(1), Jan 1971, 219-225. Engl.

Surgical work in East and Central Africa is carried out by three categories of personnel: surgeons, medical officers, and medical assistants. The bulk of new patients are first seen by dressers or medical assistants in rural health centres. Although there is no exact data on the proportion of work carried out at different levels, much surgical work is actually done at these centres. Problems presented are different from those seen in Europe, even where the cause is similar, because cases are often advanced when first seen by medical personnel. In teaching medical assistants, undergraduates, and postgraduates in surgery in Zambia, task analysis was undertaken to define the objectives and the three levels of education in behavioural terms. The important thing is to teach medical assistants when to refer patients to more highly trained personnel. Assistants are trained in admission wards, resuscitation rooms, and in the casualty department because experience there is most similar to field work.

0460 Long, E.C. *Rural health program in Guatemala.* n.p., 1972. 11p. Engl.
Unpublished document. Paper presented at the Airlie House Conference of Latin American Population Officers, 1972.

The rural health programme in Guatemala includes health promotion, preventive and curative medicine, and family planning services. The system attempts to deliver care through nontraditional techniques, which include use of auxiliary health workers, but goes beyond that to a system of simplified curative medicine and family planning programmes. Health posts are planned for the approximately 300 municipal capitals in the country. Training and deployment of supervisory teams (consisting of a doctor, a registered nurse, and a driver) are important parts of the job of helping personnel in remote areas. A communication network allows units in remote areas to keep in contact with a reference centre. Evaluation of the system is planned, using a "before" and "after" experimental design for measuring selected health parameters in a number of communities. Training of the rural health technician, who is responsible for care at health posts, is discussed in detail.

0461 Martens, E.G. *Health education and community development.* Ottawa, Canadian Health Education Specialists Society, Technical Publications No. 3, Jan 1969. 7p. Engl.

The goals of the community health worker programme in northern Canada are to encourage social participation in health activities, to increase the effectiveness of professional health workers, and to raise living conditions and health standards of the Indian and Eskimo population. The trained health worker, employed full time by the Department of National Health and Welfare, works under the guidance of a field nurse. Selection of candidates and organization of the training sessions have been described in this paper. A formal evaluation of the programme concluded that most community health workers have been able to work successfully in their communities. One hundred community health workers had been trained by 1969, and 85 were still on the job. Seven references are listed.

0462 Martens, E.G. Canada, Department of National Health and Welfare. *Health education in Medical Services Branch, Department of National Health and Welfare, Canada.* Ottawa, Department of National Health and Welfare, May 1967. 9p. Engl.
Unpublished document. Talk given at the New England Health Education Spring Meeting, Stowe, Vermont, May 1967.

This talk (given by the Director of the programme) on the health education programme given by the Canadian Department of National Health and Welfare, to the native peoples and the population above the 60th parallel begins with a brief history of the medical services since 1880. The greatest problems confronting the present programme are distance and language and cultural differences. Highlights of the present programme include development of workshops, and training Indian and Eskimo people as community health workers. Also discussed are the development of the programme at both the national and regional level, selection procedure for the trainees, and training methods. Evaluation of the programme concluded that it has been a success and recommended its continuation.

0463 Martens, E.G. *Training public health auxiliary workers in community development.* Chapel Hill, University of North Carolina, May 1963. 10p. Engl.
Community Development Seminar, Chapel Hill, N.C., 5-9 May 1963.
Unpublished document.

The paper evaluates the first programme in Canada, established in 1961, to train Indians as public health auxiliary workers. Special attention was given to three phases of the programme: selection of candidates, training, and supervision and encouragement on return to the reserve. Selection was based mainly on leadership qualities; training involved many members of the local medical staff and included methods of community health education. Trainees later became employees under the supervision of the nurse in charge of the community, with the help of a steering committee selected by the community. Much discussion in the course was devoted to the role of the health worker in the sociocultural setup of the Indian community. The results of the programme were encouraging and a similar one was designed for Eskimos in 1963.

0464 Messinezy, D.A. *Starting a health personnel training programme for Ethiopia.* Bulletin of the World Health Organization (Geneva), 6, 1952, 351-368. Engl.
This article reviews the results of a WHO-assisted training programme for health personnel in Ethiopia. Course outlines for dressers (nursing aides), sanitary inspectors, nurses, and medical assistants are given. A preliminary study indicated 5 000 auxiliary health personnel would be needed to staff hospitals and clinics and that 250 fully qualified physicians would be required. It was decided to begin by offering a series of short courses of increasingly advanced levels. Education by demonstration was stressed since the training was essentially practical in nature. Twenty-five references are listed.

0465 Moghaddam, R. *Land reform and rural development in Iran.* Land Economics (Madison, Wisc.), 48(2), May 1972, 160-168. Engl.
Land reform in Iran has been accompanied by the formation of the Revolutionary Corps for literacy, health, and development in rural areas. In creating the health corps, medical college graduates were mobilized, trained, and sent for 2-year periods to rural districts where they were assisted by high school graduates.

0466 Nigeria, Ministry of Health. *ABU (Ahmadu Bello University) medical auxiliaries training school, Kaduna.* Lagos, Ministry of Health, n.d. 1v.(various pagings). Engl.
Unpublished document.
This brief report describes fees, basic course syllabus, and length of training period for medical auxiliaries being trained in Nigeria to staff rural health posts. A list of reading materials is given.

0467 O'Neill, J.V. Westinghouse Learning Corporation, Health Services Division, Bladensbury, Md. *Paraprofessionals in health programs.* Focus on Health (Bladensburg, Md.), 5, 1971, 1-31. Engl.
The United States' experience with paramedical personnel of various types and levels is discussed briefly, with special attention to job descriptions, education and training instruction, and the legal aspects of certification and licencing. New careers have opened for paramedical workers in family planning services and family health work.

0468 Otoo, S.N. *Training and utilization of medical auxiliaries.* Ghana Medical Journal (Accra), 9(1), Mar 1970, 58-63. Engl.
The medical auxiliary is a paid health worker with limited but approved formal education, working under a physician's supervision. He may be trained to diagnose and treat common illnesses, recognize major illnesses for referral, give emergency medical care, and take part in health education. Each country must decide on the standards of a basic education syllabus and qualifying examination for its auxiliaries. It is desirable to produce only one type of medical auxiliary. Candidates may be recruited directly from the school and should have certain personal qualities, i.e. conscientiousness, initiative, etc. Other means of selection are aptitude tests and probationary period in a medical institution. Candidates should come from the area of work, and permanent training facilities with residential accommodation should be provided within the region. The duration of training courses should be 1-2 years, and a list of basic subjects is presented. In Ghana, each health area may ultimately have a health post staffed by a medical auxiliary, public health inspector, midwife, and community health nurses treating the visible illnesses. The place of a medical officer in the rural health administration is stressed. Ghana's rural health services might get underway if the potential of a satisfied, efficient medical auxiliary were exploited. Nineteen references are listed.

0469 Panyavanija, P., Lee, N. *Hill tribesmen make good medics.* American Journal of Nursing (New York), 69(1), Jan 1969, 126-130. Engl.
Three Thai tribesmen selected by villagers as persons they thought most able and interested, were given an experimental training programme as auxiliary health workers. Training began with a checklist of diagnosis of patients' symptoms and a corresponding list of care and treatment. During 3 months of training, modern concepts, such as the existence of microorganisms, and the effects of malnutrition were introduced with much time devoted to outpatient clinics.

0470 Pene, P. *Health auxiliaries in Francophone Africa.* Lancet (London), 1(7811), 12 May 1973, 1047-1048. Engl.
Health workers of all varieties have always been too scarce to cover the health needs of francophone Africa. Many states have decided to use auxiliary health workers, e.g. *medecins africains* in Senegal, *medecins malgaches* in Madagascar, and *assistants medicaux* in Zaire. These licensed physician assistants are beginning to disappear; in 1973 the Central African Republic was the only state planning to train medical assistants. In Cameroon, Congo, Ivory Coast, Dahomey, Gabon, Guinea, Upper Volta, Mali, Niger, Senegal, and Chad, *medecins africains* are grouped in a category with physicians. The number of medical assistants practicing in francophone Africa in 1973 was estimated to be around 300. Medical assistants should be more like a male nurse than a doctor. These personnel, in the position of *prevot de sante*, can provide primary care to rural communities, take charge of the health team, etc. There are about 10 000 auxiliary nurses in francophone Africa and with a minimum of additional training they

could be situated in rural areas as assistants to the *prevot de sante*. High priority should be placed on training auxiliary midwives and auxiliary technicians should be trained for work in mobile health units. Priority should be given to raising the standard of auxiliary health workers and adapting their training to tasks they must perform.

0471 Pequignot, H. *USSR: Role of the feldsher.* World Health (Geneva), Jun 1972, 28-31. Engl.

In the USSR schools for medical assistants (i.e. feldshers) admit students who have had only 8 years of schooling. In isolated rural health centres, a feldsher and a midwife are in charge. In urban health centres the feldsher's role is similar to that of a nurse. The public health feldsher assists an epidemiologist; the laboratory feldsher is similar to a laboratory technician; and in factories, feldshers are specialists in occupational health. These auxiliaries are capable of examining a sick or healthy person, of performing the routine tasks of preventive medicine, and of giving simple treatment. They can render immense service in an area where there is a shortage of doctors. In the USSR feldshers are not employed because of a doctor shortage but as a complement to the professional medical force. The unanswered question is how successful this system would be in the absence of qualified doctors.

0472 Rhodesia, Government of Rhodesia. *Health assistants (training) regulations, 1972.* Salisbury, Rhodesia, Government Gazette Notice No. 992 of 1972 (Act 24/71), Rhodesia, Oct 1972. 2005-2017. Engl.
See also entry 473.

Qualifying grounds for selection of trainees for the position of Medical Assistant in Rhodesia are outlined.

0473 Rhodesia, Government of Rhodesia. *Medical assistants (training) regulations, 1971.* Salisbury, Rhodesia Government Gazette Notice No. 705 of 1971 (Act 24/71), 731-744. Engl.
See also entry 472.

Section 69 of the *Medical, Dental, and Allied Professions Act, 1971, (ACT 24/71)*, Government of Rhodesia, provides regulation for certification of medical assistants in Rhodesia. Terms of reference are given and requirements are cited for medical assistants' schools. Entrance requirements for students, training curriculum, and outline of subjects to be included on examinations are listed.

0474 Rosa, F.W. *Training health workers in Gondar, Ethiopia.* Public Health Reports (Washington, D.C.), 77(7), Jul 1962, 595-601. Engl.

At the Haile Selassie I Public Health College and Training Center in Gondar, Ethiopia, teams composed of a health officer, a community nurse, and a sanitarian are being prepared to staff rural health centres. Their training emphasizes simple management of prevalent diseases and common medical emergencies, the approaches and techniques of preventive medicine, mass methods, control of environmental hazards, skills necessary to obtain community cooperation, and health education of the public. (Author summary.)

0475 Rosinski, E.F., Spencer, F.J. *Assistant medical officer: the training of the medical auxiliary in developing countries.* Chapel Hill, University of North Carolina Press, 1965. 199p. Engl.

A study based on visits to medical schools, hospitals, and health centres in five developing countries of Africa and the South Pacific examines the function of an assistant medical officer whose training is between that of a medical doctor and a registered nurse. Procedures for selection of candidates, aspects of the educational programme, duties, and legal status of the graduate officer are discussed.

0476 Sai, F.T. *Rural health model: Danfa, Ghana.* In Hughes, J.P., ed., Health Care for Remote Areas: An International Conference, Oakland, Kaiser Foundation, 1972, 107-125. Engl.
See entry 155 for complete proceedings.

The Danfa Comprehensive Rural Health and Family Planning Project was started in response to the Ghana Medical School's philosophy that doctors should be trained to meet the needs of the community. The project was designed as a service, training, and research laboratory for the medical school, to be part of the community health services for rural areas around Accra. Through Danfa Health Centre, the project was designed to provide comprehensive health care emphasizing maternal and child health service, nutrition, health education, communicable disease control, and improved environmental health and family planning services. The centre was completed in 1970, and is staffed by a health centre superintendent (a male nurse with 10 years experience and some retraining in diagnostic methods), midwives, midwifery assistants, and community health nurses. Physicians visit the centre once or twice a week. Activities of the centre include medical care, home visits by a health team, nutrition and education classes for women, environmental sanitation instruction, etc. Medical students are involved in field research activities and are instructed by the Health Centre Superintendent. Research goals of the Danfa project include investigation of the rural community, examination of the role of traditional medical practitioners and traditional midwives in health services, considering ways for effective implementation of the government's family planning policy in rural areas, etc.

0477 Santhanam, M.L., Sastry, K.R. Institute of Rural Health and Family Planning, Gandhigram. *Development of an aptitude test for selection of trainees for health education course.* Gandhigram, Institute of Rural Health and Family Planning, 1968. 11p. Engl.
Unpublished document. See also entry 453.

An aptitude test for applicants to the health education course in Gandighram, India, was constructed with the following four sections: personal data (age, marital status, etc.), knowledge of diseases and family planning and skill in handling situations, personality of the individual (social adjustment, extroversion/introversion, ascendance/submission, neurotic behaviour), and reactions to certain practical and real situations. Scoring and administration of the tests are described. Eleven references are listed.

0478 Sein, M.M. *Training of workers in disciplines ancillary to medicine and their contribution to surgery in Burma.* Journal of the Royal College of Surgeons of Edinburgh (Edinburgh), 16(1), Jan 1971, 187-192. Engl.

Training programmes for Burma's health workers reach beyond the health centre into the community. Training of workers is provided at the Institute of Paramedical Sciences, the National Health Laboratory, the Institute of Sick Nursing, the Health Assistant School, the Medical Corps Centre, and the Medical School. Care for rural populations began in 1951 with the founding of rural health centres, manned by health assistants from the Health Assistants' School. There are over 1 300 health assistants in Burma; in addition to their work in the health centres, they participate as members of the village "Security and Administrative Committee" as advisers on administrative work, sanitation, etc.

0479 Senecal, J. *Training of paramedical personnel in the developing countries.* Israel Journal of Medical Sciences (Jerusalem), 4(3), May-Jun 1968, 665-670. Engl.

Fourth Rehovoth Conference on Health Problems in Developing States, Rehovoth, Israel, 15-23 Aug 1967.

See entry 96 for complete proceedings.

The term "paramedical personnel" is defined as workers in all professions allied to medicine, including veterinarians and dentists with training equivalent to the M.D.'s and those with less training, e.g. nurses, midwives, sanitation technicians, etc. It does not, however, include auxiliary personnel, who are not qualified in a technical field but who should assist and work under the direction of fully qualified practitioners. In understaffed countries the auxiliary must often work on his own, without supervision. Titles given to various categories of worker are often ambiguous and do not reflect levels of training, qualification, or functions, as each country's problems and needs influence the roles of workers. To arrive at a uniform classification system for all countries it is essential to specify for each category of worker the level of primary and secondary education, length and content of professional training, and qualifications attained. Six references are listed.

0480 Sidel, V.W. *Feldshers and "feldsherism": the role and training of the feldsher in the USSR.* New England Journal of Medicine (Boston), 278(17), 25 Apr 1968, 934-939, and 278(18), 2 May 1968, 987-992. Engl.

The Soviet feldsher is a medical worker trained to give emergency medical treatment and first aid, to make a preliminary diagnosis of an illness, and to take care of patients until the arrival of a physician. His duties include prophylactic measures among the population, some nursing work in urban and rural areas, etc. In rural areas, feldshers work in a feldsher-midwife station and practice relatively independently of physicians. The rural feldsher's work emphasizes home visiting, child care, early diagnosis, preventive medicine, and health education. The feldsher's status is that of technician, but in the rural areas where a physician is not available his role is more honoured. Training takes place in middle-medical schools for 2 1/2 or 3 1/2 years depending on the student's previous education. The presence of the feldsher in a clinical role permits a considerably lower physician-patient ratio than would otherwise be required. Forty-six references are listed.

0481 Sims, P. *Training of clinic staff in the Zambia flying doctor service.* East African Medical Journal (Nairobi), 49(10), Oct 1972, 755-762. Engl.

Basic medicine was taught to the clinical assistants of the Zambia Flying Doctor Service. Teaching was experimental and results showed all methods of teaching increased in the knowledge and ability of the clinic staff. The Service provides care to rural areas of Zambia. Ten clinics, wholly staffed by visiting personnel, have been established in the more isolated areas. Radio communication is a help. Clinical staff includes: two clinic assistants, a nurse (untrained), and a dresser. Training course content for the staff and teaching methods used are described and evaluated.

0482 Solon, F.S. *Rural internship in community medicine.* Santo Tomas Journal of Medicine (Manila), 25(4), Jul-Aug 1970, 171-203. Engl.

Delivered as the 125th Luis Guerrero Memorial Lecture, University of St. Thomas, Faculty of Medicine, Manila, 20 Jul 1970.

In developing countries, medical training must provide students with community experiences in rural areas, as is done by the Cebu Institute of Medicine in the Philippines. These community programmes succeed when members and leaders of the community participate in the planning and implementation. Students learn to adopt new techniques for bedside treatment of patients in rural homes. Referral to hospitals is done cautiously, since patients who cannot afford to travel or leave work will not receive follow-up care. Analysis shows insufficient income greatly affects family health in rural Philippine communities. The need for health education is stressed.

0483 Spoustova, V., Sandtner, P. *O Profil stredniho zdravotnickeho pracovnika. (Types, education and training of paramedical workers).* Reprint; source unknown, 49-50. Czech.

The prevailing opinion in Czechoslovakia is that too many categories of middle-level paramedical workers are being turned out by the colleges of hygiene. A 12th category, the dental nurse, has recently been introduced. Each branch of the medical profession seems to want to train its own supporting staff. Categories could be reduced to five and the borderline between disciplines made clearer. Good basic training should enable students to adapt to any discipline. A two-level system of instruction and grading would permit selection of the more talented students to go on to further training in one of the five disciplines, whereas less talented students after a specially devised 2nd year of instruction could be employed as "lower-level paramedical workers." Selection of students for teaching, managerial, and research positions would be on successful completion of practical work. They would go on to full- or part-time university training. Highly qualified workers would then perform jobs requiring the skills they acquire in their training while the less demanding tasks would be done by the auxiliaries.

0484 Standard, K.L., Ennever, O. *Community health aide training programme in a developing country (Jamaica - West Indies).* Reprint; source unknown, 4p. Engl.
See also entries 437 and 614.

The Department of Social and Preventive Medicine, University of the West Indies, reports on: (1) a 4-month experimental training programme for Community Health Aides drawn from a suburban low to middle socioeconomic community; and (2) a 3-month training programme in a rural area. The overall aim was to give the aides a basic minimum training so that they could function as auxiliaries under supervision, relieving highly trained personnel to utilize their skills and training more effectively. The aides have worked in various positions, namely: in comprehensive health care programmes, in physiotherapy, as field workers in research projects, and in family planning. Evaluation of the programme indicates that these workers have performed satisfactorily and that a community health aide can be a very useful member of the health team in our developing communities.

0485 Swiss Tropical Institute, Basel. *Swiss Tropical Institute, Basel.* Tropical and Geographical Medicine (Haarlem), 19(2), Jun 1967, 118-124. Engl.
See also entry 450.

An extension of the Swiss Tropical Institute in Basel, Switzerland, is the field laboratory and Rural Aid Centre in Ifakara, Tanzania. Besides training its own staff, the centre in Ifakara is a training centre for paramedical personnel. It cooperates in this capacity with the Dar-es-Salaam School of Medicine. The centre buildings are designed as models for students' own health centres. Courses for auxiliary workers and health aides are given by African teachers. Demonstrations exhibit constructive ideas for trainees to introduce to rural villagers. Theory is reinforced by field visits and clinical observations. Such training of local people in their own country prevents the alienation of young graduates from their own culture.

0486 Tanzania, Ministry of Health. *Mwanza programme on public health, Ministry of Health, second half-yearly report for 1973.* Tanzania, Ministry of Health, Feb 1974. 7p. Engl.
Unpublished document.

The Mwanza (Tanzania) public health programme is predominantly a public health teaching scheme in various schools for medical auxiliaries. It started in 1969, supported by the Ministry of Health and utilizing staff from the Nijmegem University. The project introduces public health administration concepts into continuing education programmes for rural health workers and supervisors. The constantly evolving curriculum of medical auxiliaries related to the scheme is outlined.

0487 USA, Department of Health, Education and Welfare. *Community health medic of the Indian health service: progress report as of January 1973.* Tuscon, Arizona, U.S. Department of Health, Education, and Welfare, 1973. 16p. Engl.

The United States Indian Health Service was organized in 1955, primarily to overcome critical staff shortages and facility deficiencies. Experience showed that the effectiveness of health programmes among Indian people was directly related to the extent of their own involvement. Centres for training and health programme systems were established in Tucson, Arizona, to increase health resource effectiveness and Indian involvement. The Office of Research and Development of Indian Health Services undertook to adapt and test the concept of "physician assistant" for the delivery of health services to Indians. The position of Community Health Medic, which requires 2 years of training, was legally established in 1970. The report describes the implementation of this concept.

0488 Vaughan, J.P. *Are doctors always necessary? A review of the need for the medical assistant in developing countries.* Journal of Tropical Medicine and Hygiene (London), 74, Dec 1971, 265-271. Engl.

The need to train the medical assistant, an auxiliary to the general physician, has been outlined with regard to the desperate need for medical manpower in developing countries. The arguments for and against the training of medical assistants should be seen against the background of the demographic characteristics of the population in developing countries, the diseases they suffer from, and the resources available to deal with these disease problems. The traditional "Western" standards of medical care are not well adapted to serve the majority of people living in the rural areas in developing countries. A review of the Medical Assistant in several countries of Africa, the USSR, Fiji, and Papua and New Guinea has been made. From a review of the literature and from experience, general conclusions have been drawn concerning the training and role of the Medical Assistant in developing countries. Fifty-eight references are listed. (Author summary.)

0489 Vogel, L.C. *Public health college at Gondar (Ethiopia).* Tropical and Geographical Medicine (Haarlem), 20, Dec 1968, 406-410. Engl.

Ethiopia is a rugged country where disease patterns vary with topography. Although prominent diseases are mostly preventable, the demand for curative services is increasing. In response to these conditions a system of health centres was established, emphasizing disease control, hygiene, sanitary control, maternal and child health, and health education. The Gondar Public Health College and Training Centre has trained personnel to staff rural health centres and health stations, yet graduates shun work in the interior. Problems with the programme are mentioned, pointing out that progress will be slow until the educational, economic, and social level of the people improves.

0490 Walker, V., Williams, E. *Evaluation of community health aide programme in St. James.* Kingston, Jamaica, University of the West Indies, Department of Social and Preventive Medicine, 20 Jun 1973. 5p. Engl.
Unpublished document.

A training programme carried out by the Department of Social and Preventive Medicine of the University of the West Indies, as a result of which 150 community health aides graduated and began working in St. James parish, Jamaica, is evaluated. The object of the programme was to alleviate the work load of professional staff. Training lasted 8 weeks and emphasized basic communication and health skills. The identification by aides of cases previously neglected because of lack of community outreach activities resulted in increased attendance at public health clinics. Where aides were closely supervised their performance was superior to that of others. Some barriers to complete acceptance of aides by the community exist, e.g. older people do not feel the younger aides can teach them anything new, and middle class residents prefer to be treated by a private doctor. However, many people have been helped, and extension of training to include, for instance, midwifery and the giving of insulin injections, together with increased government efforts to provide adequate housing, would do much to improve the service to the community.

0491 WHO, Brazzaville. *Auxiliary health personnel: report on a seminar, Brazzaville, 6-13 October 1971.* Brazzaville, WHO, 26 Jan 1972. 40p. WHO/AFR/E&T/53. Engl., Fren.

The auxiliary health worker is defined in relationship to the total health team. Obstacles to effective use of auxiliary personnel are identified. These include perception of auxiliaries as a threat by local traditional healers and local politicians, bad planning and organization, inadequate supervision, poor training based on faulty understanding of the work to be done, outdated and excessive legislation, and poor quality teaching. Seminar participants decided that systematic policy formation is difficult to achieve. Needs should be defined in the context of national plans. Training should take place after the jobs have been analyzed and training objectives defined. Attention must be given to developing more training centres and to better selection of persons for training as auxiliary workers.

0492 WHO, Brazzaville. *Contribution to studies on African health demography: establishments for training medical and paramedical staff, report of a survey.* Brazzaville, WHO, 5 Aug 1971. 1v.(unpaged). WHO/AFR/EU/4. AFR/E & T/51. Engl.

A WHO study has shown that there is an extreme shortage of medical and paramedical staff in most African countries. This document describes facilities for medical and paramedical staff training in the African region as of 1971. Results of the survey indicate numbers of students being trained in the following categories: physician, dentist, pharmacist, sanitary engineer, medical assistant, professional midwife and nurse, sanitarian, medical laboratory technician, auxiliary midwife and nurse, auxiliary sanitarian, and auxiliary technical laboratory personnel. Studies of this type of training establishment for medical and paramedical staff, if repeated at regular intervals, should indicate the probable evolution of health personnel in Africa.

0493 WHO, Geneva. *World Health.* World Health (Geneva), Jun 1972. 35p. Engl.

This entire issue is devoted to auxiliary health workers, whether called medical assistants, medical aids, health centre superintendents, health assistants, feldshers, limited physicians, health extension workers, physician assistants, or medex. Separate articles trace the history of the auxiliary worker movement, experiments in Algeria, in Africa, in the Central African Republic, the USSR, and the U.S.

0494 WHO, Geneva. *Training of medical assistants and similar personnel: seventeenth report of the WHO Expert Committee on Professional and Technical Education of Medical and Auxiliary Personnel.* Geneva, WHO Technical Report Series No. 385, 1968. 26p. Engl.

There is a need for medical assistants (auxiliaries to a physician) in total health planning. The type of assistant will vary in each country. Some considerations for building a training programme are admission criteria, training objectives, curriculum, teaching methodology, staff, etc. Examples illustrate training programmes and the medical assistants' functions in six countries (Sudan, USSR, U.S.(Army), Algeria, Burma, and Venezuela). The medical assistant should not be allowed to undertake private practice but may be given additional training for promotion and offered career incentives.

0495 WHO, Geneva. *Medical, dental and pharmaceutical auxiliaries: a survey of existing legislation.* Geneva, WHO, 1968. 143p. Engl.

This survey illustrates the wide variety of patterns in the organization, classification, and definition of the auxiliary professions in 18 countries. Particular attention has been paid to such aspects as admission to training programmes, duration and content of training, examination syllabuses, and professional duties. The survey covers feldshers, social workers, dieticians, psychologists, speech and hearing therapists, health inspectors, chiropodists, optometrists and opticians, physiotherapists, etc., in addition to the various categories of auxiliary personnel employed in hospitals, dental clinics, and pharmacies.

0496 WHO, Geneva. *Expert Committee on Professional and Technical Education of Medical and Auxiliary Personnel: report on the first session.* Geneva, WHO Technical Report Series No. 22, Dec 1950. 35p. Engl.

This report on professional and technical education of medical and auxiliary personnel covers, *inter alia*, general terms of reference and discussions of international aspects of the problem of training medical and other personnel. Recommended in this somewhat outdated document are standards for assessing schools of public health, use of preventive and social-medical techniques, interdisciplinary cooperation, extension of WHO work, international exchange of workers and information, etc. Increased production and improved distribution of teaching material is suggested. Twelve references are listed.

0497 WHO, Manila. South Pacific Commission, Noumea. *Report of the refresher course on integrated rural health for assistant medical officers in the South Pacific, 2 Nov-11 Dec* Manila, WHO and the South Pacific Commission, Noumea, 1963. 170p. WHO/WPR/318/63. Engl.

This paper records a refresher course for individual Assistant Medical Officers. The course objectives were "to introduce the concept of integrated rural health services, to give knowledge and understanding of the principal duties in this respect and to give an opportunity for acquiring the experiences and skills necessary for the efficient execution of those duties." The lectures covered rural health services, surveying public health, maternal and child health, nutrition, tuberculosis, leprosy, environmental sanitation, health education, and agriculture and health. Appendices present teaching material used during the course. Evaluation of the course indicated a high degree of appreciation on the part of students.

0498 Wood, C.H. *Availability of health manpower.* In Hughes, J.P., ed., Health Care for Remote Areas: An International Conference, Oakland, Kaiser Foundation, 1972, 46-65. Engl.
See entry 155 for complete proceedings.

Progress in the health field in developing countries depends on acceptance of the medical auxiliary. In planning for the use of medical auxiliaries, priorities must be carefully assessed and job requirements carefully examined. This paper provides statistics from Tanzania on duration of training and cost and benefit analyses for various categories of health workers. Manpower targets for Tanzania are outlined.

IV.2 Primary nursing care

IV.2.1 Professional

See also: 0021, 0030, 0038, 0368, 0397, 0408, 0417, 0427, 0441, 0464, 0521, 0570, 0571, 0593, 0594, 0599

0499 Dosunmu, N.E. *Nursing as a career in Nigeria.* Nigerian Nurse (Lagos), 4(2), Apr-Jun 1972, 6-10. Engl.

Training opportunities for nurses in Nigeria are reviewed. Basic training includes four types of programmes. The 3 1/2-year general nursing programme takes place in a school of nursing attached to a hospital or university teaching hospital. After training there, the candidate qualifies for the Nursing Council Examination; students passing this are designated as staff nurses. In the 2 1/2-year midwifery training programme the student enters the Maternity Hospital Schools of Midwifery. On graduating she is designated as staff midwife and is registered as a Nigerian Certified Midwife. The 3 1/2-year community nurse programme includes public health nursing, health education, and midwifery. Other programmes, their admission requirements, and courses are described.

0500 Finland, Ministry for Foreign Affairs, Department for International Development Cooperation. *Report on advanced training course in the nursing team approach to rural health problems.* Helsinki, Ministry for Foreign Affairs, 1972. 10p. Engl.

This report outlines the planning, organization, and content of a course to study needs and problems of training health personnel in developing countries. It includes the plan of a 6-week course in public health nursing, as conducted in Helsinki. The team approach was both the main subject and method of study. Participants' comments on the value of the course in relation to health services in developing countries are included.

0501 Hughes, J.M., Joubert, C. *Paramedical personnel in the first echelon of medical care: West African experience.* Ghana Medical Journal (Accra), 11(4), Dec 1972, 365-367. Engl.

This report describes the experience in Ghana, where well-trained nurses were used in the first echelon of medical care. The aluminium smelter at Tema has a small in-plant clinic, and a hospital nearby. Nurses operate the in-plant clinic, with physician supervision from the hospital. The hospital provides definitive medical care, and includes a clinical laboratory and pharmacy. Results of a 12-month study suggest that nurses at the in-plant unit dealt effectively with the majority of problems encountered and, when required, physician referrals were usually made promptly. The system has several advantages: physicians have more time for complex problems; patients are satisfied with the health care encounter; and career satisfaction is gained by nursing personnel. Three references are listed.

0502 Hugo, E. *Training for community health work: nursing students.* Journal of the Christian Medical Association of India (Mysore City), 47(5), May 1972, 228-230. Engl.

Integration of community health into the 3-year general nursing curriculum means including the following aspects of health care: environmental sanitation, infant care, immunization, prenatal care, health education methods. The nurses understanding of human behaviour is an essential aspect of community health programmes.

0503 Romulo, C.P. *Nursing in contemporary Philippine society.* Philippine Journal of Nursing (Manila), 36, Nov-Dec 1967, 307-310. Engl.

The Philippines are in need of rural medical and nursing care. Other areas demanding attention are nurse training and the provision of better student accommodations. It is also pointed out that the departure of many professional nurses, leaving the Philippines in search of higher pay, is a great loss to health services in their homeland.

0504 Sabas, L.E. *Exploring the field of school nursing in the Philippines.* The ANPHI Papers (Philippines), Jul-Sep 1966, 15-24. Engl.

The role of nurses in schools, their salaries, qualifications, functions, and responsibilities (especially in health instruction) are outlined. It is recommended that a study be made of the job expectations of teacher nurses, that in-service training, seminars, and workshops be planned to meet these needs, and that schools of nursing plan more for the education of teacher nurses. Ten references are listed.

0505 Samater, H.N. *Some health problems in the Somali Republic.* International Journal of Nursing Studies (New York), 6, Mar 1969, 3-15. Engl.

Health problems in Somalia include inadequate medical facilities in the remote parts of the country, the need to expand maternal and child welfare services, the need for a nutrition advisory service, and the need for control of tuberculosis and malaria. Medical care in the remote parts of the country would be greatly increased with the use of mobile dispensaries and a transportation service for patients. Many health problems could be controlled through health education. Locally trained community nurses can teach health education through community discussion, home visits, and demonstration of sanitation and other health methods, with appropriate technical aids. More time should be allocated to health education instruction in the nurses' basic curriculum. Nine references are listed.

0506 WHO, Alexandria. *Review of the education and training of nurses to meet the needs of the region.* Alexandria, WHO, 15 Aug 1969. 38p. WHO/EM/RC19/Tech. Disc./2. EMRO/69/865. Engl.
Unpublished document.

A review of the education of training of nurses to meet the needs of WHO's Eastern Mediterranean Region emphasizes the necessity of extending training beyond auxiliary levels. Needs of governments, the population, and the nursing profession are examined. To ensure meeting needs on all levels, population growth, morbidity, mortality, and other factors must be considered. Nursing education must be upgraded and wages and responsibility on the job must be increased. Plans for nurse training and deployment must be worked out in the context of national health and development planning in each country and within the region. References are listed.

0507 WHO, Geneva. *Planning and programming for nursing services.* Geneva, WHO Public Health Papers No. 44, 1971. 123p. Engl.

There is a need for nurses in senior administrative positions of health services. As a member of a planning team, the nurse must know the concepts related to health planning, the relationship of national health planning to national development planning, the scope of health planning, and the major steps of the planning process. The latter include: establishing the preconditions of planning, analyzing the current health situation, determining priorities and alternatives, selecting the health plan (interpretation of its nursing component), developing a plan of action for the nursing component, and evaluating it.

IV.2.2 Nonprofessional

See also: 0076, 0321, 0397, 0464, 0492, 0561, 0563, 0565, 0566, 0611

0508 Argentina, State Secretariat for Culture and Education. *Reglamento para la ensenanza de la enfermeria profesional no universitaria y para la formacion de auxiliar de enfermeria. (Regulation governing the non-University training of nurses and nursing auxiliaries).* Buenos Aires, State Secretariat for Culture and Education, 1v.(various pagings). Span.
Unpublished document.

The decision of the Government of Argentina to establish a training program for auxiliary health workers (nursing assistants) results from the need experienced by other Latin American countries to train personnel to perform simple medical tasks to increase health services to rural communities. The program, described in detail, includes the purposes, objectives, and plan of study. The curriculum is divided into several areas with a limited number of study hours for each subject within the area. The physical and biological sciences embrace the study of seven disciplines involving 355 study hours of theory and practical training. The professional and social/humanistic studies involve 2045 and 450 hours respectively. Internal governing regulations of the school and detailed development of the course are also included.

0509 Chen, P.C. *Medical auxiliary in rural Malaysia.* Lancet (London), 1(7810), 5 May 1973, 983-985. Engl.

Steps to reduce rural poverty and ill health in Malaysia include the establishment of a rural health service, with a network of health centres and a tiered staffing system, relying heavily on auxiliary health workers. Indigenous midwives, given training in simple hygiene, are included in the health programme. Future plans include retraining midwives in child health, and training assistant nurses in midwifery for their role as community nurse-midwife. Five references are listed.

0510 Higgins, M.M. *Report on the further development of the assistant nurse/midwife program in Nepal.* n.p., Aug 1971. 9p. Engl.
Unpublished document.

A draft report by a WHO nursing consultant proposes further development of Nepal's Assistant Nurse/Midwife (ANM) programme. The Bharatpur Assistant Nurse/Midwife Training School is described. Part of the school, which can train 20-25 students, is a 25-bed hospital that usually takes in 30-35 patients, some of whom are maternity cases. Other schools described are the Biratnagar ANM Training School, and the Nepalganj ANM Training School. Achievements of the programme include a workshop in Kathmandu for three senior tutors to review programme development objectives, the use of pretesting for more effective candidate selection, and improved transportation for students.

0511 Masters, D. *Is your talent being wasted?* Saving Health (London), 12(2), Jun 1973, 26-28. Engl.

An appeal is made to Western medical workers to help care for the health needs of the developing world. Advantages of the experience are described. In Zaire, Africa, a state-recognized school trains auxiliary nurses but, although missionary nurses are on hand to train students, the school may close because the law requires the presence of a doctor. This is one example of an urgent need. Details of the kinds of problems expatriate physicians and health personnel face in translating their previous training to local health problem solving is illustrated several times. Needs expressed are urgent and an appeal is made for Western medical personnel to help train and treat persons where the need is obviously great.

0512 Montag, M.L. *Education of nursing technicians.* New York, John Wiley and Sons, Inc., 1971. 146p. Engl.

There is an increased qualitative and quantitative need for nurses, due to expanded preventive medicine programmes, scientific discoveries, increased life expectancy, health and welfare programmes, etc. Two categories of nurses, professional and practical, are recommended. Existing schools (1951) for both are discussed with respect to admission requirements, curricula, financial support, accreditation and so on, concluding that experimentation in nurses training is required. Nurses can give the bulk of nursing care to patients, functioning between the professional worker and the one trained on the job. Training must aim at a combination of social understanding and technical competence. Community colleges and technical institutes are recommended as preparatory institutions. A sample curriculum of 2 years is presented, and the preparation of administrators and teachers for these programmes is given some attention. References are listed.

0513 WHO, Geneva. *Auxiliary personnel in nursing: a survey of existing legislation.* Geneva, WHO, 1966. 19p. Engl.

This WHO monograph provides comparative analyses of legislation related to nurses as auxiliary health workers. Reference is made to laws governing nursing auxiliaries in 13 countries including Peru, Brazil, and Sierra Leone.

0514 WHO, Geneva. *Use and training of auxiliary personnel in medicine, nursing, midwifery and sanitation.* Geneva, WHO, 1961. 26p. Engl.
Ninth report of the Expert Committee on Professional and Technical Education of Medical and Auxiliary Personnel.

In a WHO committee report on four categories of auxiliary health workers, i.e. medical assistants, auxiliary nurses, auxiliary midwives, and auxiliary sanitarians, recommendations for training curricula are emphasized. Auxiliary health workers are defined as technical workers with less than full professional qualifications in their field. Before training programmes for auxiliaries begin, studies should be made to assess the need for auxiliary and professional personnel. Administrators must take responsibility for continually revising curriculum and adapting it to field requirements. The morale of auxiliaries should be maintained by providing them with opportunities for further training leading to professional status. Guidelines are presented for training methods and course content; the selection, qualification, and registration of staff; location of training schools; the training of teachers; supervision and follow-up of auxiliaries at work; and aspects of auxiliary development involving international cooperation.

IV.3 Primary family planning and midwifery care

IV.3.1 Professional

See also: 0417, 0456, 0539, 0540, 0589, 0590, 0593, 0599, 0601, 0649

0515 Acolatse, P. *Training and practice of the professional midwife in Ghana.* In Report of the Anglophone West African Working Party, Accra, Ghana, 7-16 Dec 1972, London, International Confederation of Midwives, Appendix M, 48-50. Engl.
See entry 525 for entire report.
There are 17 300 professional midwives in Ghana. Since a decree in 1972, traditional birth attendants and auxiliary midwives are no longer enrolled on official lists of Unqualified Midwives as they were previously. Because of the lack of professional midwives legal recognition should be given to traditional birth attendants and all qualified nurses enrolled as auxiliary midwives. There is no legal training or practice of midwifery without Government approval in consultation with the Nurse and Midwives Council. Yet change in orientation as well as training continues. More and more it involves a concept of total family health.

0516 Bannerman, R.H. *Maternity care in the developing countries.* In Report of the Anglophone West African Working Party, Accra, Ghana, 7-16 Dec 1972, London, International Confederation of Midwives, 14-19. Engl.
See entry 525 for entire report.
Taking a complete view of health care it must be seen that the midwife and other categories of midwifery personnel are important members of the health team. Despite the number of expert reports dealing with maternal care needs, about 70% of women in the Third World receive no professional services during the maternity cycle. The author asks four questions, for which answers are suggested: (1) what is wrong with our professional performance as health workers?; (2) how can we set ourselves on a proper course?; (3) how can we apply swiftly, smoothly, and wisely the organizational, scientific, and technological know-how of the developed countries to the Third World?; and (4) what reforms must citizens of the Third World make in their social and cultural institutions to achieve social maturity, economic and political stability, and good health? The Third World must make greater use of auxiliary health personnel. Professional midwife roles must be adapted to those of supervisor of auxiliary midwives and traditional birth attendants. Training should provide practical field training for every auxiliary.

0517 Betts, K.G. *Training and practice of the auxiliary midwife in Sierra Leone.* In Report of the Anglophone West Africa Working Party, Accra, Ghana, 7-16 Dec 1972, London, International Confederation of Midwives, Appendix N, 51-54. Engl.
See entry 525 for entire report.
Auxiliary midwifery training has been taking place in Sierra Leone since 1940. The history of this early work is sketched. It shows how illiterate village women were taught practical skills during 12 months of instruction with demonstrations. The need for trained personnel in the country continues to outdistance the country's ability to provide personnel it needs. In 1970 a new plan was developed through which a Village Maternity Assistant programme was superseded by a Maternal and Child Health (MCH) Aid Programme. This programme aims to provide every village with an MCH Aide. The training, requirements, and job definition of the MCH Aide is provided. Her definition is "a female person who has trained for a period of eighteen months in an officially recognized programme under the direction and supervision of a midwifery sister and a health sister in maternal and child health activities of a normal nature but is able to detect the abnormal and potentially abnormal and direct such patients to the nearest hospital for medical aid". Four training centres are established to train MCH aides. Evaluation of the aide includes assessment of the aide's records of her practical experience and determining how safe it is to allow her to work at the village level knowing by her own assessment her own limitations.

0518 Bowers, J.Z., Maier, J. Josiah Macy, Jr. Foundation, New York. *Training and responsibilities of the midwife.* New York, Josiah Macy, Jr. Foundation, 1967. 268p. Engl.
Macy Conference on the Training and Responsibilities of the Midwife, Bellagio, Italy, 9-13 May 1966.
Convened for the purpose of gathering information on the actual and potential role of the midwife in the world today, the conference discussed reports from 15 nations concerning such questions as the midwife training programme, responsibilities of the midwife, utilization of the midwife in family planning (especially in intrauterine device insertion) and child care, and future plans for midwifery practice. The relationship of the midwife to other health workers and to government agencies was also discussed.

0519 Central Family Planning Institute, New Delhi. *Orientation training of medical and paramedical personnel in oral contraceptives: programme, 27 June-3 July 1968, 28 Oct-2 Nov 1968.* New Delhi, Central Family Planning Institute, 1968. 2v. (various pagings). Engl.
Unpublished documents.
A training programme for medical and paramedical personnel in charge of an oral contraceptive pilot project in India is discussed. The course objectives, methodology, curriculum, and evaluation are outlined. Included are the proceedings of two separate sessions.

0520 Eliot, J.W. *Quaker service community health education program in Togo: report of training programs, Sep 1969-Feb 1970.* Philadelphia, American Friends Service Committee, 1970. 78p. Engl. Unpublished document.

Nine training courses held in Togo from September 1969 to February 1970 are documented. Each training course was held for matrons, i.e. the auxiliary midwives who carry out maternal and child health work in rural areas. *Sage-femmes* (trained midwives) were involved in the training programmes. Reports from the planning conferences held prior to these training sessions outline course content and methods of training for Togolese auxiliary midwives.

0521 Fendall, N.R. Pakistan Family Planning Council, Islamabad. *Training of clinic personnel.* In Sadik, N., Anderson, J.K., eds., Population Control: Implications, Trends and Prospects, Islamabad, Pakistan Family Planning Council, 1969, 318-332. Engl.
Pakistan International Family Planning Conference, Dacca, 28 Jan-4 Feb 1969.

It would be useful if family planning personnel could take on other responsibilities such as family guidance. High-level trained personnel are scarce, however, and if they are to fulfill these supervisory, advisory, and consultative roles, other tasks will have to be performed by lesser skilled personnel. A recent experiment in Denver, Colorado, proved that nurses could be retrained to assume greater responsibility in relation to innovations. This concept can be applied in other departments, particularly in training agricultural extension workers and community development officers to serve as clinic extension workers. Programme organization and structure, urban-rural considerations for the location of the clinic, training requirements and context, and other aspects, are discussed.

0522 Fensome, J.E. *Community Nurse Training Centre Kaduna, Northern Nigeria.* International Nursing Review (Geneva), 10(5), Sep-Oct 1963, 33-34. Engl.

The Community Nurse Training Centre in Kaduna, northern Nigeria, trains Grade II midwives in a 24-month session. Some graduate midwives receive postgraduate community nurse training, which includes home nursing, domiciliary midwifery, health education, home visiting, the administering of smallpox vaccination, triple antigen for whooping cough, tetanus and diphtheria, BCG vaccination, etc. Many of the trainees work in rural areas. Training in Kaduna provides trainees with opportunities to work with the variety of tribal groups that migrate into the urban area. Home visiting is an important aspect of training.

0523 Haward, L.R. *Midwifery in Hong Kong.* Midwives Chronicle and Nursing Notes (London), 86(1022), Apr 1973, 114-115. Engl.

Maternity services in Hong Kong employ about 2 000 midwives. Most births are delivered in hospitals or maternity centres. Maternity centres, where 45% of births occur, provide free maternal and child care. There are eight training schools for professional midwives in Hong Kong. Trainees are given examinations by the Hong Kong Midwives Board. Training takes 1 year for registered nurses; girls who are not registered nurses can pass the course after 2 years of training. Few opportunities for domiciliary midwifery exist in Hong Kong because only about 4% of confinements take place in the home. Until recently, Cantonese language texts have been imported from China and have presented data of little relevance for Hong Kong's problems. However, local scholars are working to provide more relevant texts for Cantonese-speaking students.

0524 International Confederation of Midwives, London. International Federation of Obstetrics and Gynaecology, London. *Report of conference and meetings held at the Central Midwives Board, London, 4-6 Sep 1972.* London, The Central Midwives Board, Sep 1972. 7p. Engl. Unpublished document.

This report summarizes the results of a study group with the conclusions that midwives everywhere must undergo recognized education programmes and be licensed to practice midwifery. Their tasks include supervision during pregnancy, labour, and the postpartum period, and infant care including preventive measures. Their responsibilities extend to health counselling, health education, and family planning. West African working parties are briefly mentioned.

0525 International Confederation of Midwives, London. *Report of the Anglophone West African working party, Accra, Ghana, 7-16 Dec 1972.* London, International Confederation of Midwives, 1972. 57p. Engl.
Individual papers have been abstracted separately under entries 515, 516, 517, 528, 529, 531, and 538.

This report deals with the role of family planning in midwifery. The International Confederation of Midwives hopes to assist countries restructure midwifery training curriculum to help incorporate family planning training into training for all categories of midwives.

0526 International Confederation of Midwives, London. *Report of the International Confederation of Midwives Conference on family planning in midwifery training, London, 18-21 May 1971.* London, International Confederation of Midwives, May 1971. 40p. Engl. Unpublished document.

This conference was concerned with the selection of candidates and the content of midwifery education, the midwife's appropriate role in countries with a high population, preparation of midwives for family planning, closer cooperation of midwifery schools with local health services, economic problems connected with the population explosion, resources available in developing countries for family planning, etc. Individual speakers described current progress in Thailand, Ghana, the USA, India, and Chile.

0527 International Federation of Obstetrics and Gynaecology, London. International Confederation of Midwives, London. *Report of working party on midwifery training in European countries.* London, International Federation of Obstetrics and Gynaecology and the International Confederation of Midwives, 8-9 Sep 1969. Engl.
Report of a joint study group on the training and practice of midwives and maternity nurses.

A working party on midwife training recommends the following: (1) that the WHO definition of a midwife extend to certain fields of gynecology, family planning, and child care; and (2) that midwife practice include prenatal care, labour, postnatal care of mother and child, family planning, and detection of abnormalities. Recommendations for training and postgraduate education that might later be useful in developing countries, as well as in Europe, are included.

0528 Korsah, K.K. *Developments in the training of midwives and organisation of a national maternity service to include all categories of midwives.* In Report of the Anglophone West African Working Party, Accra, Ghana, 7-16 Dec 1972, London, International Confederation of Midwives, Appendix J, 40-42. Engl.
See entry 525 for entire report.

A history of midwifery in Ghana is given. Gradually their training and numbers have increased. Training at the Korle Bu School and at the Okomfo Hospital are described. About 100 candidates present themselves at each of the two Ghana Central Midwives Board examinations annually. Organization of maternal hospitals and services are described as well as family planning services. Although traditional birth attendants are not officially recognized they treat the majority of pregnant women. The majority of the rural population depends on these traditional birth attendants. Government should not hinder the setting up of clinics or restrain midwives from setting up practice in specific areas.

0529 Samarasinghe, J. *Role of the midwife as a family health worker.* In Report of the Anglophone West African Working Party, Accra, Ghana, 7-16 Dec 1972, London, International Confederation of Midwives, Appendix L, 45-47. Engl.
See entry 525 for entire report.

The midwife has a role to play in family health. Family health maintenance includes physical, mental, emotional, and social well-being. This goal involves all team health workers, but the particular role of the midwife is described. Midwives in Ghana work with the maternal and child health division and her work is preventive in nature. Her role begins when pregnancy is discovered; prenatal care, introduction to family planning methods, observation for abnormal developments during confinement, postnatal care, record keeping, and health education are functions performed in conjunction with work of other health team members. Professional midwives will want to participate in training of auxiliary midwifery personnel. In Ghana women hold important positions in society and the health and happiness of the whole family depends on the care given by and to the mother. The midwife assures childbearing women of a safe delivery and promotes family health in general.

0530 Shillman, J.B. *Summary of family planning and other health training in AID recipient African countries, April 1970.* n.p., Apr 1970. 12p. Engl.
Unpublished document.

The author summarizes family planning and other health training in USAID recipient countries of Africa. Seven references are listed.

0531 Sosanya, R.O. *I Midwifery practice by the traditional birth attendant. II Training of the professional midwife in Nigeria.* In Report of the Anglophone West African Working Party, Accra, Ghana, 7-16 Dec 1972, Appendix C, London, International Confederation of Midwives, 20-25. Engl.
See entry 525 for entire report.

There is a need for better trained midwives in Nigeria. The Association of Midwives of Nigeria has provided concrete suggestions, many outlined here. Better equipped training schools, improved transportation for emergency care, development of a health (i.e., preventive) programme, and increased educational requirements for persons entering midwifery schools are suggested as solutions. Traditional midwifery practices are described in detail.

0532 Stiernborg, M. *Family planning in Ceylon: implementation and evaluation of the family planning training given to the public health staff.* Stockholm, University of Stockholm, Institute of Education, 1969. 164p. Engl.

Evaluation of the training of public health nurses, public health midwives, and public health inspectors in Sri Lanka's family planning programme indicated a need for more efficiency in the training programme. The full report of this evaluation begins with a brief history of Sri Lanka's family planning movement from 1953 to 1965. The report reviews educational theory behind health training and examines the important components in a training situation. The actual family planning training course, as implemented in two different training centres, is examined closely. Detailed inspection of training at one of these centres was carried out, and the principal faults discovered in the training programme were summarized. These faults include the lack of job descriptions for family planning personnel, overlap between lessons, a lack of teaching aids and textbooks, insufficient time for field work, etc. Changes that were effected as a result of this evaluation are described at length. These include the framing of job descriptions, production of teaching aids and job aids, restructuring of course content, increasing of time allotment for group work and field training, and systematic evaluation of individual trainees and of the teaching procedures. Thirty references are listed.

0533 Viel, B. Pakistan Family Planning Council, Islamabad. *Training of motivational personnel, training requirements, mode and contents.* In Sadik, N., Anderson, J.K., eds., Population Control: Implications, Trends and Prospects, Islamabad, Pakistan Family Planning Council, 1969, 293-304. Engl.
Pakistan International Family Planning Conference, Dacca, 28 Jan-4 Feb 1969.

The paper notes that the training of motivational personnel is an important subject in family planning programmes. In Latin America, family planning programmes have been adapted to the social and cultural characteristics of the population. Family planning in the developed areas is entrusted entirely to the medical professionals. In the less developed areas, there is still a search for the appropriate personnel to perform this function. A major problem is the cultural belief that children are a result of the inevitable. Other topics discussed are Chile's experience in training medical, paramedical and nontechnical personnel for family planning, motivation techniques, places where family planning information reaches the public, and resistance to family planning.

0534 WHO, Geneva. *Midwife in maternity care: report of a WHO Expert Committee.* Geneva, WHO Technical Report Series No. 331, 1966. 20p. Engl.

Midwives' functions relate to the mother (prenatal examinations, health education, delivery, and postnatal care), to the infant (examination for abnormalities, observation of general progress), and to the family and the community (health education). Midwives should have secondary school education, coordinated with nursing training, and including family planning courses. Local training centres must be provided for midwives so they can assist in child care, nutrition programmes, etc. Auxiliary midwives may work under midwife supervision or independently. Traditional birth attendants are being trained and brought into the cadre of health personnel, with continued supervision. A team approach to maternity care, with the midwife providing a link between the family and the health team, is desirable. Midwives with postbasic training must participate at national, intermediate, and local levels in planning maternity and child health services.

0535 WHO, Geneva. *Expert committee on midwifery training: first report.* Geneva, WHO Technical Report Series No. 93, 1955. 21p. Engl.

This report discusses various types of midwives, from traditional birth attendants and auxiliary midwives to fully professional midwives, and their functions. Training course curricula, school development, and criteria for students' selection are suggested. Legislation to protect mother, child, and midwife are recommended, with examples from various developed and developing countries.

0536 WHO, Geneva. *Midwives: a survey of recent legislation.* Geneva, WHO, 1954. 52p. Engl.

Originally appeared in the International Digest of Health Legislation, Geneva, WHO, vol 5, 1954, 431-482.

Laws limiting the scope of midwifery state which acts must or must not be performed, which drugs and equipment the midwife may use, as well as the circumstances under which a midwife must call in medical help. Admission requirements (including age of admission) and training vary considerably in the 30 countries studied, and certain countries are more liberal with respect to use of drugs and methods of anaesthesia. Where health services are well organized, midwife training is coordinated with nurse training. Certain countries have only gradually restricted midwifery to qualified personnel, but where such qualified personnel are insufficient, laws should be framed allowing midwives without prescribed training to continue to practice.

IV.3.2 Nonprofessional

See also: 0055, 0264, 0269, 0454, 0492, 0509, 0514, 0517, 0519, 0521, 0525, 0530, 0531, 0532, 0533, 0534

0537 Alam, A.S. Pakistan Family Planning Board, Lahore. *Evaluation of lady family planning visitors' training in West Pakistan: review of the first training course of the new paramedical cadre (1967).* Lahore, Pakistan Family Planning Board, 1967. 22p. Engl.
Third Biannual Seminar on Research in Family Planning, Dacca, Mar 1967.

Family planning in West Pakistan's rural areas is being carried out by married, matriculate women given 2 years of training at a centre in Lahore, Hyderabad, or Karachi. These female family planning visitors receive 8 months of field training in their native district. Trainees work under the supervision of a female doctor. The staff required, recruitment of trainees, the training course, and methods of student evaluation are described.

0538 Barmadia, B. *Training and practice of the traditional birth attendant.* In Report of the Anglophone West African Working Party, Accra, Ghana, 7-16 Dec 1972, London, International Confederation of Midwives, Appendix 0, 55-56. Engl.
See entry 525 for entire report.

There are three schools in Liberia giving midwifery training to traditional birth attendants (TBA). The programme of training and number of students trained are given, as is the general history of midwifery training for Liberia. Students keep experience records by which evaluation is made of skill in handling cases. The TBA must have her license renewed annually through the Liberian Midwives Council. The Government gives monthly salaries to midwives it employs but the majority are self-employed and are permitted to charge a maximum of U.S. $5 per patient. Midwives report cases of communicable disease.

0539 Brey, K.H. *Missing midwife: why a training programme failed.* South Asian Review (London), 5(1), Oct 1971, 41-52. Engl.

In 1956, the Government of India officially sponsored a programme to train indigenous dais (midwives). The programme received international assistance from UNICEF and USAID after 1967. Poor results raised questions about some of the assumptions upon which the programme was based, e.g., that there are indigenous midwives to train. Programme records and international field studies were examined for this paper. Questionable assumptions upon which the programme rests include the following: that there is such a thing as an identifiable group of female birth attendants to train; that most Indian births are attended by the indigenous dais; that the indigenous dais can be recruited and adequately trained; that the dais exercise considerable influence within the community; and that the dais can be counted on to actively support family planning. Further research is required if the programme is to continue.

0540 Hefnawi, F., Mahmoud, A.H. *Utilization of various types of health personnel (doctor, nurse, midwife, and auxiliaries) in the management of people using different birth control methods in hospitals, clinics, health station, home settings.* Egyptian Population and Family Planning Review (Cairo), 3(1), Jun 1970, 145-160. Engl.

Utilization of health personnel in family planning programmes is discussed in relation to the settings, methods of contraception, and phases of service. Eleven references are listed.

0541 Huxtable, K.A. *Study of the general gynecological experience and the knowledge, attitudes toward, and experience in family planning of the lady doctors and lady health visitors in the West Pakistan government health service in 1965.* Chapel Hill, N.C., University of North Carolina, School of Public Health, Dec 1966. 39p. Engl.
Unpublished document.

Research designed to study knowledge of attitudes toward and experiences in family planning among women physicians and female health visitors in West Pakistan in 1965 showed that family planning activities before the national family planning programme began occupied very little of these worker's time. One-quarter of the women interviewed spent less than 1 hour a week on work related to planning. Although physicians showed satisfactory knowledge of contraceptive methods, female health visitors were less well informed. Almost all women felt family planning should be practiced in Pakistan. Only 30% of the physicians had had experience inserting an IUD. Given that 60% of the physicians had performed tubal ligation, and considering the fact that physicians and female health visitors both recommended the operation, increased government support might be given to make tubal ligation more readily available.

0542 Institute of Rural Health and Family Planning, Gandhigram. *Introducing the Institute of Rural Health and Family Planning, Gandhigram: genesis, organization and current finances of the Institute.* Gandhigram, Institute of Rural Health and Family Planning, 1969. 16p. Engl.
Unpublished document. See also entries 82 and 454.

Functions of the Gandhigram Institute of Rural Health and Family Planning are outlined. These include research in methods of identifying, training, and utilizing leaders for the family planning programme, a service division evolving work programmes for family planning workers and developing methods of reporting and channeling data, and a training division that coordinates all training programmes administrated by the Institute and provides an audiovisual service.

0543 Kaul, S.J. *Comparison of field performance of medical vs. paramedical personnel in the IUD programme in Mymensingh and Lahore.* Pakistan Journal of Family Planning (Karachi), 3(2), Jul 1969, 75-89. Engl.

A survey in Lahore and Mymensingh districts of Pakistan reveals that the IUD insertion performance of paramedical personnel is reasonably comparable to that of medical personnel. Full-time family planning personnel generally give better service than part-time workers. Better training and supervision of auxiliary health workers is necessary as well as adequate follow-up of IUD insertions.

IV.4 Primary dental care

IV.4.1 Professional

See also: 0362, 0582, 0605

0544 Revzin, M.E. *Vietnam dental education project: a five-year report.* Journal of the American Dental Association (Chicago), 84(5), May 1972, 1049-1062. Engl.

In 1966, the American Dental Association conducted a survey of resources for dentistry education in South Vietnam. The purpose of the investigation was to assess ways American support could be used to upgrade dental education in South Vietnam. Dental education at the University of Saigon was to be enhanced with a view to increasing the number of practicing dentists in the country. Aid was provided in the form of American advisors and faculty, building and equipment funds, education abroad, and financial support. Vietnamese students showed an interest in preventive medicine and other aspects of the training they received.

IV.4.2 Nonprofessional

See also: 0492, 0495, 0573, 0605

0545 Barmes, D.E., Schamschula, R.G. *Dental education in Papua-New Guinea. Part II: Integrated dental officer and dental nurse courses.* Australian Dental Journal (Sydney), 12, Feb 1967, 34-41. Engl.

Dental auxiliary and dental nurse training programmes have been started to extend dental care services to remote areas of Papua and New Guinea. Curricula for courses for both types of workers are given; they include technical subjects as well as preventive dentistry, anthropology, sociology, public health, and health education. Training for rural work is reflected in such things as emphasis on equipment maintenance in remote areas. The subjects of diagnosis and referral are dealt with jointly within the context of practical difficulties in referring primitive and isolated groups to services away from their own areas. These same problems make the programme emphasis on preventive dentistry important. The future environment in which trainees will work is one of the main determinants of the contents of this training programme.

0546 Fendall, N.R. *Dental manpower requirements in emerging countries.* Public Health Reports (Washington, D.C.), 83(9), Sep 1968, 777-786. Engl.

The training and use of dental auxiliaries in newly emerging countries are proposed as the solution in such countries to the prevalence of dental disease, the paucity of professional dentists and dental schools, and the competing demands on their economies. Statistically valid dental health surveys of many countries do not exist, but scattered evidence from Jamaica, Guatemala, Thailand, Senegal, and Kenya, among others, indicates that caries and periodontal infections are widespread, and malocclusion, malignant neoplasms of the mouth, and calcium defects are not infrequent. The ratio of dentists to population varies from 1 to 15 000 in Jamaica to 1 to 250 000 in Kenya. Only 130 to 150 dentists are graduated each year from Africa's seven dental schools; half the countries of the world have no dental school and no prospects of attaining one. The cost of producing one professional dentist is prohibitive — $23 000 per dentist in Guatemala, for example. Auxiliaries can fulfill many basic dental needs of both children and adults in these countries. A program with three consecutive but overlapping phases is suggested. Phase one is to produce a small corps of superbly trained dentists. Phase two is to supplement this corps by giving existing paramedical and auxiliary health personnel 6 weeks of practical chairside training to increase outreach. Phase three is to develop specific cadres of trained dental auxiliaries. Single skill auxiliaries can be trained in 2 years. A dental surgeon and six such auxiliaries can serve an estimated 25 000 persons. Multiple skill auxiliaries with 8 years of general education need 3 years of technical training, preferably in an institution where graduate dentists and dental hygienists are also prepared. The auxiliary's role is both as assistant to the dentist and, where supervision is remote, as his substitute. Producing two types of auxiliaries, one oriented to the dental care of children, mostly preventive, and the second to the curative care of adults, would permit the organization of dental health services on a rational priority basis. Seventeen references are listed. (Revised author's summary.)

0547 Gereda, R. Universidad de San Carlos de Guatemala, Facultad de Odontologia San Carlos, Guatemala, Guatemala. *Actualizacion del programa de promotores rurales en salud oral en el Departamento de Huehuetenango, Guatemala, C.A. (Updating of the programme for rural oral health promoters in Huehuetenango, Guatemala).* San Carlos, Universidad de San Carlos de Guatemala, Facultad de Odontologia, March 1974. 9p. Span.

In Guatemala 64% of the population live in 3 903 communities of less than 2 000 inhabitants. Oral health delivery services are unevenly distributed in the Republic: in the interior the dentist/patient ratio is 1:43 114 whereas in the capital it is 1:3 717. In view of this, a pilot programme was undertaken in 1969 in the province of Huehuetenango to train 18 indigenous leaders chosen from 10 municipalities and six villages as "oral health promoters." The main objectives were to evaluate the training and utilization of a new type of rural health promoter who would become the liaison agent between the community and the regional health centres. His job would be to carry out preventive and curative oral activities. The document gives details of eight courses representing a total of 201 hours of theoretical and practical training, given between 1969 and 1973.

0548 Malik, S.M. *Preparation of dental auxiliaries in Sudan.* Khartoum, Sudan, Khartoum Civil Hospital, Dental Department, n.d. 4p. Engl. Unpublished document.

In the Sudan, dental auxiliaries are similar to dental nurses, although they are called dental assistants. The School of Dental Assistants in Khartoum, its student enrollment, curriculum, and examinations, the responsibilities of graduates in rural areas, and their salary are discussed.

IV.5 Primary laboratory care

See also: 0185, 0392, 0492, 0495, 0574, 0575

0549 Cornejo, L.Z. *El internado en Tecnologia medica. (Medical technology and the intern).* Valdivia, Chile, Universidad Austral de Chile, Escuela de Tecnologia Medica, Reprint, n.d., 18-20. Span.

The purpose of this curriculum is to train the student to put into practice at rural hospital laboratories skills acquired in the basic and professional sciences. The document describes the technical functions of the medical technologist in accordance with standard laboratory practice. The intern is an integral part of the health team and as such must be given the opportunity to assume his role and responsibilities within the team. Functions of the health team at the rural hospital level and its relationship with the generalized programmes of the rural health schools are described, as well as the functions of the medical technologist at different hospital levels determined by the laboratory analysis facilities.

0550 Cornejo, L.Z. *Consideraciones sobre la ensenanza de la tecnologia medica. (Teaching of medical technology)*. Valdivia, Chile, Universidad Austral de Chile, Escuela de Tecnologia Medica, n.d. 7p. Span.
Unpublished document.

This document discusses some of the problems that characterize the establishment of schools of medical technology, as they relate to objectives and occupational field requirements. Criteria used by the School of Medical Technology of the Universidad Austral de Chile for selecting students and interns are presented.

0551 National Convention of Medical Technologists, Santiago. *Analisis critico del rol asistencial de tecnologos medicos: adecuacion de su formacion profesional y su proyeccion futura. (Critical analysis of the medical technologist's role: his training and future prospects)*. Santiago, National Convention of Medical Technologists, 12-14 Aug 1972. 10p. Span.

The conclusions reached by the National Convention of Medical Technologists in Santiago de Chile in August 1972 established the overall role of the medical technologist within the health team and at the rural level, and concentrated on the quality and content of his training and his future prospects. The medical technologist's functions, which vary according to where they are performed and to the degree of sophisticated equipment available, i.e. at the rural health post, peripheral consulting office or hospital, are set out in detail. This professional training should emphasize his auxiliary role but should be based on the dual concepts of theory and practice that tell not only the "how" but the "why" of things. In view of the ever-increasing need for this category of worker, recommendations are made in such policy areas as grading and definition of status within the professional corps, widening the scope of activities to include anaesthesia, sterilization techniques, etc., and recognition of the teaching and administrative roles of the medical technologist.

0552 WHO, Geneva. *Training of health laboratory personnel (technical staff): fourth report of the WHO Expert Committee on Health Laboratory Services*. Geneva, WHO Technical Report Series No. 345, 1966. 81p. Engl.

The functions and responsibilities of various categories of technical laboratory personnel are defined. A training programme is outlined, including methods of instruction, curriculum, selection of candidates, teacher qualifications, and official examinations. A detailed 40-week programme for the training of certified assistant technicians is presented.

IV.6 Primary environmental health

See also: 0040, 0192, 0492, 0564, 0584

0553 Andrade, J. *Cursos en tecnologia de la salud: situacion en Venezuela para 1973. (Courses in health technology: situation in Venezuela in 1973)*. Caracas, Ministry of Health and Social Welfare, 1973. 21p. Span.
Unpublished document.

Finding solutions to the problems of providing medical care in developing countries necessitates analyzing the whole epidemiological pattern and ascertaining the critical socioeconomic factors involved, in order to find ways to influence them. The size of a country's economy dictates its capacity to provide basic health services. The problem is aggravated for poorer countries by a rapid increase in population. A comparison of two countries with similar populations – Malawi, with a per capita GNP of U.S. $51, and Zambia with six times that figure – illustrates the superiority of Zambia's achievements in the provision of health care and bears out the argument that countries with a per capita GNP of under U.S. $76 cannot from their own resources provide basic health services on anything but the most unsatisfactory and rudimentary scale, whereas those with GNP's of between U.S. $76 and 150 provide a reasonable level of health care only with great difficulty. International help is needed to enable the poorest nations to develop basic health services, not only for humanitarian reasons, but because of their effect on the economy through increased efficiency of the work force and, in the long term, their influence on population growth through improved maternal and child health.

0554 Mendia, L. *Environmental health in developing countries*. Israel Journal of Medical Sciences (Jerusalem), 4(3), May-Jun 1968, 415-424. Engl. Fourth Rehovoth Conference on Health Problems in Developing States, Rehovoth, Israel, 15-23 Aug 1967.
Se͏ try 96 for complete proceedings.

F ..s common to all human environments are water supply, sewage disposal, solid waste disposal, and housing. These are interrelated; it is not possible to establish any single priority for the solution of the multiple problems. Often religions and traditional systems interfere in the process of safeguarding the environment. Public health personnel must be aware of each others' roles so that cooperation can take place. The importance of educating health personnel in environmental subjects must be recognized. Both experts and paraprofessionals should be trained.

0555 Owens, P.N. *Training of sanitary engineers and other environmental health specialists in Latin America.* American Journal of Public Health (New York), 56(11), Nov 1966, 1948-1953. Engl.

Training of sanitary engineers and other environmental health specialists in Latin America has undergone profound change both in content and methodology. Development banks, UNESCO, USAID, and private foundations have helped place full-time faculty in teaching positions and have encouraged projects in which the university studies the community and its environment. Although undergraduate programmes have already begun, texts are in demand. Professional graduate programmes in industrial management have taken the form of short courses. Nine references are listed.

0556 Pan American Sanitary Bureau, Washington, D.C. *Seminario interamericano sobre adiestramiento de personal auxiliar de saneamiento. (Inter-American seminar on the training of auxiliary sanitation personnel).* San Jose, Costa Rica, Pan American Sanitary Bureau, 1960. 120p. Span.

The Pan American Sanitary Bureau is the Secretariat of the Pan American Health Organization. This seminar was held in San José, Costa Rica, from 3-21 August 1960, under the auspices of the Administration for International Cooperation, the Panamerican Sanitary Bureau, and the governments of 18 Latin American and Caribbean countries. Many of the mortality and morbidity cases are attributed to lack of sanitary facilities at the rural level. Throughout Latin America more than 90 million rural inhabitants do not have access to potable water and more than 100 million to sewage disposal facilities. The objective of the seminar was to provide an opportunity to the delegates from the different ministries of Public Health and the universities to revise, discuss, and develop personnel training programmes for auxiliaries in the field of environmental sanitation. Working conditions, pay, status of the sanitary inspector, recruitment and selection of candidates, and minimal qualifications of those seeking to graduate as sanitary inspectors are detailed. Each participating country presented a paper on its past and present environmental sanitation programmes, number of inspectors available and in training, methods of training, etc., with comparative data to show their respective progress.

IV.7 Teaching aids

IV.7.1 Rural health care

See also: 0367, 0466

0557 African Medical and Research Foundation, Nairobi. *Tuberculosis - Tanzania.* Nairobi, African Medical and Research Foundation, Nov 1972. 2p. Engl.
Unpublished document.

This review of the tuberculosis situation in Tanzania includes suggestions for identification and treatment of cases. Detailed instructions for collection of sputum specimens and staining techniques are included.

0558 Argentina, Department of Social Welfare. *Manual de procedimientos para el auxiliar de enfermeria o agente sanitario: programas de salud rural. (Procedural manual for the auxiliary health worker: rural health programmes).* Buenos Aires, Department of Social Welfare, Aug 1969. 111p. Span.

The Ministry of Health in Argentina realizes that to deliver integrated health care services to the inhabitants of rural communities, it must rely on the qualified and controlled performance of the auxiliary health worker. This manual, written in simple language, teaches the health worker elementary principles of hygiene; use and maintenance of medical instruments; early detection and treatment of common diseases; vaccination techniques; and first aid. Most of the mechanical tasks to be performed are graphically illustrated, as are pregnancy and maternal and child care methods in a rural environment. Finally, environmental sanitation and proper utilization of resources (rain water, wells, rivers, etc.) as a means of preventing disease are discussed.

0559 Belbin, R.M. Organization for Economic Co-operation and Development, Paris. *Discovery method: an international experiment in retraining.* Paris, Organization for Economic Cooperation and Development, Apr 1969. 85p. Engl.

This report describes four experiments using the discovery method for older workers. The Austrian project was concerned with stonemasons, the United Kingdom project with locomotive drivers, and the Swedish study with the reading and interpretation of engineering drawings. In the United States, three case studies covered workers in machine shops, data processing, and electrical work. The author claims that these experiments prove the discovery method to be more suitable than traditional methods, especially for older workers. Moreover, it permits a shorter training period. With this method, tasks and problems of various grades are presented to the trainees according to their level of knowledge and progress. It is in solving the problems that the trainee can find out how things work and why.

A progressive series of tasks and problems are presented to the trainee enabling him to master the increasingly difficult and involved skills and knowledge. The author concludes that the success of the method depends on the careful definition of the requirements of specific jobs and on their translation into an ordered series of tasks and problems. The training designer is, therefore, the key person in the programme, and the wide use of this method depends upon increasing the number of such persons in each country. (Book abstract.)

0560 **Canada, Department of National Health and Welfare.** *Treatment manual for community health auxiliaries.* Ottawa, Department of National Health and Welfare, 1973. 20p. Engl.

This manual lists common illnesses and the treatment used for each. It has been prepared for use by the community health auxiliaries to help them in their day-to-day work. The doctors and nurses will give more instructions when they talk with the auxiliaries on the radio or telephone and when they visit. *The Guide to Treatment for Nurses and Lay Dispensers* also will give the auxiliaries more information on illness, medicines, and treatment. Requisitions or requests for medicines should be made to the field nurse or to the zone office. This manual should be kept near the medicines, ready for use. The books, *Fundamentals of First Aid* and *Patient Care in the Home* used during the training course will help to remind the auxiliary about these subjects. The *Family Health Manual* and *Sanitation Manual* will also help the community health auxiliary in his work.

0561 **Canada, Department of National Health and Welfare.** *Guide for field orientation of community health workers.* Ottawa, Department of National Health and Welfare, Medical Services Branch, 1970. 21p. Engl.

A community health worker programme for Indians and Eskimos of Canada aims to increase the number of health workers in the field, link professional health workers with the local community, encourage local participation, and assist the native population in reaching health standards comparable to the remainder of the population. The training programme, divided into four parts, involves 2 months orientation with the field nurse in the local health centre, a more formal 8-week training period at a selected centre, 6 months continued on-the-job training, and a second part of formal training lasting 4 weeks. A curriculum outline, general comments on planning the course, and sample forms for health worker evaluation are included.

0562 **Canada, Department of National Health and Welfare.** *Methods manual for community health workers.* Ottawa, Department of National Health and Welfare, 1970. 30p. Engl.

This methods manual presents techniques of community organization for community health workers. Communications, interviewing, working with committees, groups, and local governments are subjects dealt with in simple terms. Ideas from group dynamics and modern educational and social change theory are included.

0563 **Canada, Department of National Health and Welfare.** *Sanitation manual for community health workers.* Ottawa, Department of National Health and Welfare, Medical Services Branch, 1965. 101p. Engl.

This manual reviews subjects discussed at the training course for community health workers. These subjects include: basic principles of sanitation in relation to germs, diseases, and water; the disease-carrying activities of several domestic insects and animals, including flies, mosquitoes, bedbugs, lice, ticks, cockroaches, and rats; and under the heading of water, subjects like pollution, water supplies, water purification, human waste disposal, and sanitation with dogs. The appendix gives a list of filmstrips, flip charts, etc. on sanitation that are available from the Department of National Health and Welfare, and also a suggested programme for the community health worker.

0564 **Canada, Department of National Health and Welfare.** *Family health manual.* Ottawa, Department of National Health and Welfare, Medical Services Branch, n.d. 1v.(various pagings). Engl. Unpublished document.

This manual covers basic principles of hygiene and personal well-being. Separate chapters deal with general principles of hygiene (family health, maternal and child health), problems of teenagers, alcohol abuse, dental hygiene, and treatment of venereal diseases, rabies, and trichinosis. Ways of achieving physical, mental, and social health are discussed.

0565 **Chile, National Health Service.** *Manual de enfermeria. (Nursing manual).* Santiago, National Health Service, 1972. 105p. Span.

The purpose of this manual is to complement the training of nurse auxiliaries, and to serve as a practical guide at the hospital or in the field. It covers the majority of emergency situations with which the nurse auxiliary may have to contend in the absence of a health professional. Mechanical operations and emergency first aid care are graphically illustrated, e.g., artificial respiration, transportation of sick and wounded, treatment of fractured limbs, etc. The sequence of actions to be performed by the nurse auxiliary is well detailed, indicating what must be done in every case and what must be remembered in order to provide the best possible health care. An immunization programme for infants and preschool age children is also included.

0566 **Colombia, Ministry of Public Health.** *Programa para la formacion del auxiliar de enfermeria. (Nursing assistant training programme).* Bogota, Ministry of Public Health, Nov 1973. 1v.(various pagings). Span. Unpublished document.

To compensate for the shortage of professional medical personnel, the Ministry of Public Health of Colombia established, in 1974, a training programme for

IV Primary Health Manpower – Training and Utilization

nursing assistants. The programme involves two main areas: maternal and child care, and medical and surgical activities. The document lists the different admission requirements (age, level of education attained, etc.). The 18-month training period will be divided into two stages: theoretical training, lasting 12 months (1 880 hours); and supervised practice, lasting 6 months. The medical-surgical stage includes 187 hours of theoretical training, 187 hours of demonstration, and 826 hours of practice. The maternal and child care stage involves 645 hours: 118 hours of theory, 117 hours of demonstration, and 410 hours of practice. These nursing assistants will be assigned to health delivery centres throughout the country. The document lists the curriculum of the programme and ends with a description of the functions and activities of the nursing assistant.

0567 **Colombia, Ministry of Public Health. Colombian Association of Faculties of Medicine, Bogota.** *Manual de normas administrativas y promocion de servicios. (Manual of administrative procedures and promotion of health care delivery services).* Bogota, Ministry of Public Health, Nov 1973. 83p. Span.

This manual has been prepared for the rural health promoter. It describes health care procedures and administrative standards conducive to the smooth, uninterrupted delivery of health care services and their accompanying benefits to the community. The two main chapters deal with: (1) administrative organization; and (2) promotion of services. The first chapter includes the following topics: areas of medical attention covered by the programme; general administration; areas of personal responsibility; supervision of services; and the use of radiocommunication and ambulance services. The second chapter discusses the promotion of health care services. This includes: home visits; environmental sanitation; first aid; and maternal and child care. All practical procedures are graphically illustrated and extensively developed. Seventeen references are listed.

0568 **Colombia, Ministry of Public Health.** *Manual para el adiestramiento de promotoras rurales de salud. (Training manual for rural health promoters).* Bogota, Ministry of Public Health, Jan 1969. 237p. Span.

Due to uneven distribution of health professionals throughout Colombia, a great percentage of the rural population lacks the most elementary health care services. The purpose of this manual is to impart basic knowledge of health care methods to the rural health promoter, whose function is the practice of simple means of disease prevention, the delivery of first aid services, the reduction of maternal and infant morbidity and mortality, and the education of the community.

0569 **Cruickshank, R., Standard, K.L., Goldthorpe, G., Cook, R., ed(s).** University of the West Indies, Mona, Jamaica. *Manual for community health workers.* Mona, Jamaica, University of the West Indies, Department of Social and Preventive Medicine, 1968. 212p. Engl.

The Department of Social and Preventive Medicine of the University of the West Indies launched a programme to give initial training to a group of community health aides to: assist in training leaders to organize courses for community health aides in rural areas; and assist medical officers of health and public health staff to develop training courses at the parish level for various groups of community health aides. This manual, designed for the training of community health aides over a 3-month period, is of value to any organization desiring to train such auxiliary health workers. It discusses Jamaica's demographic and social features, the structure of government and social agencies before dealing specifically with the community health worker's goals within the community, and ways of achieving them. The following topics are discussed in a direct, simple manner with appropriate illustrations: nutrition and food preparation; basic anatomy and physiology; basic nursing theory; personal hygiene; and community health, i.e. sources of safe drinking water, restaurant inspection, waste disposal, insect vector control. Instruction in maternal and infant care, family planning, child growth and development through to adolescence, marriage, and old age, is aimed not only at the future community health aide, but also at other health-workers-in-training or laymen interested in improving community health. In evaluating the course it was recommended that more time be spent in practical work in the field; that educational qualifications of health aides be such that in addition to being able to read and write, they should be able to interpret new meanings for health and illness apart from superstition and mystery; that the aides should live in the community; that duties should include assisting the trained nurse, interpreting symptoms, and reporting them to the appropriate authority, and, in the clinic, weighing and measuring babies, preparing simple dressings, assisting a male doctor during pelvic examinations, etc. Community work would include follow-up of broken appointments, basic home care such as giving bed baths, first aid care, and so on.

0570 **Fountain, D.E.** *L'infirmier comme diagnosticien. (The medical assistant as diagnostician).* Kinshasa, Ecole d'Infirmiers Auxiliares de Vanga, n.d. 161p. Fren.

This booklet has been designed to assist nurses in Zaire perform all aspects of their work in hospitals and centres. Information on health education, hygiene, prophylaxis, diagnosis, and treatment is included.

0571 **Fream, W.C.** *Aids to tropical hygiene and nursing.* London, Bailliere, Tindall and Cassell, 1964. 220p. Engl.

In this concise illustrated textbook for nurses the following are topics examined: nutritional disorders in the tropics; parasitic worms; diseases spread by insect vectors; tropical hygiene and diseases associated with poor hygiene; animal and other diseases that occur in man; diseases and conditions of the skin; poisonous bites and stings; and climatic conditions. Diseases linked to protein deficiency such as kwashiorkor, beriberi, pellagra, sprue, obesity, cholera, etc., are discussed. Malaria, tetanus, leishmaniasis, trypanosomiasis, smallpox, leprosy, yaws, and venereal diseases are covered as well.

0572 **Ghana, Ministry of Health.** *Manual for health assistants.* Accra, Ministry of Health, Jun 1964. 171p. Engl.

This programme was compiled by Ghana's Health Education Unit for training health assistants (auxiliary health workers) to work in health posts (health centres), in cooperation with the health inspector and the community health nurse. The health assistant is in charge of the post (under the supervision of a medical officer who is in charge of the region) and is responsible for treating patients at the health post, visiting homes and schools, etc. The health inspector looks after environmental sanitation and health education where people work, whereas the community health nurse looks after women and children of pre-school age. The manual explains in simple terms the causes, symptoms, and treatment of fevers, convulsions, abdominal pain, jaundice, etc. and tells when these must be referred to the hospital. Basic facts about nutrition, i.e. valuable sources of vitamins, minerals, and protein, and the principles of diet and meal planning are discussed. Lists are given for equipment, supplies, sanitation procedures, the care and administration of medicines, and first-aid methods. Sample record sheets for daily register of patients, monthly morbidity return, drug register, etc., are included. Aspects of health education covered are: methods of communication; teaching methods and aids; community organization; and general considerations in programme planning. In the area of maternal and child health services, instructions for advice to be given to expectant and nursing mothers on infant feeding, child development, breast feeding and weaning, and vaccination are given. Simple steps toward environmental sanitation, i.e. refuse disposal, housing facilities, water purification, and vector control, are stated. Brief consideration is given to dental hygiene and the treatment of some dental conditions. The nature of communicable diseases, principles of immunity and control measures, as well as specific facts and recommended procedures for smallpox, chickenpox, malaria, tuberculosis, leprosy, yellow fever, measles, whooping cough, poliomyelitis, etc., are dealt with at length.

0573 **Halestrap, D.J.** *Simple dental care for rural hospitals.* London, Medical Missionary Association, 1971. 26p. Engl.

A recent survey of dental work in church hospitals in rural areas of Uganda, Rwanda, and Burundi revealed auxiliary workers were untrained and usually dealt with toothache by extraction. Only a few workers had had any training in administration of local anaesthetic and in some hospitals no attempt was made to administer anaesthesia at all. Consequently it was felt some workers could benefit from further instruction in simple dental work. The instruction presented here was drafted and pretested. Pretesting helped simplify diagrams and keep vocabulary understandable for workers, most of whom use English as a second language. The aim of the small text is to provide a guide for use by rural hospital workers in developing countries.

0574 **Hanning, L.** Nigeria, Laboratory Assistants Training School. *Notes on general laboratory procedure.* Kaduna, Laboratory Assistants Training School, Nov 1962. 60p. Engl.
Modified and revised by C.E.W. Hoar.

Notes on general laboratory procedures have been prepared for use by laboratory assistant trainees at the Laboratory Assistants Training School in Kaduna, Nigeria. Procedures described will enable assistants to take charge of outpost laboratories.

0575 **Keitzman, B.** *Medical guide for dispensary attendants.* Kano, Nigeria, Sudan Interior Mission, Dec 1961. 37p. Engl.
Unpublished document.

This handbook has been compiled for dispensary attendants in the Sudan. Diseases are classified according to the chief organ system involved, with instructions to the reader to seek further information in other texts if necessary. Auxiliaries are reminded that they are not expected to recognize or treat all diseases. Information on rare diseases is included, however, in case the dispensary attendant is the only one nearby who can possibly deal with the case. For each illness, symptoms and treatment methods are described.

0576 **Kwansa, E.V., Cannon, J.A., Belcher, D.W., Hosu-Porbley, M.** *Perception and comprehension of health education visual aids by rural Ghanaian villagers.* Ghana Medical Journal (Accra), 11(4), Dec 1972, 387-396. Engl.

This study describes the perception and comprehension of health posters by 1 060 rural villagers in the Greater Accra Region. Features of effective visual aids were determined. Picture style and colour preferences are also described. A set of three criteria by which to predict the effectiveness of a picture in communicating an intended message were found to be: (1) familiarity; (2) realism; and (3) simplicity. Change in health behaviour is dependent upon effective communication. When communication is left to untested posters and teaching aids, misinterpretations result among rural villagers if they are comprehended at all. Nine references are listed. (Author abstract.)

0577 **Latham, M.** FAO, Rome. *Human nutrition in tropical Africa: a textbook for health workers with special reference to community health problems in East Africa.* Rome, Food and Agriculture Organization, 1965. 268p. Engl.

This book is designed to teach the health worker how to scientifically identify the nutritional problems of the community and to suggest specific ways to solve them. The topics covered include public health aspects of nutrition, basic nutrition, disorders due to malnutrition, foods, practical solutions to nutritional problems, diets, toddler recipes, and home preservation of food. The appendices provide useful information on recommended intakes of nutrients, conversion tables, and a food composition table. References are listed.

0578   Nigeria, Ministry of Health. *Standard treatments in dispensaries, 1965.* Kaduna, Government Printer, 1965. 1v.(various pagings). Engl.

This text of standard treatment is designed for use by dispensary attendants in northern Nigeria. The handbook describes practical procedures appropriate to conditions encountered in dispensaries. A list of standard equipment necessary for all dispensaries is included. The manual was drawn up after consultation with specialists, medical officers, and a World Health Organization consultant.

0579   Ortega, R.B. Peru, Department of Health. *Manual de normas y procedimientos para auxiliares de enfermeria de puestos sanitarios de la zona de salud sur Altiplanica, Puno. (Manual of methods and procedures for auxiliary health workers in health posts of the Altiplano, Puno).* Puno, Ministerio de Salud, Zona de Salud Sur Altiplanica, 1972. 290p. Span.

For 80% of the inhabitants of Puno (Peru) living in rural areas, standards of health, nutrition, sanitation, etc. are all very low with correspondingly high rates of infant mortality, maternal mortality, and morbidity. Traditional customs, ignorance, and illiteracy are to some extent responsible for this situation. In Puno's health area there are two hospitals, two health centres, 14 dispensaries, and 46 rural health posts. The rural health posts are manned by an auxiliary health worker. Almost all rural health posts are provided with minimum equipment. The rural health post is responsible for first aid, vaccinations, health education, and statistical records in an area occupied by about 3 000 people. This manual, in direct and simple language, explains the functions and duties of the auxiliary health worker, emphasizing the importance of administrative practices such as registration of births and deaths, recording of activities in the health post, etc. The most common diseases likely to be encountered by the health worker are described. First-aid care methods are graphically described. A list of minimum supplies to be kept at the rural health post as well as samples of the forms used by the auxiliary health worker for reporting to the health centre are included. Thirty references are listed.

0580   Philippines, Bureau of Health. *Handbook for rural health unit workers.* Manila, Bureau of Health, 1963. 32p. Engl.
Unpublished document.

This is a handbook for rural health unit workers in the Philippines, outlining the legal background and work goals of the rural health programme for the country. Health services were established in rural areas after the Philippine Congress passed Act Number 1082 in 1954. Other acts related to rural health followed this legislation and are outlined in the handbook. The legislation called for employment of more physicians, midwives, nurses, and sanitary inspectors to live and work in remote areas. The overall objective is to reduce the rate of preventable disease in the country. The legislation created Senior Health Units and Junior Health Units, which used fewer staff. A part of the programme's goal is to consolidate health units in the Provinces under the Bureau of Health. The handbook lists contents for the medical kits used by physicians, nurses, midwives, and sanitary inspectors. Organizational charts, copies of health care legislation, and duties of each category of worker are provided.

0581   Stolten, J.H., Elman, A. *Health aide.* Boston, Little, Brown and Company, 1972. 373p. Engl.

This textbook is designed to help student health aides efficiently perform the responsibilities of their future profession. The author explains in easily understandable terms the basic skills necessary in caring for bedridden and ambulatory adults and for the general care of infants. Chapters cover skills such as maintaining safety and cleanliness in the patient's room, bathing the patient, caring for infants, and providing recreation. The basic functions of the health aide are also discussed. Although it has been compiled specifically for health aides in the USA, the textbook is valuable for hospitals, public health agencies, nursing homes, and private homes as a training manual and as a practical reference source.

0582   Universidad de San Carlos de Guatemala, Guatemala. *Desarrollo resumido del programa oral. (Condensed oral education programme).* Guatemala, Universidad de San Carlos de Guatemala, n.d. 1v.(various pagings). Span.
Unpublished document.

This document provides information for the student oral health promoter on preventive dental care, clinical treatment of the patient, extractions, anaesthesia, proper handling of equipment, etc. Aims of the programme, length of the course, materials required, teaching personnel, timetables, etc. are indicated. An elementary therapeutic guide identifying the most common oral diseases with appropriate means of treatment and a sample for recording the oral health promoter's daily activities are included.

0583   Venezuela, Ministry of Health. *Manual normativo para auxiliares de enfermeria y otro personal voluntario. (Training manual for auxiliary health workers and other voluntary personnel).* Caracas, Department of Health and Social Welfare, 1971. 212p. Span.

In Venezuela, as in most developing countries, health care services for rural populations are either difficult to deliver or nonexistent. The training of auxiliary health workers is an attempt to improve health care delivery to rural areas. This manual is a course in simplified medicine to train such personnel. It covers the symptoms and treatment of most common diseases, pregnancy recognition and care, methods of environmental sanitation, and first aid for various types of injuries, with illustrated procedures. Upon the completion of this 19-week course, the auxiliary worker is posted to a rural health centre, where he receives weekly visits from the rural zone doctor. Since auxiliary workers are in short supply, members of the Armed Forces, the National Guard, and permanent firefighting brigades are given the course as well.

0584 Wilkie, W. *Jordan's tropical hygiene and sanitation.* London, Bailliere, Tindall and Cox, 1965. 437p. Engl.

This is a handbook on hygiene for health inspectors and other subsidiary health staff, in tropical and subtropical zones. It contains practical instruction on sanitation services, construction techniques and housing, food hygiene, water quality, disease control, pest control, and methods of health education.

IV.7.2 Family planning and midwifery

See also: 0519

0585 Center for Population Planning, Ann Arbor, Michigan. *Leadership group practice session 1, 2, and Myun-Eup family planning workers training course information, education, organization.* Ann Arbor, Mich., Center for Population Planning, n.d. 1v.(various pagings). Engl.
Unpublished document.

This paper instructs family planning workers in Myun-Eup, Korea, on how to plan and organize meetings. The following topics are discussed: the objectives of the family planning programme; the objectives of the job; and the planning and carrying out of educational encounters with the public to encourage the use of birth control. Group practice sessions on planning meetings, preparing materials for education and publicity, and answering questions are outlined. A copy of the training examination is included.

0586 Center for Population Planning, Ann Arbor, Michigan. *Family planning workers pre-service training course group practice sessions: 1) know your subject; 2) meeting your public; 3) planning your meetings; 4) preparation of mass media and education materials.* Ann Arbor, Mich., Center for Population Planning, n.d. 1v.(various pagings). Engl.
Unpublished document.

The practice sessions aim at preparing the family planning workers in Turkey to deal with people in home and group situations, to organize publicity and education campaigns, and to prepare educational materials, both graphic and written. The emphasis is on public relations and knowledge of the subject. Test questionnaires and hypothetical personal encounters are included.

0587 Colombia, Ministry of Public Health. Colombian Association of Faculties of Medicine, Bogota. *Manual materno infantil y control de enfermedades transmisibles. (Manual of maternal and child care and control of communicable diseases).* Bogota, Ministry of Health and the Colombian Association of Faculties of Medicine, Nov 1973. 93p. Span.

This manual describes in detail the functions of and procedures to be followed by auxiliary health personnel in promoting and protecting the health of mother and child, not only during pregnancy, but after the birth, growth, and development of the child up to school age. It aims primarily to safeguard the health of women and children, not only because they constitute more than half the population of Colombia, but also because they are more susceptible to malnutrition and communicable diseases. The seven chapters are devoted to: anatomy of genital organs and physiology of reproduction; prenatal care; normal delivery; growth and development of the child; child accident prevention; control of communicable diseases; family planning including birth control methods; and the content and organization of a local programme. Twelve references are listed.

0588 East Pakistan Research and Evaluation Centre, Sweden-Pakistan Family Welfare Project, Dacca. *Manual of publicity for Thana officers.* Dacca, East Pakistan Research and Evaluation Centre and the Sweden-Pakistan Family Welfare Project, n.d. 17p. Engl.

This manual for Thana family planning officers in East Pakistan (now Bangladesh) describes the role of publicity in raising the awareness necessary for people to adopt change. Topics discussed include the following: whether publicity is effective; how its effectiveness can be measured; the manual's purpose; what steps to take in planning a publicity effort; how to establish effective communication, e.g. through the use of posters and other media; and how to use a publicity planning map. The manual was designed to help set up a good continuing publicity effort in the Thana family planning officer's area. Steps outlined are put forth in an order that communication experts consider logical, but amenable to adaptation to local circumstances.

0589 Ebrahim, G.J. *Newborn in tropical Africa.* Nairobi, East African Literature Bureau, 1969. 111p. Engl.

This handbook on obstetrics and pediatrics first discusses infant morbidity in the tropical zone of Africa, then goes on to provide instructions concerning prenatal care, pregnancy disorders, midwifery, feeding difficulties, congenital defects, and routine care of the newborn. Forty-six references are listed.

0590 Gray, H.H. Christian Council of Nigeria, Lagos. *Treatment handbook for health centres in West Africa.* Lagos, Christian Council of Nigeria, 1973. 58p. Engl.

The handbook is intended to help dispensary attendants and midwives in caring for patients primarily in West Africa. It provides brief descriptions of many diseases but no details on diagnosis. The introduction contains instructions on good maintenance of a dispensary and a maternity home, team work, care of the sick, health education, children's drug dosage, etc. Other health topics discussed include preventive medicine and vaccines, family planning, diseases of the nervous system, and special instructions for midwives.

0591 Huang, T.T. *Ways of family planning.* Taiwan, Provincial Department of Health, Sep 1968. 28p. Engl.
Unpublished document.

This is a booklet for lay women on family planning, produced by the Committee on Family Planning, Taiwan Provincial Department of Health. Emphasized is family planning practice reinforced by other forms of planned living, such as sound family nutrition and economic budgeting. Reasons for family planning, information on pregnancy and health care during pregnancy, and choices of family planning methods are discussed. The booklet concludes that quality of life, in general, can be improved through planning.

0592 Huang, T.T. *Training for family planning workers.* Taichung, Taiwan Provincial Department of Health, Dec 1967. 26p. Engl.
Unpublished document.

Outlined are procedures, curriculum, and training examinations for Taiwan township level, county/city level, and provincial level family planning workers. Examples are given of oral and written examinations for township level family planning workers.

0593 India, Ministry of Health and Family Planning. *Guidelines for training select nurse personnel in IUCD techniques.* India, Ministry of Health and Family Planning, Department of Family Planning, n.d. 12p. Engl.
Unpublished document.

Guidelines for training nursing personnel in IUD insertion are outlined. Training is designed for qualified trained nurses who should supplement the work of lady doctors with regard to IUD insertion work. Curriculum to be covered includes patient selection by history and pelvic examination, aseptic techniques for insertion and removal of IUD's, follow-up methodology and care of complaints and complications, and record keeping.

0594 Institute of Child Health of the University of Lagos, Lagos. *Manual of procedures of the Gbaja family health clinic.* Lagos, Nigeria, University of Lagos, Institute of Child Health, n.d. 87p. Engl.

A pilot project in the use of nurses to operate a comprehensive maternal and child health/family planning clinic in Nigeria.

Specific procedures carried out in a maternal and child health/family planning clinic in Lagos, Nigeria, are presented. The clinic, operated by nurses under a doctor's supervision, was designed to provide total continuous care for children up to 6 years of age, to offer family planning advice and services, and to give parents health education and food demonstrations. The clinic's screening procedures, registration, weighing and measuring, entry and exit table procedures, immunization scheme, family planning, home visiting, and so on are described in detail. Directions in all instances are simple and explicit, making this manual a necessity for nurses working at the Gbaja Clinic and a useful sourcebook for others interested in establishing a similar health clinic.

0595 Institute of Rural Health and Family Planning, Gandhigram. *Curriculum for 7 days orientation training in family planning for medical officers of primary health centre.* Gandhigram, Institute of Rural Health and Family Planning, 1968. 7p. Engl.
Unpublished document. See also entries 596 and 598.

The training course in family planning for medical officers of primary health centres is described. Contents listed include group processes, the operational objectives, function and setup of centres, districts and blocks, the study of the ongoing family planning programme, work preparation and implementation, field visits, analysis of job functions, use of a community approach in work, records maintenance, conducting and organizing training camps, a review of contraceptive methods, methods of staff evaluation, and principles of supervision.

0596 Institute of Rural Health and Family Planning, Gandhigram. *Curriculum for 10 days orientation training in family planning for lady health visitors and auxiliary nurse midwives.* Gandhigram, Institute of Rural Health and Family Planning, 1968. 6p. Engl.
Unpublished document. See also entries 595 and 598.

Curriculum outline for a 10-day orientation training course in family planning for female health visitors and auxiliary nurse midwives is described. Course contents include how the female health visitor and auxiliary nurse midwife can integrate her functions in family planning with maternal and child health work; goals and organization of the National Family Planning Programme of India; the setup of family planning personnel at district, block, and state levels; methods of family planning programme work at the village level; working with the community and with audiovisual teaching aids; a review of family planning methods; supervision and coordination of family planning work with health and block staff work; and use of educational opportunities in clinics.

0597 Institute of Rural Health and Family Planning, Gandhigram. *Training (curriculum for*

health assistants in family planning). Ghandhigram, Institute of Rural Health and Family Planning, Feb 1966. 1v.(various pagings). Engl.
Family Planning Communication Action Research Projects, Fourth Workshop, Lucknow, 14-19 Feb 1966.

Minimum skills and knowledge needed by health assistants in family planning, and a training programme to prepare such personnel are described, based on research by the Institute of Rural Health and Family Planning, Gandhigram, India. General principles applicable to the training of any professional public health worker are listed. The Institute's method for developing a field-oriented training programme is practical rather than academic and reduces the period of training to the minimum.

0598 **Institute of Rural Health and Family Planning, Gandhigram.** *Curriculum for 30 day orientation course for the district extension educators XI batch: objectives.* Gandhigram, Institute of Rural Health and Family Planning, n.d. 10p. Engl.
Unpublished document. See also entries 595 and 596.

An outline of the curriculum for a 30-day course on planning, implementing, and evaluating the family planning programme is given. The course was designed for district extension educators in India. Course content included the following topics: the district extension educator's job, functions of district and primary health centres, communication techniques, family planning methods, demography, report writing, leadership, group dynamics, educational methods, use of audio-visual aids, record keeping, planning training camps for village leaders, counselling techniques, staff supervision, and seminar planning.

0599 **Manisoff, M.T.** Planned Parenthood-World Population, New York. *Family planning: a teaching guide for nurses.* New York, Planned Parenthood-World Population, 1969. 104p. Engl.

This guide is intended as a teaching aid for nursing school educators and nurses responsible for in-service education at health and welfare agencies and hospitals. It will also be helpful to individual nurses interested in preparing themselves more broadly in family planning. Topics treated include definition of terms, history and philosophy of family planning, population problems, birth control, poverty, health rationale for family planning, family planning as a public health function, anatomy and physiology of reproduction, and methods of birth control. A bibliography is appended that could help instructors to select relevant materials for their lectures or, where the programme permits, to teach the entire unit as a course by itself.

0600 **Pakistan Academy for Rural Development, Comilla.** *Thana family planning officers' training manual.* Comilla, East Pakistan, Jul 1966. 43p. Engl.
Unpublished document.

The Thana family planning officer's training manual is based on the experience in Comilla Kotwali Thana in East Pakistan (now Bangladesh). It supplements other literature prepared by the Family Planning Department. Special emphasis is placed on the organization and functions of the staff of Thana family planning offices and IUD clinics. The manual gives clear instructions for starting a Thana family planning programme including choosing a location for the office, training office staff, involving local leaders, etc. Instructions are provided for mass distribution of conventional contraceptives, for setting up, publicizing, and promoting a family planning programme, and for evaluation of the programme.

0601 **Perkin, G.W., Mullins, C.** Pakistan Family Planning Council, Islamabad. *Use of programmed instructions in family planning training programmes.* In Sadik, N., Anderson, J.K., eds., Population Control: Implication, Trends and Prospects, Islamabad, Pakistan Family Planning Council, 1969, 333-350. Engl.
Pakistan International Family Planning Conference, Dacca, 28 Jan-4 Feb 1969.

The paper discusses the development of programmed instruction for a family planning training programme designed for midwives and nurses in Thailand. It begins with the applications and benefits of this technique. The self-instructional course, *Methods for Family Planning*, covers introduction to the methods, i.e., the loop and oral pills, as well as tests, answer keys, and instructions for scoring. The materials were translated into Thai and used as part of the 5-day training course in family planning. Data on the test performance of midwives and nurses have been analyzed. The paper concludes that the course will provide uniform training designed to equip the midwives and nurses with skills and knowledge required for their job responsibilities. The appendices provide samples of the instructional material.

0602 **Rahman, S., Begum, S., Begum, J.** East Pakistan Family Planning Board, Dacca. *Lady family planning visitor's course.* East Pakistan Family Planning Board, Dacca, n.d. 16p. Engl.

A training course of 1 year was set up by the East Pakistan Family Planning Board to train Lady Family Planning Visitors for East Pakistan (now Bangladesh). The requirements for admission to the training course, training facilities, the course's content, the content and procedures for examinations, and a detailed syllabus are provided. The syllabus gives the details of numbers of hours for lecture and discussion and demonstration for each topic introduced in training. Training of Lady Family Planning Visitors was initiated to alleviate the need for female personnel to insert IUD's for women residing in rural areas of what is now Bangladesh.

0603 **Sweden Pakistan Family Welfare Project, Lahore.** *Training schedules: family planning doctors, Thana family planning officers, family planning supervisors, family planning assistants, union*

Abstract 0603

council secretaries, dais. Lahore, Sweden Pakistan Family Welfare Project, n.d. 6p. Engl.

Training schedules for family planning doctors, Thana family planning officers, family planning supervisors, family planning assistants, and union council secretaries indicate course content, duration of training, and training organization. Physician training, of 10-days duration, provides clinical practice in contraception emphasizing IUD use. Thana supervisors and their assistants receive 2-weeks training as an introduction to their work. Dais training involve 18 days of training in midwifery, family planning, and field work processes connected with work within the National Family Planning Programme.

V Formal Evaluative Studies

V.1 Health manpower

See also: 0026, 0074

0604 Alexander, C.A., Shivaswamy, M.K. *Traditional healers in a region of Mysore.* Social Science and Medicine (Oxford), 5(6), Dec 1971, 595-601. Engl.
A survey of 628 traditional healers in rural Mysore State, India, showed positive attitudes toward public health programmes but revealed a lack of cooperation between healers and the government health system. The status of healers is very high among people they serve. Traditional healers belong to professional organizations that protect their interests. Traditional healers in the study expressed positive approval of the government's family planning programme though most had no contact with it. Traditional healers in Mysore State handle about eight times the number of patients treated by organized government health care in the area.

0605 Colombia, Ministry of Public Health. *Estudio de recursos odontologicos. (Study of dental manpower resources).* Bogota, Ministry of Public Health 1972, Recursos Humanos Serie 1, Numero 3. 136p. Span.
This is a statistical resume relating to dentistry in Colombia. Although well documented, it does not mention what odontological human resources are available at the rural level. Eighty percent of dentistry professionals reside in Colombia's three main cities; only 7% are located in cities having 25 000 – 50 000 inhabitants. The document states that this low figure shows a lack of interest on the part of the professional to establish himself in a small community. It must be assumed, then, that oral health care available to the rural dweller is nonexistent or very limited. The activities, qualifications, and training of auxiliaries and technicians are also discussed.

0606 Cunningham, C.E. *Thai 'injection doctors': antibiotic mediators.* Social Science and Medicine (Oxford), 4, Jul 1970, 1-24. Engl.
Thailand has experienced a proliferation of uncontrolled and unlicensed rural "doctors" who inject antibiotics and do much rural curing in comparison with government physicians or herbal and occult practitioners. Changing attitudes toward medicines, village values about treatment, a gap between villagers and official health personnel, professionalization and urbanization of the modern medical profession, and an open drug market contribute to this phenomenon. Twenty-eight references are listed. (Journal abstract.)

0607 Gadalla, F.R. *Study of duties and responsibilities of physicians in maternal child health centres, in U.A.R.* Journal of the Egyptian Public Health Association (Cairo), 41(4), 1966, 183-201. Engl.
Since 1912, the number of maternal and child health centres in Egypt has increased greatly; in 1962, the Ministry of Public Health expected to staff over 2 500 rural health centres by 1970. This paper is a report on the research findings of a study determining the function of the physician in the rural maternal and child health centre. Questionnaires sent out to the physicians requested data on their duties and the problems they encountered; the findings were to be used in the preparation of a curriculum for physician training. As a result of the study, it was recommended that physicians working in these centres be given administrative training, since their attitude is crucial to the work of nursing and auxiliary health personnel. Seven references are listed.

0608 Hughes, J.M. *Ghana: paramedical personnel at VALCO.* In Hughes, J.P., ed., Health Care in Remote Areas: An International Conference, Oakland, Kaiser Foundation, 1972, 80-86. Engl.
See entry 155 for complete proceedings.
At the site of the VALCO project conducted by the Kaiser Foundation in Tema, Ghana, nurses provided primary medical care for workers. They were providing a complete range of care for injured workers, and referring patients to physicians when such action was necessary.

0609 Iran, Ministry of Health. *Health Corps: 7 years progress.* Iran, Ministry of Health, n.d. 31p. Engl.
The Health Corps was considered one of the pillars of the Revolution of the Shah and the People of Iran in 1963. The Health Corps was designed to bring health facilities to rural Iran by moving qualified physicians from cities to villages. Young doctors were required to spend 2 years in rural service. They were to be backed up by selected high school students with 6 months of intensive training in rural health programmes. The

Corps then settled in strategic villages and subcentres and conducted a predominantly preventive campaign, building sanitary facilities, vaccinating people, etc. Legal, organizational, and statistical aspects of Health Corps activities are briefly outlined.

0610 Neumann, A.K., Bhatia, J.C., Andrews, S., Murphy, A.K. *Role of the indigenous medicine practitioner in two areas of India: report of a study.* Social Science and Medicine (Oxford), 5(2), Apr 1971, 137-149. Engl.

Interviews of 72 rural indigenous medicine practitioners in India in a southern district (Kerala State) and a northern district (Punjab State) are reported, as well as the results of observations of their work while diagnosing and treating a total of 542 patients. The practitioners were located in the vicinity of two primary health centres. The stereotype of the indigenous medicine practitioner as one using traditional herbs, oils, and incantations and having little or nothing to do with modern medicine is not supported by this enquiry. The training of the men was extremely varied and ranged from an apprenticeship of a few months to 6 years of formal training in a recognized school of indigenous medicine. The practitioners were present in a ratio of about 1:1 500 of rural population and outnumbered modern (allopathic) physicians by 10:1. They treated all types of illnesses and appeared to be well regarded by the villagers. Many had stethoscopes, and the majority used modern medicine. About one-third of the patients seen in the North by the indigenous practitioners were given injections. Half of these were penicillin or streptomycin. It is suggested similar studies be carried out in India and elsewhere and the entire question of the role of indigenous practitioners and their relationship to modern medicine, especially in rural areas, be subject to critical review. Included in this is the question of the role these men might play in disseminating family planning information and supplies. Fifteen references are listed. (Journal summary.)

0611 Peng, J.Y., Nor Laily, A.B., Ariffin, M. *Village midwives in Malaysia.* Ann Arbor, Michigan, University of Michigan, School of Public Health, Department of Population Planning, Population Reprint Series, Reprint No. 50, 1972. 4p. Engl.

Results of an informal questionnaire administered to Malaysian village midwives recruited for a training programme showed positive attitudes toward provision of family planning services for married women. Most midwives interviewed expressed willingness to participate in the government programme. Integration of family planning services into rural health units in Malaysia began in 1971. Ten references are listed.

0612 Prachuabmoh, V., Muangman, D., Baumau, K., Rosenfield, A.G. *Comprehensive health planning: health manpower survey.* Chapel Hill, N.C., Carolina Population Centre, Sep 1969. 5p. Engl. Unpublished document.

Underutilization of health personnel can be studied by means of a household survey to evaluate villager attitudes to health care. Sample questions for a survey conducted in Thailand are given. Health workers' attitudes were evaluated at the same time by means of a questionnaire and through personal contact.

0613 Roemer, R. *Legal systems regulating health personnel: a comparative analysis.* Milbank Memorial Fund Quarterly (New York), 46, Oct 1968, 431-471. Engl.

An international comparison is made of legislation governing licensure of health personnel. Licensure processes affect health personnel, development of educational programmes, and development of occupation groups. Examples are taken from Sweden, Japan, Colombia, the United Kingdom, the Federal Republic of Germany, Poland, France, and the United States. In all but the United States a national health agency plays an important role in licensure. Systems interrelate with existing educational processes. Problems of standards arise as the number of new types of auxiliary staff increases. Worldwide demand for health services encourages lowering of standards and rapid deployment of staff. This means that a closer look must be taken at licensing practices in relation to standards of health care, occupational role definition, and long-term national manpower planning processes. One hundred and fifty-two references are listed.

0614 Standard, K.L., Marsh, M.C., Ennever, O. *Evaluation: community health aide programme, part II.* Kingston, Jamaica, University of the West Indies, Department of Social and Preventive Medicine, Apr 1968. 7p. Engl. Unpublished document. See also entries 437 and 484.

A 3-month experimental project to demonstrate that community health aides can successfully be used as outreach adjuncts to health teams in the West Indies is reviewed and evaluated. Ideally, such auxiliary health workers, while reflecting the values and attitudes of the communities they will service, should be sufficiently literate to be able to grasp new concepts concerning the causes of health and illness that formerly were interpreted in terms of superstition and mystery and be able to communicate these new concepts to the community in ways that would influence attitudes and stimulate awareness of the importance of maintaining good health standards. The programme emphasized the concept "man in his total environment," in addition to training in practical health skills. All eight trainees found employment in health work at the end of the course. Functions and duties of the community health aide are listed.

0615 Tribhuvan University, Kathmandu. *Proposal for health manpower research project.* Kathmandu, Nepal, Tribhuvan University, Jul 1972. 12p. Engl. Unpublished document.

Health manpower training in Nepal has been related to the educational traditions inherited from the British colonial system and ad hoc training efforts. New approaches to training are being developed that will attempt to meet consumers' needs and to solve problems such as the lack of continuing education for health personnel. Appropriate consultants, university support, and government participation are considered.

V.2 Organization and administration

See also: 0168, 0305, 0309, 0317, 0318, 0320, 0333, 0666, 0667, 0669, 0670, 0686

0616   Abelin, S., Larsson, Y., Segersky, U.B. *Medical services and public health in Tanzania: report with proposal for a Swedish assistance project.* Stockholm, Swedish International Development Authority, Health and Nutrition Unit, 14 Feb 1972. 30p. Engl.
Unpublished document.

As the result of a request for Swedish assistance in developing rural health centres, the historical background of Tanzania's health sector from 1961 to 1971 is reviewed. This report, setting out proposals for a Swedish aid project, establishes that although the number of medical institutions has increased, the supply of health personnel, with the exception of nurses, has not kept pace with demand. The increase in population, inflation, and bureaucratic problems impede progress, and curative services consume more of the available resources than do preventive services, so that urban areas have benefitted while the situation in the rural areas has not changed. However, increasing concern with rural development is seen as an indication of rethinking of priorities by those responsible for medical and public health services and support for selected key targets such as construction and equipment of health centres and a school for medical aides, training and education of health personnel, and provision of doctors is advocated. Statistical data are appended.

0617   Adesuyi, S.L., Horn, J.S., Shehu, U., Salawu, F.A., Austen-Peters, A.O. *Priorities in health care.* In Akinkugbe, O.O., Olatunbosun, D., Esan, G.J., eds., Priorities in National Health Planning: Proceedings of an International Symposium, Ibadan, Caxton Press (West Africa) Ltd., 1973, 11-40. Engl.
See entry 123 for full report of symposium.

The chapter covers five papers on priorities in health care. The first paper lists the priorities as: training of health manpower; control of communicable diseases; environmental health programmes; and expansion of basic health services in Nigeria. It claims that although the concept of medical assistants did not work in Nigeria, the country has the necessary infrastructure to train more doctors to meet the demand. The second paper explores the health care system of the People's Republic of China and suggests that developing countries should adopt aspects of China's system, which would improve their own standards of health care. Paper three analyzes the health delivery system in Nigeria and advocates the introduction of an integrated system. The fourth paper lists some common health administration problems and common diseases in Nigeria and suggests ways to combat them. Paper five discusses the medical manpower needs in Nigeria. Subsequent discussion focusses on priorities in health care, medical assistants, health care delivery in the People's Republic of China, rural health care, and medical social workers.

0618   Akim, N.B. Tanzania, Ministry of Health. *Impressions of a Tanzanian delegation on Cuban health services.* Dar es Salaam, Ministry of Health, 16 Oct 1972. 15p. Engl.
Unpublished document.

A 2-week visit to Cuba for the purpose of studying rural health services included visits to 13 health establishments (hospitals, convalescent centres, medical schools, etc.). Cuba has a well-developed health service with special campaigns against malaria, tuberculosis, leprosy, etc., and immunization programmes. General health progress is the result of a high standard of living. Given the same conditions, the author believes Tanzania could achieve similar health standards.

0619   Arnhold, R.G., Pike, M.C. *Patients and prescriptions: understanding medical instructions. (A study in an East African dispensary).* Journal of Tropical Pediatrics and Environmental Child Health (Kampala), 14, Mar 1968, 10-11. Engl.

In Uganda free medical care is given in government clinics. The staff have a small number of drugs to be dispensed directly and additional drugs are dispensed by a pharmacy with written instructions. A medical student interviewed parents of children being treated at the Mulago Hill Dispensary to test their understanding of instructions for prescribed medications. About 20% of the parents misunderstood at least some of the directions. A more detailed survey was designed to find out the reasons for this high rate of misunderstanding and particularly to see if the use of different labels would improve understanding. Four different labels were tested. These were used 2 days each during an 8-day period in random order and 795 parents were interviewed. Literate parents consistently did better, but in general one in four parents did not understand how to administer the drugs. The simple system of writing only numbers gave as good results as systems where words were used, for both literate and illiterate parents.

0620   Ashitey, G.A., Wurapa, F.K., Belcher, D.W. *Danfa rural health centre: its patients and services 1970-71.* Ghana Medical Journal (Accra), 11(3), Sep 1972, 266-273. Engl.

In 1970 evaluation methods were used to study the operation of the Danfa Rural Health Centre, located north of Accra, Ghana. The project is divided into three parts, with each part providing a different type of service to its respective area. Task analyses were made for project workers. Detailed job descriptions were drawn up from which training changes could be made. The age-sex characteristics of those using the services were studied. Timed patient-flow studies indicate that the average time spent by a patient at the centre was 4 hours. The typical patient was young and suffered from a disease that could be readily diagnosed and treated by paramedical staff, using relatively few drugs. Most health centre visitors live within 3 miles of the centre; there is little contact with preschool children and pregnant women in villages that are farther than 3 miles from the centre. As a result of the study, staff retraining was begun and two mobile clinics were started for women and preschoolers living away from the centre. Five references are listed.

0621 Bice, T.W., White, K.L. *Cross-national comparative research on the utilization of medical services.* Medical Care (Philadelphia), 9(3), May-Jun 1971, 253-271. Engl.

A health services system is comprised of two conceptually distinct yet mutually dependent subsystems, a public health (or environmental health services) system, and a medical care (or personal health) system. Assuming that there is fundamental agreement among nations concerning the goals of medical care systems, then the variability in means employed to achieve them provides a rationale for carrying out cross-national comparative utilization research. Research on the utilization of medical services is concerned with medical transactions occurring between patients and health professionals and facilities within medical care systems and with the outcomes of these transactions. This paper examines four types of cross-national studies, methodological problems in utilization research, and the relationships between research and evaluation and decision-making. Seventy-eight references are listed.

0622 Chang, W.P. *Appraisal of health problems and definition of priorities in planning of health development: outlines of the presentation for a panel discussion.* Addis Ababa, Haile Selassie I University, Faculty of Medicine, May 1969. 9p. Engl.
Unpublished document.
Fifth Annual Medical Conference of the Ethiopian Medical Association, Ethiopia, 29 May 1969.

In order to define priorities for health development in Ethiopia, present resources and current health problems have to be analyzed. Communicable preventable diseases overwhelm curative resources and result in health problems for great numbers of people. The population is very scattered. Reaching people with services is difficult in rural areas, many of which are accessible only in the dry season. A great need for trained manpower exists there. Problems will not be solved by building large hospitals. Rather, the more effective and economic approach to health care delivery in a country such as Ethiopia, with numerous health problems and limited resources, is the preventive one. This calls for the use of lower- and middle-level medical personnel, backed up by adequate financial support, supervision, administrative techniques, and professional career structuring. Statistical data on medical facilities, manpower supply, and project needs are included in this article. Three references are listed.

0623 Colombia, Ministry of Public Health. *Estudio de instituciones de atencion medica (Anexo): informe general. (Study of health care delivery facilities (Annex): general information).* Bogota, Ministry of Public Health, Institute for Special Health Programs, Series II, No. 3, Nov 1971. 49p. Span.
See also entry 6.

This document presents the results of the Colombian government's survey of medical institutions. The study embraces all hospital institutions and the majority of outpatient services. All aspects of manpower resources, financing, organization and administration, and registration methods were meticulously researched. An analysis of the data indicates the necessity for changing registration methods since basic information on the activities of medical institutions was not being compiled.

0624 Courtejoie, J., Herman, F. *Une experience d'education sanitaire en Afrique centrale. (An experiment in health education in Central Africa).* Revue Medicale de Liege (Liege), 21(11), 1 Jun 1966, 265-267. Fren.

The vital importance of pretesting audiovisual aids used in health education is emphasized. The authors tested material, developed in Nigeria, in the Mayumbe area of the Central Zaire province of Zaire. Two main obstacles were encountered: a lack of total comprehension of the scenes, i.e. many people interpreted various factors without relating them to each other; and an inability to identify with the Nigerians represented in the pictures. To simplify the causal sequence, the number of pictures was increased. Pictures drawn from photos of local village scenes were used. The results were tested on different groups of women. It was discovered that the women preferred being represented as they would like to live, rather than as they presently live. They identified with what appealed to them. Despite current trends toward developing educational material with cross-cultural validity, the process of pretesting, though time consuming, is considered worthwhile because it enables the educator to avoid misunderstanding and to gain a deeper insight into the psychological and cultural factors that condition the success of any health education programme.

0625 Dahlin, L. *Medical services and public health in Zambia: report with proposal for Swedish assistance.* Stockholm, Swedish International Development Authority, Health and Nutrition Unit, Jan 1973. 31p. Engl.
Unpublished document.

This report comments on Zambia's health situation and health administration. Statistics are given for physical resources available as of 1971, i.e. hospitals, health centres, and dental and maternal and child health services. An examination of medical manpower reveals a shortage of all categories of personnel. The first and second National Development Plans strove, with externally financed assistance, to extend preventive services, training schemes, and medical facilities in rural areas. The report supports a request for Swedish assistance with the training of health personnel, central planning, nutritional problems, and maternal and child health care in accordance with the objectives of Zambia's Ten Year National Health Plan. Full details of the plan, including statistical data concerning health centres, staffing, and financing, are given.

0626 Del Mundo, F., Soriano, L.R. *Observations on health attitudes and preparation for illness among 150 rural families in the Philippines.* Journal of the Philippines Medical Association (Manila), 41(9), Sep 1965, 657-666. Engl.

Health improvement for the Philippines' rural poor began by organizing a network of rural health units. This was preceded by a study of 150 rural families to ascertain their attitudes toward and preparedness for illness, and their reactions to medical assistance. Despite alarmingly low income, 70% of rural families were interested in and concerned with health matters. Only 4% showed apathy, and the rest were health conscious but needed more information and incentive. Five references are listed.

0627 Dempsey, J.J., Grant, J.A. *Viewing program evaluation as a component of the administrative process: the RAGPIE model.* Perspectives in Maternal and Child Health (Boston), Series B (4), Sep 1971, 1-6. Engl.

The advantages and disadvantages of the RAGPIE (resources, activities, goals, planning, implementation, evaluation) evaluation model, which considers programme evaluation to be an integral part of the administrative process, are discussed. The RAGPIE model has proved itself to be of use in programme administration, service coordination, teaching, research, and consultation. Five references are listed.

0628 Dunlop, D.W. *Development of an output concept for analysis of curative health services.* Social Science and Medicine (Oxford), 6, 1972, 373-385. Engl.

This paper focusses on a major theoretical issue in medical economics: the conceptualization of output commonly employed in analyses of health services. Homogeneous concepts, such as patient days, are viewed as inadequate; convenient measures, such as the number of trained manpower or beds per unit of population are discarded as analytically unsound. It is suggested that in order to improve upon the present conceptualization, it is important to consider that the output of a health services firm is not homogeneous, but rather consists of a set of individuals who have: (1) contracted one or more given diseases; (2) have received various diagnostic and treatment services specific to the contracted disease; and (3) have responded in varying degrees to the services received. A brief note discusses an analysis of health services in Uganda, in which the output concept presented here was employed. Thirty-three references are listed. (Journal abstract.)

0629 Evans, T. WHO, Manila. *Public health administration, final report.* Manila, WHO, 3 Sep 1962. 86p. WHO/WPR/382/62. Engl.
Unpublished document.

A report on public health administration in the Philippines by WHO short-term consultants examines: (1) training programmes for rural health personnel; (2) organization, administration, and programmes of the rural health services; (3) integration of the health services with rural health services; and (4) coordination of rural health unit programmes with official and voluntary organizations in the medical, health, and related fields. Appended are copies of information sheets for completion by rural health unit staff, interview guide for use in assessing the national rural health programme, interview guide for use of regional training centre staff, a map showing itinerary of the assessment team, and notes on the environmental health aspects of the rural health services. Preservice and inservice training of rural health personnel should be the subject of a formal study. The team was only able to give rough indications of training needs for health team members other than sanitation workers. Closer relationships are recommended between regional and provincial health staff and the staff of training centres.

0630 Fry, J. *Medicine in three societies: a comparison of medical care in the USSR, USA and UK.* New York, American Elsevier Publications, 1970. 249p. Engl.

This publication compares and contrasts systems of medical care in the USSR, USA, and U.K. The author collected data for the study in the 1960's during his visits to the USA and USSR where he was able to study all levels and forms of medical services. The contents deal with the philosophy of medical care and with the components and levels of administration. In all systems, there are first-contact services providing primary care with specialist services available at hospitals. A section is devoted to each level and an analysis made of the ways in which the three systems provide these services. Two specific topics, maternity and child care and mental illness, are then taken to examine how care is provided in each system. The training and structure of the greater medical profession is described and finally some personal thoughts are given on future needs. The difficulties of attempting to compare the three systems are recognized.

0631 Habicht, J.P., Guzman, G., Reyna-Barrios, J.M. *Outpatient curative medical care provided by a paramedical staff: needs, practicability, and quality control.* Bethesda, Md., National Institute

V Formal Evaluative Studies

of Child Health and Human Development, National Institutes of Health, n.d. 45p. Engl. Unpublished document.

The principles, background, and organization of curative outpatient medical services are presented for a programme in four Guatemalan rural communities. These services were provided under physician supervision by paramedical personnel trained in history-taking, diagnosis, and therapy. High quality ambulatory care was achieved at moderate cost. Since curative services had high priority in the eyes of the villagers, the workers were able to introduce preventive measures along with curative work. Villagers' medical needs were investigated, various kinds of care were evaluated in terms of practicability, and the system was maintained to provide information on methods of improving it. The care was provided through dispensaries at a cost of U.S. $2.26 per inhabitant per year, including all medicines, which represents a saving of 50% on costs before the system was instituted. Ten references are listed.

0632   Hilario, J. *Valor economico de saude. (Economic value of health).* Revista Brasileira de Malariologia e Doencas Tropicais (Rio de Janeiro), 18, Jan-Mar 1966, 189-198. Portuguese.

The relationship between health and productivity is well known. Poor health contributes to low productivity, low productivity to low salaries, poor nutrition, education, and living conditions, which in turn lead to even lower productivity, thus perpetuating the vicious circle of poverty and underdevelopment. An analysis of Brazil's health problems illustrates how these factors serve to maintain the permanent underdeveloped condition of the country. Some 40-60% of the population consume goods and services produced by the rest of the population, but because of preventable endemic and epidemic disease and chronic malnutrition, they die before reaching an age where they become part of the productive labour force. These figures compare unfavourably with those of, for example, the United States and Sweden, where less than 10% of the population die before the age of 20. The serious housing problem (a shortage of 7 million housing units), together with the fact that 50% of existing dwellings do not have running water or sewage disposal facilities, contributes in large measure to the country's high morbidity rates. The author suggests that health care is a government responsibility and recommends greater recognition of the right of the individual to better health, living, and working standards.

0633   International Hospital Federation, Washington, D.C. *Summaries of papers presented to the Eighteenth International Hospital Congress discussion group on health services in remote and sparsely populated areas, Montreal, 17-22 June 1973.* Washington, D.C., International Hospital Federation, 1973. 15p. Engl. Unpublished document.

Health services in remote and sparsely populated areas is the topic of conference papers from Australia, Brazil, Canada, Chile, Colombia, Fiji, Norway, and Tunisia. Brazil reports that the proliferation of government and private agencies responsible for health care delivery, each acting independently of the rest, and the lack of a total health care programme, is hampering development of the Amazon region and its integration with the rest of the country. In Tunisia, lack of trained manpower is a problem. This is overcome in Fiji where the Health Services is part of the Civil Service, by deployment of medical staff. Colombia reports control of yellow fever through vaccination campaigns and advances in research of viral diseases transmitted by anthropods. The problems of communication and supply are overcome by the use of air ambulances (Australia, Canada, Fiji). In Fiji the public mass media is used to disseminate health education.

0634   Jones, G., Boonpratuang, C. *Effect of population growth and urbanization on the attainment of public health goals in Thailand.* Bangkok, National Economic Development Board, Manpower Planning Division, May 1972. 72p. Engl. Unpublished document.

Research indicates that Thailand requires increased government spending for rural areas, lower attrition rates, and reduced population growth, if health services are to be effective.

0635   Karunaratne, W.A. *Zambian health services and its development.* n.p., n.d. 12p. Engl. Unpublished document.

Zambia's health services are described. Figures for existing health resources (hospitals, hospital beds, graduate doctors) and special services (dental, mother and child health services, etc.) are presented. Health problems such as malnutrition, and preventable diseases such as leprosy and malaria, which account for nearly 50% of morbidity, could be lessened by educating people. Development plans for 1972-76 (including general objectives, organization, expenditure, and personnel training) are briefly stated.

0636   Katsuta, K., Takeshita, K., Nakao, A., Shibata, T., Hozumi, M. *(Four years medical observations in a remote village at Fukuoka-ken).* IRYO (Medical Journal of the National Hospitals and Sanatoriums of Japan) (Tokyo), 22(3), Mar 1968, 387-393. Japanese.

The Hobashira Clinic was established in July 1962 in a remote village at Fukuoka-ken, Japan. Its parent hospital is the National Kokura Hospital. During the next 4 years, statistical observations were made. In the first year after opening the Hobashira Clinic, the average number of outpatients per day was 23.7. The number of outpatients then decreased year by year as the population in the village decreased. From 1966 the average number of outpatients per day was less than 20. In the parent hospital in 1962 the average number of outpatients per day per physician was 33.4, and the average number of patients increased year by year up to 35.9 in 1966. Patient's payment per day in the Hobashira Clinic was 220 yen less than that of the outpatient clinic in the parent hospital. During 4 years 68 cases from the

Hobashira Clinic were transferred to the parent hospital. Each physician must spend about 3 weeks in a year in the clinic to perform medical duties there. In other words, in the parent hospital one physician is always absent during the year.

0637 Korn, J. Institute for Development Research, Copenhagen. *Report from the health sectors in Kenya and Tanzania.* Copenhagen, Institute for Development Research, IDR Internal Paper E 73.2, Mar 1973. 31p. Engl.
Unpublished document.

This report reviews present and planned health programmes in Kenya and Tanzania and participation by donor agencies in these plans. Kenya's planning stresses the rural health sector and includes family planning. The following have assisted in Kenya's health sector: World Health Organization, International Bank for Reconstruction and Development, Food and Agriculture Organization, the Netherlands, Finland, etc. Danish aid has financed several training health centres, especially the Community Nurse Training School in Eldoret, graduates of which are essential to health delivery programmes. The author proposes further Danish assistance to the Eldoret School, a survey of existing health facilities, and a seminar on Kenyan rural health. Tanzania emphasizes the development of rural health services as well. Plans for staff training include physicians, medical assistants, nurse-midwives, and a cadre of mother and child health aides (Kenya's Community Nurse) to bring family planning to rural areas. As in Kenya, international aid finances construction of rural health centres, mental hospitals, provision of equipment, etc. Danish aid includes a bilharziasis control project, two schools for health auxiliaries, two district hospitals, etc. Among the author's proposals for future Danish aid are an onchocerciasis eradication programme and a plague diagnostic unit. Twenty-one references are listed.

0638 Litman, T.J., Robins, L. *Comparative analysis of health care systems: a socio-political approach.* Social Science and Medicine (Oxford), 5(6), Dec 1971, 573-581. Engl.

There has been increased interest in a comparative analysis of national health care systems. Analyses have suffered from inattention to the sociopolitical factors that shape health care development and operation. Although application of a carefully translated, highly standardized set of questions on health and health care to a sample population living under a diversity of sociopolitical conditions may provide valuable information on the health status of people and on health services, idiosyncratic features of the systems studied may be ignored. Sociopolitical factors must be considered early and taken into account in the design of the study. Fifty-four references are listed.

0639 Lucas, A.O., Ebie, J.C., Ransome-Kuti, A.O., Okojie, C.G., Graham-Douglas, M.S. *Preventive vs. curative.* In Akinkugbe, O.O., Olatunbosun, D., Esan, G.J., eds., Priorities in National Health Planning: Proceedings of an International Symposium, Ibadan, Caxton Press (West Africa) Ltd., 1973, 43-78. Engl.
See entry 123 for full report of symposium.

The chapter deals with five papers on preventive and curative medicine. The first paper reviews the causes for the gap between the stated ideal and actual performance of the health services of developing countries, under four major headings: conceptual problems, information systems, organization and administrative problems, and technical and scientific problems. The second paper outlines the development of the health services in the Mid-western State of Nigeria, supporting it with hospital and health statistics. It advocates the adoption of the health centre concept in the state. Paper three examines the first 15 causes of child morbidity, as found in Lagos University Teaching Hospital. All are infectious diseases and indicate the poor environment of the children. It proposes the establishment of the family health clinic as a means of promoting community health. The fourth paper lists examples of typical patients in the rural areas of Nigeria: an 18-month-old boy infested with worms, a child with measles, and a boy with intramuscular guineaworm abscesses. It claims that these common diseases emphasize the need for preventive medicine more than curative medicine in such communities where doctors are in short supply. Paper five examines provision of the Nigerian Second National Development Programme and suggests the establishment of a medical manpower board that will ensure adequate training of the necessary manpower. The general discussion centred attention on the dichotomy between preventive and curative medicine, additional training for nurses, the adequacy of hospital equipment and drugs, the importance of health education, maintenance of standards in the hospitals, and community health programmes.

0640 Margulies, H. *Medical manpower for rural areas.* Washington, D.C., U.S. Department of Health, Education and Welfare, 21 Mar 1969. 9p. Engl.

The author begins with reminiscences of the inadequate health services available in his native rural Jackson County, South Dakota in 1928, comparing them to those in some developing countries today. He observes that the U.S. is rapidly becoming an urbanized society and the rate of producing trained physicians is not increasing rapidly enough to keep up with the population explosion. This creates a problem for rural areas because, despite the many innovative efforts to entice physicians to establish a rural practice, new physicians are concentrated in the urban areas. However, the problem of inadequate rural health services is not hopeless if the small communities will take advantage of those people in their communities who have some background and experience in health service. Such local services, aided by modern technology, can have a very positive effect on the health service problem in rural America. In addition, the passing of recent federal legislation aimed at area-wide planned health services can further alleviate this recognized problem.

0641   McKeown, T. *The next forty years in public health.* Population Studies (London), 17, 1964, 269-292. Engl.

The author discusses principal causes of morbidity and mortality and predicts future trends. Methods to deal with these problems are suggested, i.e. control of inheritance in man and control of environmental agents. Medical services are examined critically in relation to contemporary needs and suggestions are made concerning possible changes.

0642   Medalie, J.H., Mann, K.J. Kiryat Hayovel Health Centre, Jerusalem. Hadassah Medical Organization, Jerusalem. *Evaluation of medical care: methodological problems in a 6-year follow up of a family and community health center.* Journal of Chronic Diseases (London), 19, 1966, 17-33. Engl.

Methodological problems are reviewed for a 6-year follow-up of a family and community health centre in a new immigrant housing section in Jerusalem. The purpose of the programme was to integrate previously uncoordinated services, to make them more efficient and economical. Kinds of services and kinds of illnesses presented are reviewed for the period under examination, against national figures for the same period. Although most of the major predetermined objectives of the centre were achieved, it was not possible to estimate the exact contribution of the health centre to the significantly improved local health status. Forty-two references are listed.

0643   Omran, A.R. *Impact of economic development on health patterns in Egypt.* Archives of Environmental Health (Chicago), 13, Jul 1966, 117-124. Engl.

Egypt's major medical, sanitary, sociocultural, and administrative problems before 1952 are summarized and illustrated by specific examples. After 1952, the death rate decreased, the size of lower age groups increased as a result of the reduction in infant and preschool mortality, and there was an increase in life expectancy, indicating significant social and medical change. Since 1952 there has been an almost complete absence of major epidemics. As regards endemic diseases, fewer deaths have occurred from tuberculosis, and young children have been successfully protected from schistosomiasis infection. Sanitation services have increased the supply of clean water to villages. As a result of increased budget, facilities, manpower, rural health services, and endemic disease centres, significant changes have taken place in health services. An extensive project is underway to set up some 2 500 rural health units headed by a physician, each serving 5 000 rural inhabitants. It is concluded that a comprehensive health index, sensitive to early changes in health levels, is still in great demand. Sixteen references are listed.

0644   Pakistan, Health Department of West Pakistan. *Report by the health study group: March 1970.* Lahore, Superintendent, Government Printing, Punjab, 1971. 99p. Engl.

This report, put out by the Department of Health, West Pakistan, contains a section entitled "Rural Health Programme". During the Second Five Year Plan, a network of rural health centres, each consisting of a central unit and three secondary units and servicing a population of 50 000, was set up. The preventive approach was stressed. The objective of the plan was to establish 150 such health centres, but only 62 were actually established. Despite the aim of the Third Plan (1965-70) to provide 500 centres, there were still only 86 by 1971. Lack of personnel rather than lack of funds was responsible for this failure. It is concluded that, since revitalization of rural health is essential to urban health and the health of the nation, the training of personnel to man these centres should be of high priority. One hundred and twenty-one references are listed.

0645   Pan American Health Organization, Washington, D.C. *Delivery of primary care by medical auxiliaries: techniques of utilization and analysis of benefits achieved in some rural villages in Guatemala.* Washington, D.C., Pan American Health Organization, 1973. 45p. Engl.
Unpublished document.
PAHO Advisory Committee on Medical Research, Twelfth Meeting, Washington, D.C., 25 Jun 1973.

A comparative study of two forms of curative-preventive medical programmes for rural areas in Guatemala indicated that one form uses nonphysician, auxiliary personnel, whereas the other uses physicians to deliver care. Data on extent of coverage, case loads, referral rates, and costs show that infant mortality can be halved and preschool mortality quartered by providing medical services through nonprofessional primary care personnel. Nonphysician care was acceptable to Indian and non-Indian populations in rural Guatemala. Cost comparisons show nonphysician care greatly reduces the cost of care, even for highly supervised nonphysician programmes. Additionally, rural medical programmes can serve as nuclei for community development projects in general. Seven references are listed.

0646   Rabin, D.L. *International comparisons of medical care.* Milbank Memorial Fund Quarterly (New York), 50(3), Jul 1972, 1-99. Engl.

Six papers present in brief the results of scientific inquiry into health services and health services systems. Two purposes of the investigation were (1) to develop methods of comparison of health services in different populations and (2) to establish the fact that patterns of health services have measurable differences and similarities. Salient features of the study are organization and development, methods, ecological results, resources and systems, behavioural results, and methodological results.

0647   Raman, M.V. *Study of some aspects of mortality and medical facilities in India.* Indian Journal of Public Health (Calcutta), 12(1), Jan 1968, 1-15. Engl.

India's registration system for vital statistics suffers from qualitative and quantitative defects. Estimates of vital rates are made from time to time from continuing rounds of the National Sample Survey. From 1958 to 1968 there was a decline in the death rate and an increase in life expectancy. However, in the absence of corresponding changes in the social and economic situation, the declining mortality trend cannot long be sustained. Health progress depends on economic progress. Urban death rates are found to be as high or even higher than rural ones. Private native practitioners meet some of the needs in rural areas. Twenty-three references are listed.

0648 Ranganna, M.G., Prasad, B.G., Bhatnagar, J.K. *Study of medical care services provided by the primary health center, Sarojini Nagar, Lucknow, India.* Medical Care (Philadelphia), 6(5), Sep-Oct 1968, 412-418. Engl.

In 1968 there were 4 898 primary health centres providing care to rural areas in India. These centres integrate preventive and curative approaches to care, decentralize services, and ensure maximum community cooperation. This study attempts to determine productivity of staff, attitudes of patients toward the services and staff of the primary health centre at Sarojini Nagar, Lucknow, and the extent to which services are used by the people. The centre evaluated is not altogether typical in that it provides more than the usual services and staff. Observations were recorded for 1 month of the average daily work load of various sections of the centre and staff, the morbidity pattern among those seeking treatment, and the time spent by each patient at the centre. Data from outpatient, inpatient and laboratory registers for 1966 were analyzed. A questionnaire was used in an attitude survey carried out in five villages within a 5-mile radius of the centre, to determine distances travelled by patients to obtain treatment, means of transport, reasons for use or nonuse of services, etc. The main findings were: medical care provided by the centre is inadequate because the population to be served is too large and patients must travel too far to obtain treatment; the unavailability and poor quality of medicines, and the lack of facilities for tooth extractions, etc. cause dissatisfaction among patients. Fourteen references are listed.

0649 Roemer, M.I., Manning, O. *Strengthening of health services and training of health personnel.* Manila, WHO, Feb 1969. 150p. WHO/WPR/56/69. Engl.

Unpublished document. Assignment report, Malaysia 0035.

A WHO report on strengthening health services and health personnel training in West Malaysia emphasizes health administration, nursing, and research needs. The report includes historical material, a description of health services, the rural health scheme, and health manpower training programmes, as well as recommendations for improving rural health services. Appendices provide 90 references for further reading and survey results concerning the rural midwife in West Malaysia.

0650 Spruyt, D.J., Elder, F.B., Messing, S.D., Wade, M.K., Ryder, B., Prince, J.S., Tseghe, Y. *Ethiopia's health centre program: its impact on community health.* Ethiopian Medical Journal (Addis Ababa), 6(3), Jul 1967, 1-87. Engl.

Ethiopian Medical Association, Third Annual Meeting, Ethiopia, May 1967.

This Demonstration and Evaluation Project of the Ministry of Public Health, Ethiopia, and USAID, was started in 1961 as a 6-year study of Ethiopia's rural health centre programme. Health conditions in three selected health centre communities and three matched control communities were studied at the time the health centre programme was initiated. The study was repeated 4 years later to measure programme effectiveness. This study project relates to the work of the Gondar Public Health College and Training Centre, which trains auxiliary workers for rural health centres. Teams of health staff trained at Gondar deliver decentralized health service to remote and rural areas of Ethiopia. Evaluation study design, functional analysis of health workers' duties, health centre activities, and the study findings and recommendations are discussed. Recommendations, although not exhaustive, cover basic points, such as improving rural water supplies, upgrading organization and financial assistance to health centres, and educational training for health centre staff. Thirty-one references are listed.

0651 Swedish International Development Agency, Stockholm. *Hopitaux, Equipements, Medicaments et Preparations Chimiques a Destination de la Republique Democratique du Vietnam (RDV). (Hospitals, equipment, medicines and pharmaceuticals destined for the Democratic Republic of Vietnam).* Stockholm, Swedish International Development Authority, Health and Nutrition Unit, 1973. 20p. Fren.

Unpublished document.

Developments in the health sector of the Democratic Republic of Vietnam during and after the French colonial period are reviewed. Present needs, health administration, maternal and child health services, facilities for sick children, and medical facilities in general are described. Suggestions made by the North Vietnamese that funds offered by Norway, Sweden, Denmark, and Finland be applied to building and equipping a children's hospital and a general hospital, supplying medicines and equipment to existing centres, etc., were agreed to. The report considers that the part of the project proposal concerning supply of medicines and equipment is sufficiently well defined as to present no problems. As regards the hospitals, however, several details concerning final costs, construction phases, procedures, etc., remain to be worked out.

0652 Tekirli, N., ed(s). *Koysel bolge saglik hizmetlerini degerlendirme metodolojisi. (Methodology and evaluation of health services in rural areas).* Ankara, Tisa Matbaacilik Sanayii, 1972. 265p. Turkish.

V Formal Evaluative Studies

The report is the result of a functional system analysis of the health services in rural areas in Turkey. The research was conducted jointly by the Ankara School of Hygiene of the National Health and Welfare Ministry in Turkey, and the School of Hygiene and Public Health of the Johns Hopkins University. The project was sponsored by USAID through the Johns Hopkins University. Research was conducted to find the appropriate methodology to be used in the determination of: (1) the needs and the demands in health services of rural area population; and (2) the activities of the community health centres, which are the smallest units, in order to bring health services to the rural area population. It is hoped that the report, which exposes present weaknesses in this area, will be useful in the implementation of the health socialization program in Turkey. The research was conducted during 1966-69 in two stages. A pilot study was done at the village of Etimesut (Ankara). The basic research was done in some regions of Kars, Mus, and Diyarbakir. The report consists of the following chapters: general information on Turkey; development of health services in Turkey; functional analysis research of institutions that administer health services in Turkey; findings about villages and evaluation; findings about health organizations and evaluations; findings about the concept of illness and evaluation; findings about the treatment of illnesses in rural areas and evaluation; findings about mother and child care and family planning and evaluation; and conclusion and suggestions. Forty-eight references are listed.

0653 Tiglao, T.V. *Role of public health in community development in the Philippine setting.* Chapel Hill, University of North Carolina, n.d. 15p. Engl.
Community Development Seminar Working Paper No. 5.

A project in the Philippines began by diagnosing the community's socioeconomic, cultural, and health status. Innovations were made in the public health services, e.g. the addition of essential services, provision of supplies, in-service training for public health personnel, etc. Integration of agencies such as agricultural cooperatives and the Public Works Department resulted in improved roads, wells, farming techniques, etc. Ten years after the programmes' initiation, there were noticeable improvements in personal health practices. There was a positive correlation between community consciousness and acceptance of health innovations. Ten references are listed.

0654 Wakatsuki, T. *Role of general practitioners in villages for improvement of health services for rural population in Asia.* Varna, Fifth International Congress of Rural Medicine, 11 May 1972. 6p. Engl.
Fifth International Congress of Rural Medicine, Varna, Zlatni Pjassutsi, 11 May 1972.

In Asia, there is a great shortage of medical doctors, and most doctors are concentrated in urban areas. The appropriate form of health service seems to be that of the Soviet Union, in that it offers comprehensive health services to the entire nation, and integrates disease prevention with medical service. The People's Republic of China is also setting an example by focussing medical services on farm villages. General practitioners in Asia should conduct mass physical examinations and group health checks, and play a greater role in preventive medicine and education programmes. Practitioners' remunerations for disease prevention work should be authorized in the medical insurance system. Each country must train general practitioners and assign them to villages within 2 years after graduation.

0655 Weinerman, E.R. *Research on comparative health service systems.* Medical Care (Philadelphia), 9(3), May-Jun 1971, 272-290. Engl.

There is a pressing need for international comparative research of health services. This paper attempts to review the theoretical considerations in cross-national research on comparative health service systems, to survey the relevant publications in this field, to identify problems and needs related to such research, and to project possible lines of study for the future. Four basic goals of cross-national study are identified: (1) to rationalize the existing health service systems in relation to the values and resources of the society; (2) to provide for flexible adaption to changing human needs and scientific potentialities; (3) to establish appropriate priorities for the health service subsystem in the overall national context; and (4) to expedite the transformation of knowledge and resources to health values through the intervention of health services of optimum effectiveness and efficiency. An annotated bibliography of 64 publications is included.

0656 White, K.L., Andjelkovic, D., Pearson, R.J., Mabry, J.H., Ross, A., Sagen, O.K. *International comparisons of medical care utilization.* New England Journal of Medicine (Boston), 277(10), 7 Sep 1967, 516-522. Engl.

In spite of substantial differences in ways of life, in organization of health services, and in reported morbidity and disability, people in three widely differing communities appear to consult doctors in a similar fashion. The possibility exists that there is a propensity for consulting doctors for curative services, which may be unrelated to the number of doctors available. Different factors may influence use of preventive services. Patterns of hospital utilization vary substantially in these three communities, and the differences raise interesting questions about the ways in which hospitals are organized and used in each. Internal consistency in similarities and differences of rates observed is reassuring; most standard errors are acceptable. The consistency of hospital utilization data with what is known about national data in the three areas affords additional confidence in the methods. Validation studies indicate that the methods are responsive to the problems. Epidemiologic methods employing household interviews appear suitable for international and regional comparisons of medical-care utilization. These collaborative studies require prompt communication and frequent conferences among all participants. With the use of refinements of our questionnaires, manuals, and computer programmes, it appears practical to undertake simultaneous studies of larger populations in different regions within several countries. Such studies should permit testing hypotheses concerning relations between availability of health personnel and resources, methods of organizing medical care, and paying for services and utilization of services. (Author summary.)

0657 WHO, Geneva. *Evaluation of environmental health programmes: report of a WHO scientific group.* Geneva, WHO Technical Report Series No. 528, 1973. 64p. Engl.

A WHO technical report on evaluation of environmental health programmes reviews the historical background, the purposes of programme evaluation, programme characteristics in environmental health, problems of norms and design, and issues in the conduct of programme evaluation in environmental health. It is concluded that the plethora of approaches, terms, and conceptual systems in programme evaluation must be codified to be of general use, that evaluation practice could be improved by increasing the quantity and quality of manpower resources, that many difficulties in the conduct of evaluation studies appear to be connected with sociopsychological factors in administrative organizations, etc. Efforts must be made to train public health workers in programme evaluation. International collaboration in the field of environmental health is a necessity in dealing with environmental health problems. Definitions of terms used in the report and a selected bibliography of approximately 75 references are provided.

0658 WHO, Geneva. *Local health service: third report of the Expert Committee on Public Administration.* Geneva, WHO Technical Report Series No. 194, 1960. 49p. Engl.

This report considers the methodology of local health studies. Study of local services in the community context and in the family context are suggested as models for local administrators in charge of planning. These health surveys should be conducted by health officers and their staff with a view to educating local level personnel in particular health problems of the community. Effective administration is important for decentralizing health services. Staff at local levels must apply health education and community development principles in their work. Standards for local level service administration are set forth. Pilot studies from Mysore (India), Zutphen (Netherlands), Trujillo Alto (Puerto Rico), Zulu Reserve, Natal (South Africa), and Loughborough (U.K.) are discussed.

V.3 Planning

See also: 0637, 0640

0659 Mabry, J.H. *International studies of health care.* Medical Care (Philadelphia), 9(3), May-Jun 1971, 193-202. Engl.

In 1969, 36 sociomedical scientists met to encourage international collaboration on, and to assess sociological studies of, medical and health care within a cross-national perspective. The workshop focussed on comparative studies of epidemiologic problems, perception of and response to symptoms of illness, organization and planning of health services, health manpower and resources, the use of health services, and comparative health systems. The workshop stressed personal health services with minimal attention to public health practice and environmental health services. Participants defined the problems facing them as: (1) definition of terms, inadequacy of reported statistics, and national differences in research settings; (2) selection of concepts and comparability in recording instruments; (3) theory and definition of research goals; and (4) sampling methods and interpretations of statistical analyses. Sixty-four references are listed.

0660 Modi, J.A. *Test of a technique for planning medical procedures in preventive health examination programs.* Socio-Economic Planning Sciences (Elmsford, N.Y.), 6(2), Apr 1972, 173-185. Engl.

From a study of a new management technique (a linear programming model), it is concluded that a preventive health examination programme based on this model has the following advantages over a conventional programme: (1) in the same time available to medical staff, a model programme can be designed to cover more individuals; (2) the sum total of findings is likely to be greater; and (3) a model programme can be designed to have a high rate of detection.

0661 Navarro, V. *Methods of planning the distribution of personal health services.* In Reinke, W.A., ed., Health Planning: Qualitative Aspects and Quantitative Techniques, Baltimore, Md., Johns Hopkins University, 1972, 265-276. Engl.

Planning for personal health services involves four steps: elaboration, acceptance of the plan by those affected, implementation, and evaluation. This paper reviews the methods used in the first step: planning for adequate and appropriate distribution of health resources. Mathematical models are presented for methods based on morbidity, mortality, resource/population ratio, analysis of demand, analysis of distribution, system performance, and system structure. Twenty-two references are listed, with additional recommended readings.

0662 Price, E.W. *Non-filarial elephantiasis of the lower legs in Ethiopia: a simple method for rapid survey by school enquiry.* Tropical and Geographical Medicine (Haarlem), 25, 1973, 23-27. Engl.

In Ethiopia nonfilarial elephantiasis of the lower leg was surveyed using a simple method. Pupils of junior schools in rural areas were asked questions from which the prevalence rates for school children were determined. The validity of the method described was confirmed by correlation with actual counts of persons with elephantiasis attending market in the centre where the school was situated. The method is felt to be applicable to other conditions in which some deformity or disability is evident, e.g. goiter, poliomyelitis, and trachoma. Rapid survey by the school inquiry method is recommended for its broad applicability and its economy in time and personnel.

0663 Reinke, W.A., Baker, T.D. *Measuring effects of demographic variables on health services utilization.* Health Services Research (Chicago), Spring 1967, 61-75. Engl.

To predict demands for health services, planners must measure the impact of demographic change. This article presents a new method, the multisort technique, to improve analysis of the effects of multiple demographic variables. The technique is demonstrated in an analysis of the changing demand for physicians' services in Taiwan. Multiple regression techniques, including those that utilize dummy variables, have been used to analyze effects of demographic variables, but interactions may be overlooked entirely or inadequately identified. Analysis of variance has proved useful in handling interactions, but uneven distribution of observations among cells creates orthogonality problems. The multisort technique is an approximation procedure that simplifies computations while maintaining the analysis of variance approach. The procedure assigns cell weights in all evaluations according to the rules for evaluating main effects; thus the assessment of interactions is approximate but not tedious. Comparison of computer results obtained by the new technique with those from certain multiple regression procedures indicates that the multisort technique offers more promise in the evaluation of demographic data than previous applications of analysis of variance would indicate. The study also gives practical suggestions for combining various techniques in a total analysis. The Taiwanese data in this paper were obtained from a survey supported by the U.S. Agency for International Development. Thirteen references are listed.

0664 Revista Saude Publica, Sao Paulo. *Apreciacao do "plano nacional de saude." (Evaluation of the "National Health Plan").* Revista de Saude Publica (Sao Paulo), 2(2), Dec 1968, 95-109. Portuguese.
Editorial.

The Faculty of Hygiene and Public Health of the University of Sao Paulo examines some of the guidelines and proposals of Brazil's National Health Plan. The theoretical aspects of the plan include the definition of the health concept, the basic guidelines embracing the three main functions of a national health plan, and the principle that any national health plan must administratively and technically integrate preventive, curative, and social measures. To be able to evaluate economic efficiency of a health care delivery system, it is necessary to compare it with the general index of economic development. As health technology increases, it is necessary to increase the number of persons benefitting from the innovation in order to minimize costs. The National Health Plan divides the country into 107 health areas, ranging from population centers of less than 100 000 to over 7 000 000. Allocation of resources will be made on the basis of local per capita income and population density. Some of the negative aspects of the programme are summarized.

0665 Roemer, M.I. *Evaluation of health service programs and levels of measurement.* HSMHA Health Reports (Rockville, Md.), 86(9), Sep 1971, 839-848. Engl.

This paper reviews five levels of benefit evaluation for health service programmes: health status outcomes; estimated quality of service; quantity of services provided; attitudes of recipients; and resources made available. In addition to these five levels of evaluation there is cost measurement, which may be regarded as another type of evaluation. The most useful strategy for evaluation would be to determine the effects of health service programmes at all five levels plus their costs. Fifty-seven references are listed.

V.4 Geographic distribution of health services
See also: 0652

0666 Colombia, Ministry of Public Health. *Estudio sanitario de comunidades rurales. (Health study of rural communities).* Bogota, Ministry of Public Health, Institute for Special Health Programs, Series III, No. 4, 1973. 1v.(various pagings). Span.
See also entry 667.

Recognizing the inadequacies of basic health care, the high morbidity, and low socioeconomic status of the rural population, Colombia's Ministry of Public Health began a health survey of rural communities in 1970. To maximize the limited economic resources available for this project, it was necessary to analyze certain criteria and establish an order of priorities for the different communities. Some of these criteria were geographic location of the community and availability of basic health services. This volume presents the survey methodology employed, statistical data obtained, and an analysis of the results. The purpose of the study was to provide the national government and other health-oriented institutions with the basic information necessary in planning health and sanitation projects. Seven references are listed.

0667 Colombia, Ministry of Public Health. *Estudio sanitario de comunidades rurales: manual metodo-*

logico. *(Health study of rural communities: manual of methodology)*. Bogota, Ministry of Public Health, National Institute for Special Health Programs, Series III, No. 1, 1972. 1v.(various Span.
See entry 666 for abstract.

0668 Cordero, A.L. *Determination of medical care needs in relation to a concept of minimal adequate care: an evaluation of the curative outpatient services of a rural health centre*. Medical Care (Philadelphia), 2(2), 1964, 95-103. Engl.
A concept of minimal adequate care was proposed for health centres in Puerto Rico. Based on this concept the needs of patients at a rural health centre were determined over a 3-month period. Knowing also the average patient load, it was possible to determine the total number of physicians needed. (Journal abstract.)

0669 Gershenberg, I., Haskell, M.A. *Distribution of medical services in Uganda*. Social Science and Medicine (Oxford), 6, Jun 1972, 353-372. Engl.
The provision of medical and educational facilities serves a dual purpose. It improves the quality of the life of the individuals who can take advantage of these services by making them healthier and more knowledgeable and they enhance their productivity. Healthier, more knowledgeable, and more productive individuals, in turn, can make a greater contribution to the economic and social development of the nation. The government of Uganda has declared its dedication to the enhancement of the quality of life of all its citizens. This reflects its concern to build a socialist state. In more precise terms, what this involves is the development of educational, medical, and other facilities as well as economic opportunities that will be available to the mass of the population rather than to any particular group, defined geographically, ethnically, tribally, or economically. Given the existing economic resources of Uganda, this suggests, with regard to the establishment of schools and health services, that monies be allocated so that all of the people may shortly be able to have access to some such service. In the field of health it follows that preference be given to the construction of medical centres and dispensaries rather than fully equipped hospitals since a multiple of centres and dispensaries can be built and staffed for the cost of a hospital. The purpose of this paper is to analyze the Government of Uganda's current medical programme to determine its consistancy with the objective of making medical service available to the greatest number of people in the shortest amount of time. Since Uganda is currently engaged in writing its third 5-year development plan, this exercise may prove to be instructive. The analysis may also be relevant to the planning of health services in other less economically developed countries where, as in the case of Uganda, poverty acts as the major determinant of the extent and pattern of medical care. To provide this analysis this paper presents in Part I what might be termed a macroanalysis of Uganda's health services, discussing the distribution and adequacy of these services over the nation at large. Part II analyses in more detail the medical services that are utilized in a particular district. This analysis is largely based on materials developed in a field survey in that area. In this analysis our concern will not be the allocation of monies between major sectors of the economy. The prevailing sectoral allocation, determined largely by political as well as other realities, will be taken as given. What the subject matter of this essay then is, is how are the resources that have been allocated to the health sector being used and how might their use and distribution be improved to make health services available to the greatest number of people in the shortest amount of time. Twenty-three references are listed. (Revised journal abstract.)

0670 Lizana, J., Elorz, X. *Disponibilidades de los Laboratorios Clinicos del sur del pais. (Clinical laboratory services in Southern Chile)*. Revista Medica de Chile (Santiago), 99, 1971, 313-318. Span.
Twenty-seven laboratories providing technical services in the medical care of 1 350 000 inhabitants distributed over 100 000 kmb were asked to reply to a questionnaire about their currently used methods and instruments. Data from 21 of those laboratories showed that very few people (only 62 professionals of different levels) were performing a rather limited number of tests, frequently using inadequate methods and outmoded, inaccurate instruments. With only one exception, blood glucose was still determined titrimetrically and only one laboratory determined blood urea with urease and Nessler reagent. Checking the methodological accuracy by standard control sera is not practiced at all and the normal values used are almost universally obtained from the literature, without regard for local variables of age, sex, nutritional status, environment, etc. A plea is made for assistance from the Public Health Service to integrate and expand the services that this small group of institutions is rendering. Seventeen references are listed.

0671 Pakistan, Ministry of Health and Social Welfare. *Annual report of the Director General Health/Addl. Secy.: July 1970-June 1971*. Pakistan, Ministry of Health and Social Welfare, 1973. 110p. Engl.
Specialized programmes' activities, facilities, and changes in the Pakistani health care programme are noted. Health centres are discussed under a section entitled "Curative Services." In the Second Five Year Plan 30 health centres with 90 subcentres were established in the Punjab. Health centres were not established during the Third Five Year Plan due to revised thinking. Considering the Fourth Five Year Plan period, 11 health centres have begun to be built with 33 subcentres. Twenty-eight new health centres are to be started during the fiscal year 1971-72.

V Formal Evaluative Studies

V.5 Financial aspects

See also: 0623, 0637

0672 Abel-Smith, B. WHO, Geneva. *Paying for health services: a study of the costs and sources of finance in six countries.* Geneva, WHO Public Health Papers No. 17, 1963. 86p. Engl.
This report attempts to define and classify health costs. A pilot study is reported in which these definitions were applied in six countries with varying systems of financing health services. Separate chapters deal with the economic concepts used in the study, a definition of the medical terms, a description of the health services systems of the six countries (Sri Lanka, Israel, Czechoslovakia, Sweden, USA, Chile), sources and methods of data collection, the results of the pilot study, and proposals for future work.

V.6 Cultural aspects

See also: 0435, 0679

0673 Messing, S.D., Prince, J.S. *Health practices in Ethiopian pre-urban communities.* Journal of Health and Human Behavior (Fort Worth), 7, Winter 1966, 272-276. Engl.
Health practices existing prior to the establishment of rural health centres were studied by representative sampling and by observation. Data reported include practices relating to water, use of soap, and occasions for washing hands. Problems of obtaining reliable quantitative data are cited. One conclusion is that installation of suitable facilities are a prerequisite to improved practices and to health education. Another conclusion is that ethnographic observation is essential as a check of the reliability of quantification by questionnaire, especially in a culture not yet habituated to the imperatives of accurate responses to questionnaires and still emphasizing politeness as a dominant cultural norm. (Journal abstract.)

V.7 Epidemiological, family planning, MCH, and nutritional studies

See also: 0295, 0352, 0360, 0532, 0533, 0604, 0607, 0624, 0651, 0652

0674 Agren, G., Almgard, G., Mellander, O., Vahlquist, B. *Children's nutrition unit: an Ethio-Swedish project in the field of health.* Ethiopian Medical Journal (Addis Ababa), (1), Nov 1966, 5-13. Engl.
This article relates to a nutrition project for preschoolers in Ethiopia, sponsored by the Swedish International Development Agency (SIDA). The aim of the children's nutrition unit is to survey the incidence of malnutrition in Ethiopia, design an enrichment programme based on indigenous foodstuffs, and evaluate the physical fitness in relation to nutritional status of school-age children and adults in Ethiopia. The organization of the project motivated many sectors and fields of study: agriculture, animal farming, fishing, economic planning, industry, biochemistry, clinical medicine, public health, and sociology. The Swedish experts worked with Ethiopian counterparts. The development of a basic laboratory in Addis Ababa and field centres and stations of the project is outlined. Careful consideration was given to collection of baseline data, which were later used in the evaluation of the effects of the applied nutrition programme. A special education programme was planned to work out methods for education including use of radio broadcasts, and also in group training of health personnel, teachers, etc. The article concludes that the goals of the project are worth striving for, although they may take a few years. Five references are listed.

0675 Aouchiche, M., Kebbouche, M.L. *La lutte anti-trachomateuse: valeur et limites des campagnes de masse a travers l'evaluation d'une action menee dans le sud algerien. (Trachoma control: value and limitations of mass campaigns through the evaluation of a programme carried out in southern Algeria).* Revue Internationale du Trachome (Marseille), 49, 1972, 25-40. Fren.
For nearly 9 years, Algeria has been fighting trachoma through large-scale campaigns by following and applying the recommendations of the WHO. Of 65 000 cases of blindness, one-third were due to either trachoma or conjunctivitis. The campaign aimed at preventing corneal complications, suppressing contagion, and instituting treatment. The method of action included campaigns in schools and home treatment, emphasizing self-treatment and prevention. As a result, the severity of trachoma decreased, the morbidity rate regressed, and transmission was limited. It was found that disease perpetration is not due to the virus itself, but to its association with a number of germs of different origins. Eleven references are listed.

0676 Campbell, A.A. *Population: the search for solutions in the behavioral sciences.* American Journal of Obstetrics and Gynecology (St. Louis), 116(1), 1 May 1973, 131-152. Engl.
Recommendations presented here constitute immediate (1973) objectives of population research over the next few years, to establish the determinants and the consequences of population change, provide information needed for development of government policies, establish the determinants of fertility, and examine migration. Fifty-two references are listed.

0677 Collver, A., Have, R.T., Speare, M.C. *Factors influencing the use of maternal health services.* Social Science and Medicine (Oxford), 1(1), Apr 1967, 293-308. Engl.

A study of low-income obstetric patients shows that rates of attendance at prenatal, postpartum, and family planning clinics are associated with a variety of patients' background characteristics such as age, number of living children, and years of school completed. In addition, distance of clinics from patients' homes appeared to have a substantial effect on attendance. (Journal abstract.)

0678 Colombia, Ministry of Public Health. *Extension de servicios de atencion materna e infantil: estudio preparatorio. (Expansion of maternal and infant care services: preliminary study).* Bogota, Ministry of Public Health, Institute for Special Health Programs, 1969. 1v.(no pagination). Span.

The Colombian Association of Schools of Medicine and the Department of Public Health studied the demand for and cost of maternal and child health care services. The research programme examined population, mortality, human and institutional resources, scope of services, construction and operating costs, and projections of available manpower resources in the selected districts. Districts were included in the survey if they belonged to one of the areas programmed by the Department of Public Health, if the municipalities within the district had similar geographic, economic, ecological, and cultural characteristics, and if the population of the districts was around 100 000. Statistical data obtained in the survey are presented separately for urban and rural areas.

0679 de Mejia, M.O. Population Reference Bureau, Bogota. *Mujer, participacion y planificacion familiar. (Women, participation and family planning).* Bogota, Population Reference Bureau, 1973. 12p. Span.

Paper presented at the United Nation's Seminar on the Conditions of Women and Family Planning, Santo Domingo, Dominican Republic, May 1973.

This paper examines the status of women in Latin America since the beginning of Spanish colonization and includes information on women's progress in the civil rights field and the economic life of the Latin American countries. Family planning programmes in Latin America have not established improvement in the status of women as an objective. Only Cuba and China have formally endorsed participation of women in their social and economic development. Family planning programmes in Latin America have not considered these aspects. Their objectives are to decrease growth rates, develop responsible parenthood, reduce damages caused by induced abortion, reduce maternal death by abortion and multiple births, decrease infant mortality, and study trends and movements of demographic variables. The secondary role played by women, and their classification as inferior beings have not been considered in family planning programmes.

0680 Dutta, R. *Public health and family planning: a study of inter-relationship in India.* American Journal of Public Health (New York), 63(2), Feb 1973, 158-162. Engl.

Developing countries must give high priority to the control of population growth. These efforts may be considered temporary and of an emergency nature. Slower programmes and permanent measurers of control will be possible as socioeconomic patterns of life change. Under the assumption that socioeconomic change and the knowledge of preventive public health measures are related, research was conducted in India on the relationship between public health practice and family planning knowledge and practice. In the three rural villages studied, of those couples who had adopted public health practices more had knowledge of and were practicing family planning than those who had not adopted such health measures. This result supports the policy of integrating family planning programmes with public health efforts. Eleven references are listed.

0681 Ebanks, G.E. *Family planning among health clinic patients in Barbados.* Social Biology (Chicago), 18(2), Jun 1971, 137-147. Engl.

Statistical data from a survey of female health clinic patients in Barbados indicate that the family planning programme is affecting the fertility behaviour of these women and is partially responsible for a decline in crude birth rates. Ten references are listed.

0682 Ethiopia, Ministry of Public Health. *(Memorandum related to) request from H.E. the Minister of Health to examine the feasibility of expanding maternal and child health services.* Addis Ababa, Ministry of Health, Maternal and Child Health Division, Jan 1971. 4p. Engl.

Unpublished document.

An examination of the feasibility of expanding maternal and child health services in Ethiopia to include family guidance and child spacing services draws attention to the fact that only a small fraction of women and children use these services and that most services are in urban areas. Personnel in health centres are ready and willing to provide family "guidance" services if authorized to do so and if such guidance is requested by women visiting the centres. Some recommendations are to secure short-term consultants from abroad, to expand the number of midwifery training centres, and to strengthen the maternal and child health services throughout the country. In Ethiopia there are 542 health stations staffed by dressers with no midwifery or maternal and child health training. This leaves the rural population with only one "delivery" system: the untrained birth attendant and the faith healer.

0683 Frimodt-Moller, J., Acharyulu, G.S., Pillai, K.K. *Observations on the protective effect of BCG vaccination in a south Indian rural population:*

V Formal Evaluative Studies

fourth report. n.p., n.d. 16p. Engl.
Unpublished document.

The findings of a controlled BCG trial at Madanapalle, India, carried out from 1950 to 1955 are reported. Subjects were classified as vaccinated, unvaccinated, or Mantoux positive reactors. The effect of the vaccination was quite high during the first 5-9 years; thereafter the difference between the vaccinated and unvaccinated decreased. The protective effect at 9 years corresponded to 83%, at 12 years to 46%, and at 21 years to only 20%. The incidence in the unvaccinated negative group during the first 10 years was several times lower than that in the Mantoux positive group but thereafter increased, so that at 20 years, the group initially Mantoux negative had had the same total experience of tuberculosis as the Mantoux positive group. The author suggests that the development of tuberculosis in South Indian patients takes a longer time than observed in European cases. The incidence among the vaccinated at the end of the 20 years' observation period was higher than among the unvaccinated controls. The author suggests that the main effect of vaccination in man is the same as observed in experimental animals, namely, the slowing down of multiplication of the bacilli after primary infection. In many instances this is sufficient to prevent the development of demonstrable tuberculosis, but in others it only delays the onset of the disease. Six references are listed.

0684   Hofvander, Y., Eksmyr, R. *Applied nutrition program in an Ethiopian rural community.* American Journal of Clinical Nutrition (Bethesda, Md.), 24, May 1971, 578-591. Engl.

The work of the Ethiopian Nutrition Institute, which was established as part of Sweden's bilateral aid to Ethiopia, focusses on protein-calorie malnutrition problems. A 2-year, country-wide education programme and a supplementary food scheme are part of their programme. This paper evaluates the impact of the applied nutrition on school children in the typical rural community of Ijaji, as measured in terms of anthropometric, clinical, and biochemical findings. Results of the study of 212 children under 11 years of age, subjected for 2 years to the influence of the applied nutrition programme, can be summarized as "improvements," "no change," and "impairments." "Improvements" were evident in reduction of clinical signs of protein-calorie malnutrition, increase in upper arm muscle circumference-for-age, decrease in prevalence of various skin and scalp infections, etc. "No change" was observed in height-for-age, frequency of anemia, or frequency of Ascaris infestations. "Impairments" such as increased frequency of hookworm infestations and an increase in gamma globulin in the serum were observed. An appreciable improvement in the children's general nutrition status was therefore concluded. Forty-one references are listed.

0685   International Union for Child Welfare, Geneva. *Rehabilitation programme for destitute, displaced and orphaned children in the People's Republic of Bangladesh.* Geneva, International Union for Child Welfare, 10 Apr 1973. 16p. Engl.
Unpublished document.

In Bangladesh, the first phase of a rehabilitation programme for displaced and orphaned children included: (1) reception centres providing 4 410 displaced children as of February 1972, with temporary feeding, medical care, and continuing education, directed by social welfare personnel; and (2) a family assistance programme reuniting 1 473 children with their families, providing material assistance and counselling, training caseworkers, providing grants to widows for vocational training, and proposing solutions for children needing long-term care. The second phase proposes the following: a 6-month extension of the family assistance programme, local community homes for orphaned children of both rural and urban backgrounds, residential youth hostels near vocational centres, and a social welfare programme for widowed mothers. An estimate of costs and a list of donor organizations are included.

0686   Kapil, K.K. *Organizational procedures in integration of family planning education with maternal and child health service.* Journal of the Indian Medical Association (Calcutta), 50(9), 1 May 1968, 433-437. Engl.

In India, a range of services are provided through tax-supported maternity homes. Maternal and child health centres are either domiciliary or institutional. Domiciliary care provides education for mothers on baby care, mother craft, nutrition, and family and community health. Institutional care provides medical services and health education to mothers during prenatal, natal, and postnatal periods. Details of these programmes are described to show how family planning education and services can be integrated with services already underway. Personnel can be trained, a teaching unit can be developed following sound principles of health education, and group counciling methods can be used to conduct sessions for mothers who use domiciliary or institutional care. Maternity homes as well as maternal and child health centres offer potent settings for imparting family planning instruction to recently delivered mothers. Seven references are listed.

0687   Maichuk, Y.F. *(Treatment of patients suffering from trachoma and conjunctivitis in Sudan).* Vestnik Oftalmologii (Moscow), 79, Mar-Apr 1966, 31-36. Russ.

The first organizational methodical training centre for the control of infectious eye diseases in Sudan was set up in the northern province with the aid of WHO. The centre carried out epidemiological, clinical, and laboratory studies of trachoma and conjunctivitis among rural and urban residents. Intermittent treatment involving topical application of tetracycline was put to extensive clinical trial. Evening therapy ensured better permeability of the antibiotic, and had essential organizational advantages. Cure was effected, following a

6-month course of intermittent treatment, in 78.4% of the trachoma cases and 82.8% of the conjunctivitis cases. Following 6 more months of treatment, trachoma cures increased to 87.9%, comprising a 94.9% cure for first-stage trachoma, a 72.3% cure for second-stage trachoma, and a 94.1% for third-stage trachoma. A comparative study of two methods of intermittent treatment practiced in elementary schools, i.e. single and twice a day instillation of the drug, showed both to be equally effective. The role of sanitary education cannot be overemphasized in realizing mass health programmes. (Revised journal abstract.)

0688 Marson, W. *India's project number one.* Canadian Nurse (Ottawa), 63, Nov 1967, 45-49. Engl.
There are 446 Protestant mission hospitals and dispensaries in India. With the participation of a Canadian University Services Overseas nurse, a Christian Medical Association of India (CMAI) project was begun to encourage the addition of family planning services to these institutions. The programme began with financial assistance, relieving hospitals of the financial burden of tubal ligations, vasectomies, and intrauterine device insertions. Staff and patient education in family planning was then initiated in hospitals. More than 150 mission hospitals and dispensaries have since become involved in the CMAI Family Planning Project, and clinical and educational projects and services have expanded rapidly. With further development of priority educational programmes for staff and patients it was anticipated that interest in family planning work will grow.

0689 Otoo, S.N. *Suggestions for the re-organization of the maternal health services of Accra.* Ghana Medical Journal (Accra), 12(1), Mar 1973, 78-91. Engl.
Accra's Maternal Health Services consist of three levels: (1) services provided by traditional birth attendants; (2) extrahospital facilities for normal pregnancies, i.e. maternity homes, midwives, clinics, etc.; and (3) hospitals with resources for surgery demanded by abnormal pregnancy. Attempts to coordinate the midwives' services and services provided by the Maternity Hospital have had limited success. The Maternity Hospital has become overcrowded and efficiency has suffered. Clinic facilities have not been fully exploited, and are too few and far between. There is a need for: (1) strengthening the central advisory and inspection machinery of the Ministry of Health; and (2) a local coordinating body to ensure health coverage of the whole population. To spread the patient load more equitably, efforts are being made to provide more clinics and maternity homes and community nurses to patients attending maternity clinics. Nine references are listed.

0690 Research Triangle Institute, North Carolina. *Appraisal of the population project of the rural health research center at Narangwal, India: the integration of family planning and rural health services at the village level.* Research Triangle Park, North Carolina, Research Triangle Institute, 1971. 64p. Engl.
The Population Project of the Narangwal Rural Health Centre, India, is designed to evaluate whether contraceptive acceptance is greatest when health services are offered for women, or for women and children, or for children alone. A review committee, which briefly observed activities of the Centre, found the project potentially useful for its attempt to research input and output nationally, since social planning has occurred in India on a large scale without objective knowledge of success and failure of various approaches.

0691 Reynolds, J. *Delivering family planning services: autonomous vs. integrated clinics.* Family Planning Perspectives (New York), 2(1), Jan 1970, 15-22. Engl.
This article reports the result of a 1968/69 study to determine which type of family planning system is more effective: an autonomous family planning service or one that is integrated with other services. The study covered 12 family planning clinics clustered in four geographic areas of New York City. Each cluster consisted of one clinic in a voluntary organization, one in a health centre, and one in a hospital. Viewpoints of the community and the patients are reported. Recommendations are given for improvement of the quantity, quality, and efficiency of the major family planning delivery systems.

0692 Rosenfield, A.G., Limcharoen, C. *Auxiliary midwife prescription of oral contraceptives: an experimental project in Thailand.* American Journal of Obstetrics and Gynecology (St. Louis), 114(7), 1 Dec 1972, 942-949. Engl.
In 1969, the Thai Ministry of Public Health initiated a study in which auxiliary midwives in four rural provinces were allowed to prescribe oral contraceptives without the requirement of a physician examination. A simple checklist was utilized to rule out contraindications; pelvic examination was not required. There was no increase noted in the incidence of either side effects or complications. There was a fourfold increase in the number of pill acceptors in the four study provinces in the 6 months following initiation of the study, as compared to the 6 months before. In these provinces, this resulted in both a larger number of pill acceptors and a higher percentage of the eligible female population who accepted the pill than in the 13 control provinces, in spite of the much larger number of eligible women, health personnel, and facilities in the control provinces. In addition, the continuation rates were higher for pills prescribed by midwives than for those prescribed by physicians. At the end of 1 year of study, the Ministry of Public Health ruled that the more than 3 000 auxiliary midwives throughout the country who had received basic family planning training could prescribe the pill, with a resultant threefold increase in the number of pill acceptors nationwide, from approximately 8 800 in April 1970, to almost 31 000 in December 1971. The importance of the effective use of nurses and other

paraprofessional personnel in family planning programmes is emphasized. Seventeen references are listed. (Journal abstract.)

0693 Rosenfield, A.G. *Family planning: an expanded role for paramedical personnel.* American Journal of Obstetrics and Gynecology (St. Louis), 110(7), Aug 1971, 1030-1039. Engl.

This paper presents the case for a rational approach to family planning utilizing existing technology. Three questions are asked: (1) Is a pelvic examination necessary prior to the prescription of oral contraceptives and does it significantly reduce risk of complication of oral contraception? (2) If pelvic examination is necessary, are there significant differences between an examination conducted by a physician and one by a paramedic? (3) Can a simple checklist be prepared for use by the paramedic? It is concluded that the major reason for a pelvic examination is to take a Papanicolaou Smear, and if facilities for reading smears are available, paramedics can easily be taught to obtain the smear. When cytologic examination is impossible, the argument is put forth that there is no significant increased risk by the omission of a pelvic examination. Evidence is also presented to suggest that paramedical personnel with proper training and supervision can insert the IUD as safely as most physicians. Finally, a simple checklist is presented for use by the paramedic. It is argued that the present controversy concerning oral contraception does not affect the rationale for the prescription by personnel other than physicians. A plea is made to the medical profession to be more realistic and practical in setting standards of good medical practice. Sixty-eight references are listed. (Revised author abstract.)

0694 Roy, P., Kivlin, J. India, National Institute of Community Development, Hyderabad. *Health innovation and family planning: a study in eight Indian villages.* Hyderabad, National Institute of Community Development, May 1968. 53p. Engl.

This is a special companion report on health innovation and family planning of the Diffusion of Innovations project that was undertaken in collaboration with Michigan State University. Smallpox vaccination, cholera innoculation, malaria prevention, water treatment, bedbug killing, and modern childbirth practices were studied among residents of eight Indian villages. Characteristics of adoptors of each innovation were noted. IUD and vasectomy acceptors were studied in a comparable analysis of adoptor characteristics. Communication variables were the best predictors of adoption of health innovations for the sample as a whole. Knowledge of health extension agents contributed greatly to adoption. Standard of living was positively related to adoption. Information efforts should be continued. Change agents are important sources of information.

0695 Schultz, T.P. *Effectiveness evaluation of family planning: case study Taiwan.* Santa Monica, The RAND Corporation, Document no. P-4890, Sep 1972. 29p. Engl.

Methods for evaluating the effectiveness of family planning programmes are reviewed, with comments on the strengths and weaknesses of each. From a case study in Taiwan, it is evident that different methods of evaluation yield different implications for improving policy. Thirty-eight references are listed.

0696 Shah, K.K. *Analysis of I.U.C.D. insertions in a rural area by a primary health centre.* Indian Journal of Public Health (Calcutta), 12(4), Oct 1968, 195-197. Engl.

In Gujarat, India, in 1965 an IUD insertion programme was begun in a rural area served by a primary health centre. Women in the area were encouraged to participate in the programme. Pelvic examinations were conducted prior to IUD insertion and women were told to anticipate some side effects. Women with three children or less responded to the programme better than did women with six or more children. Initial response was better than later response. The programme's failure to continue to recruit women is a result of IUD complications after insertion. The loop proved to be a satisfactory contraceptive method for about 80% of the women who used it.

0697 Singh, S., Gorden, J.E., Wyon, J.B. *Medical care in fatal illnesses of a rural Punjab population: some social, biological and cultural factors and their ecological implication.* Indian Journal of Medical Research (New Delhi), 50(6), Nov 1962, 865-880. Engl.

In a rural village of the Punjab, India, observations revealed that medical care for fatal illnesses in infants, females, the poor, and elderly is less than for other segments of the population and death rates for these groups were higher. The importance of acute infectious diseases as a cause of death points to the necessity for preventive services especially in maternal and child health.

0698 Stanfield, J.P. *"At risk" concept.* Journal of Tropical Pediatrics (Kampala), 14, Dec 1968, 201-204. Engl.

Maternal and child health in developing countries is best dealt with at the rural level. Recent efforts based on those developed for more sophisticated areas have relied on curative and referral service. However, preventive and educational measures, along with diagnostic and curative services, are more effective. These aims were pursued in a rural maternal and child care clinic north of Kampala, Uganda. Patients, such as children suffering from malnutrition, and thus particularly vulnerable to disease, are termed "at risk". Parents of these children receive nutritional education and the future health status of the child is observed. It is too soon to assess the value of this approach, but it is one well within the reach of government health centres.

0699 Unhanand, M. *Summary report on family health work in Thailand (from the beginning of* *services until 31 December 1968).* Bangkok, Ministry of Public Health, 1969. 6p. Engl.

Unpublished document translated from Thai.

In 1968 the Research and Evaluation Unit of the Family Health Programme, of the Ministry of Public Health in Thailand, sent out questionnaires to family health clinics throughout the country. Figures were requested for the numbers of new IUD acceptors and new pill users since the beginning of service. Figures were also requested for numbers of persons receiving surgical sterilization during the previous 4-year period. Of the questionnaires, 88% were returned. Statistical data on results are provided. It was concluded that between 1964 and 1968, 4.2% of the total group of married Thai women age 20 to 44 received family health services. If all users of family planning services or methods are considered, about 12% of the eligible population can be said to use family planning services. The majority received services from hospitals in Bangkok and Thonburi.

0700 Zachariah, S. *Midwifery service in rural West Bengal.* Nursing Journal of India (New Delhi), 62(8), Aug 1971, 251-252. Engl.

Maternal and child health services in West Bengal, India, are an integral part of the general health services. In primary health centres most beds are occupied by maternity cases. Untrained midwives (dais) deliver normal births whereas abnormal births may require hospital delivery. A study was conducted to assess the attitudes of rural people toward health centre staff, their preferences for place of deliveries, and reasons for these preferences. One hundred and twenty prenatal mothers were interviewed. As educational status of husbands increased, the couple's preference for health centre and hospital services increased. Dais were sought for deliveries if they had safely delivered a previous birth for the family. Hospital and health centre delivery was preferred for safety reasons whereas delivery by dais was preferred for comfort.

Rural health centre, Brazil.

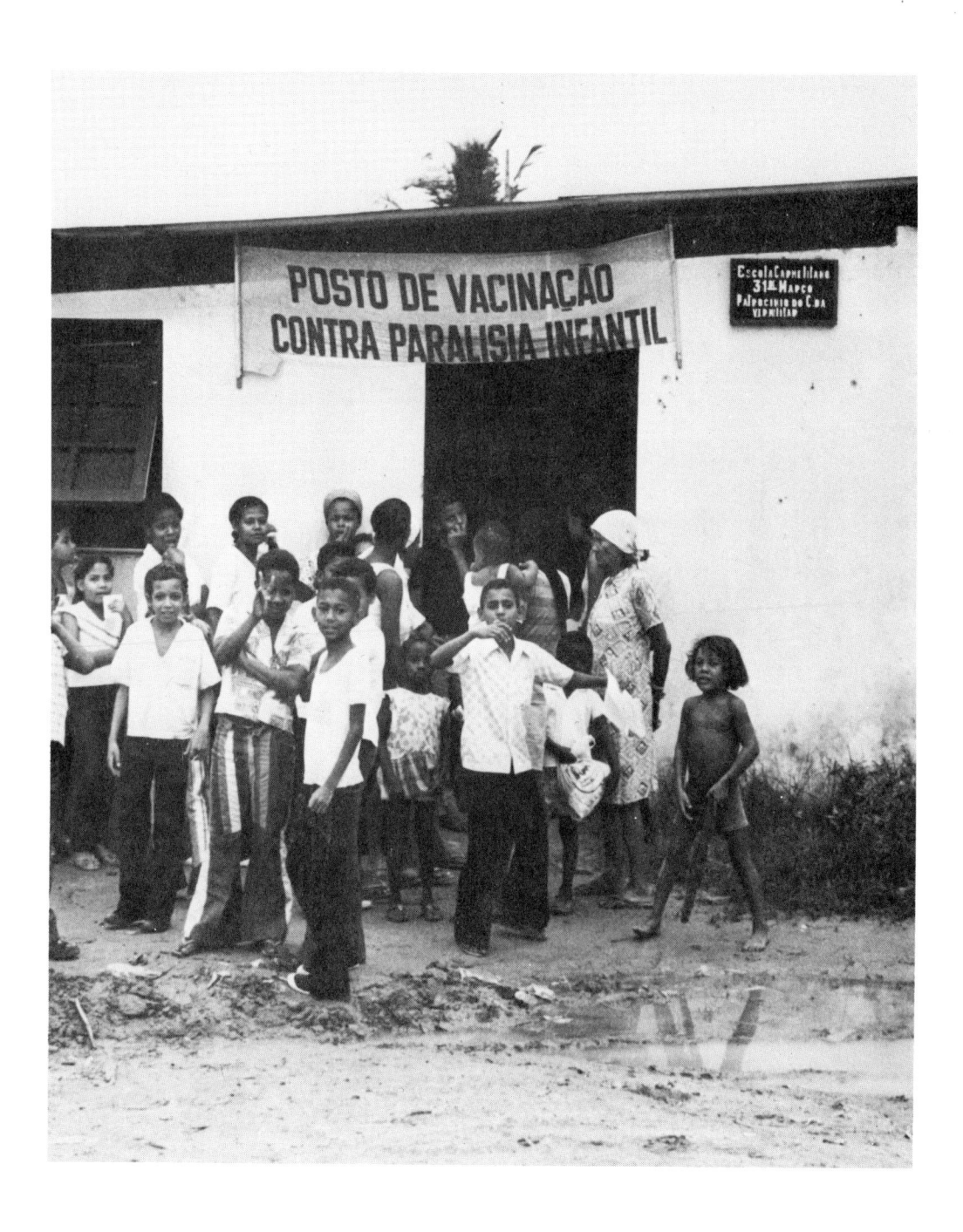

Appendix 1
Abbreviations and Acronyms

ABU – Ahmadu Bello University, Zaria, Nigeria

ALERT – All African Leprosy and Rehabilitation Training Centre, Addis Ababa

APHA – American Public Health Association, Washington, D.C.

BCG – Bacillus Calmette-Guerin vaccine

CAHP – Coordinating Agency for Health Planning, New Delhi

CENTO – Central Treaty Organization, Ankara

CIDA – Canadian International Development Agency, Ottawa

CMAI – Christian Medical Association of India, Bangalore

CMC – Christian Medical Commission, Geneva

CPC – Carolina Population Center, Chapel Hill, N.C.

CSG – Capital Systems Group, Inc., Bethesda, Md.

DANIDA – Danish International Development Agency, Copenhagen

Devt. – Development

DHEW – United States Department of Health, Education and Welfare, Washington, D.C.

Engl. – English

FAO – Food and Agricultural Organization, Rome

FP – Family Planning

Fren. – French

GPHCTC – Gondar Public Health College and Training Centre, Ethiopia

IBRD – International Bank for Reconstruction and Development, Washington, D.C.

ICA – Colombian Agricultural Institute, Bogota

IDR – Institute of Development Research, Copenhagen

IDRC – International Development Research Centre, Ottawa

ILO – International Labour Organization, Geneva

IPPF – International Planned Parenthood Federation, London

IRHFP – Institute of Rural Health and Family Planning, Gandhigram, India

ITDG – Intermediate Technology Development Group, London

IUCD – Intrauterine Contraceptive Device

IUD – Intrauterine Device

KAP – Knowledge, Attitude, and Practice (Study)

KNIPOROS – Kenya-Netherlands-Israel Project for Operational Research in Outpatient Services, Kenya

LRCS – League of Red Cross Societies, Geneva

MCH – Maternal and Child Health

Med. – Medical/Medicine

MEDLARS – Medical Literature Analysis and Retrieval Systems

MESH – Medical Subject Headings

NTIS – National Technical Information Service, Washington, D.C.

OECD – Organization for Economic Cooperation and Development, Paris

PAHO – Pan American Health Organization, Washington, D.C.

Res. – Research

Russ. – Russian

SIDA – Swedish International Development Agency, Stockholm

Span. – Spanish

Trop. – Tropical

UCLA – University of California, Los Angeles

UN – United Nations, New York

UNDP – United Nations Development Program, New York

UNESCO – United Nations Educational, Scientific and Cultural Organization, Paris

UNESOB – United Nations Economic and Social Office in Beirut, Beirut

UNFPA – United Nations Fund for Population Activities, New York

UNICEF – United Nations Childrens Fund, New York

USA – United States of America

USAID – United States Agency for International Development, Washington, D.C.

USGPO – United States Government Printing Office, Washington, D.C.

WHO – World Health Organization, Geneva

Author Index
(figures refer to abstract numbers)

A

Abel-Smith, B., 0120, 0672
Abelin, S., 0616
Abramowitz, J., 0121
Abramson, A.S., 0287
Acharyulu, G.S., 0683
Acolatse, P., 0515
Adadevoh, B.K., 0126
Adedeji, A., 0122
Adesuyi, S.L., 0617
African Medical and Research Foundation, Nairobi., 0008, 0055, 0056, 0335, 0336, 0337, 0423, 0557
Agren, G., 0674
Aguirre, A., 0376
Akenzua, S.I., 0122
Akim, N.B., 0618
Akin-Deko, G., 0057
Akinkugbe, O.O., 0021, 0057, 0123, 0377
Alam, A.S., 0537
Alexander, C.A., 0226, 0604
Ali, D.S., 0378
All India Institute of Hygiene and Public Health, Calcutta., 0058
Allen, L.R., 0379
Almgard, G., 0674
Ambwani, G.J., 0366
American Friends Service Committee, Philadelphia., 0290
American Medical Association, Chicago., 0001, 0002
American Public Health Association, Washington, D.C., 0227
Anderson, J.K., 0355
Andjelkovic, D., 0656
Andrade, J., 0553
Andrews, S., 0610
Aouchiche, M., 0675
Arbona, G., 0059, 0156
Argentina, Department of Social Welfare., 0124, 0380, 0558
Argentina, State Secretariat for Culture and Education., 0508
Ariffin, M., 0611
Arnhold, R.G., 0619
Arole, M., 0060, 0424
Arole, R.S., 0060, 0291, 0292, 0356
Asayesh, K., 0228
Ashitey, G.A., 0620
Association of American Medical Colleges, Washington, D.C., 0003
Attia, S.E., 0293

Audu, I.S., 0028
Austen-Peters, A.O., 0617
Australia, Department of Health., 0061

B

Backett, E.M., 0378
Bactat, J.L., 0022
Badgley, R.F., 0023, 0024
Baker, T.D., 0025, 0026, 0425, 0663
Balasegaram, M., 0426
Bali, P., 0244
Banerji, D., 0229, 0230
Banerji, S.C., 0381
Bangxang, H.N., 0392
Banjo, B., 0408
Bankole, M.A., 0046
Bannerman, R.H., 0516
Barkhuus, A., 0150
Barmadia, B., 0538
Barmes, D.E., 0545
Barzilai, I., 0125
Bassir, O., 0126
Baumau, K., 0612
Baxter, A.J., 0294
Beghin, I.D., 0295
Begum, J., 0602
Begum, S., 0602
Behm, H., 0231
Belbin, R.M., 0559
Belcher, D.W., 0576, 0620
Benjamin, V., 0317
Bennett, F.J., 0127, 0232, 0315, 0357, 0358, 0382
Betts, K.G., 0517
Bevan, P.G., 0383
Bhatia, J.C., 0610
Bhatnagar, J.K., 0648
Bhattacharjee, B.N., 0132
Bice, T.W., 0621
Bisley, G.G., 0062
Black, R.H., 0233
Blankhart, D.M., 0234
Bloom, S., 0023
Bodenheimer, T.S., 0338
Boletin de la Oficina Sanitaria Panamericana, Washington, D.C., 0063, 0128
Bolton, J.M., 0296
Bomgaars, M.R., 0064
Bonnet, P.D., 0213
Boohene, A.G., 0427
Boonpratuang, C., 0634

Bowers, J.Z., 0518
Braga, E., 0027
Bravo, A.L., 0199
Brey, K.H., 0539
Bright, M., 0129
Brodie, A., 0065
Brooke, D.E., 0428
Brown, R.E., 0235, 0236, 0429
Browne, S.G., 0430, 0431
Bruce, S., 0297
Bull, G.M., 0298
Bureau of Hygiene and Tropical Diseases, London., 0004, 0005
Buri, P., 0384, 0385
Burkitt, W.R., 0339, 0340
Byer, M.A., 0299

C

Campbell, A.A., 0676
Campbell, E.P., 0130
Campos, P.C., 0386
Canada, Department of National Health and Welfare., 0432, 0462, 0560, 0561, 0562, 0563, 0564
Candau, M.G., 0131
Candib, L.M., 0104
Cannon, J.A., 0576
Carty, C., 0237
Castano, A.A., 0066
Cebrian U.J., 0387
Center for Population Planning, Ann Arbor, Michigan., 0585, 0586
Central Family Planning Institute, New Delhi., 0265, 0519
Central Treaty Organization, Ankara., 0300
Chablani, T.D., 0301, 0388, 0389
Chakravarti, D.N., 0132
Chang, K.K., 0067
Chang, W.P., 0068, 0133, 0433, 0622
Chen, P.C., 0509
Chile, National Health Service., 0565
Chow, L.P., 0238, 0239
Christian Council of Nigeria, Lagos., 0590
Christian Medical Association of India, Bangalore., 0341
Christian Medical College Hospital, Vellore, India., 0390
Ciba Foundation, London., 0198
Collis, W.R., 0028
Collver, A., 0677
Colmenares, A., 0395
Colombia, Ministry of Public Health., 0006, 0029, 0566, 0567, 0568, 0587, 0605, 0623, 0666, 0667, 0678
Colombian Association of Faculties of Medicine, Bogota., 0567, 0587
Commonwealth Bureau of Nutrition, Aberdeen, Scotland., 0007
Cook, R., 0569
Cooper, E.S., 0030
Cooper, J.K., 0014
Copping, A.M., 0240
Cordero, A.L., 0668

Cornejo, L.Z., 0549, 0550
Corsa, L., 0069, 0134
Coster, M.E., 0305
Courtejoie, J., 0283, 0359, 0624
Cox, P.S., 0342
Cruickshank, R., 0569
Cunningham, C.E., 0606

D

Dada, B.A., 0122
Dadgar, M., 0302
Dahlin, L., 0625
Davachi, F., 0241
David, P., 0242
Davidson, L., 0391
Davies, A.M., 0096
Daynes, J.A., 0434
de Glanville, H., 0008, 0303, 0343
de Hertaing, I.R., 0283
de Kadt, E., 0200
de Martinez, V.G., 0066
de Mejia, M.O., 0679
de Silva, D.M., 0135
Dehne, E., 0070
Del Mundo, F., 0626
Dempsey, J.J., 0627
Deshaies, J.C., 0136
Deuschle, K.W., 0435
Diaz, S., 0203
Dimataga, A.L., 0304
Doege, T.C., 0392
Dosunmu, N.E., 0499
Dowling, M.A., 0378, 0393
Du Toit, A.E., 0305
Dunlop, D., 0214
Dunlop, D.W., 0628
Duraiswami, P.K., 0344
Dutta, R., 0680
Dyer, H., 0299

E

East African Medical Journal, Nairobi., 0201
East Pakistan Family Planning Board, Dacca., 0602
East Pakistan Research and Evaluation Centre, Sweden-Pakistan Family Welfare Project, Dacca., 0588
Ebanks, G.E., 0681
Ebie, J.C., 0639
Ebrahim, G.J., 0589
Eckersley, L.W., 0286
Eksmyr, R., 0684
el Borolossy, A.W., 0378
Elder, F.B., 0650
Elebute, E.A., 0137
Eliot, J.W., 0520
Elliott, J., 0071
Elliott, K., 0436
Elman, A., 0581
Elorz, X., 0670
Ennever, O., 0437, 0484, 0614
Esan, G.J., 0123, 0408
Ethiopia, Ministry of Public Health., 0168, 0250, 0682

Evans, T., 0629
Excerpta Medica Foundation, Amsterdam., 0009, 0010, 0011

F

FAO, Rome., 0577
Farmer, S.K., 0050
Fendall, N.R., 0072, 0073, 0138, 0139, 0306, 0307, 0308, 0438, 0439, 0440, 0441, 0442, 0443, 0444, 0445, 0521, 0546
Fensome, J.E., 0522
Ferrand, G.J., 0140
Finland, Ministry for Foreign Affairs, Department for International Development Cooperation., 0500
Fisek, N.H., 0074, 0141, 0309
Flahault, D., 0446, 0447
Flavier, J.M., 0310
Forbes, C., 0311
Fountain, D.E., 0031, 0570
Fream, W.C., 0571
Frenkel, J.K., 0202
Freyvogel, T.A., 0448
Frimodt-Moller, J., 0683
Fry, J., 0449, 0630
Fukuoka, M., 0263
Fulop, T., 0215

G

Gadalla, F.R., 0607
Gale, G.W., 0075, 0142
Galli, E.A., 0360
Garcia, A.L., 0361
Gaur, S.D., 0243
Geigy, R., 0450
Gereda, R., 0362, 0547
Gershenberg, I., 0669
Ghana, Ministry of Health., 0076, 0572
Ghana, Ministry of Information., 0032
Ghosh, S., 0244
Gilbert, D.N., 0143
Gilbert, F.F., 0407
Gill, P.S., 0144
Gilles, H.M., 0394
Gish, O., 0012, 0145, 0146
Giulani, C., 0451
Goldthorpe, G., 0569
Gonzalez, C.L., 0147, 0395
Gorden, J.E., 0697
Goswami, A.L., 0033
Gourlay, R.J., 0299
Gourley, G., 0148
Graham-Douglas, M.S., 0639
Graham, R.G., 0077
Grant, J.A., 0627
Graver, V., 0345
Gray, G.L., 0013
Gray, H.H., 0590
Greenberg, J.H., 0143
Griffith, D.H., 0078
Grzegorzewski, E., 0396
Gupta, S., 0267
Gupta, S.C., 0079

Guyer, B., 0245
Guzman, G., 0631

H

Haas, J., 0083
Habicht, J.P., 0631
Hacettepe University, School of Medicine, Institute of Community Medicine, Ankara., 0309
Hadassah Medical Organization, Jerusalem., 0088, 0642
Haile Selassie I University, Faculty of Medicine, Addis Ababa., 0397
Halestrap, D.J., 0573
Hall, M.F., 0276
Hall, T.L., 0203
Hanning, L., 0574
Hansen, J.D., 0258
Haraldson, S., 0149
Harrison, T.J., 0452
Haskell, M.A., 0669
Have, R.T., 0677
Haward, L.R., 0523
Hays, C., 0037
Heald, K.A., 0014
Hefnawi, F., 0540
Herman, F., 0624
Higgins, M.M., 0510
Hilario, J., 0632
Hill, K.R., 0034
Hilleboe, H.E., 0150, 0151
Hinman, E.H., 0152
Hobson, W., 0398
Hofvander, Y., 0684
Holz, P., 0346
Horn, J.S., 0617
Horwitz, A., 0153
Hosu-Porbley, M., 0576
Hozumi, M., 0636
Huang, T.T., 0591, 0592
Hughes, J.M., 0501, 0608
Hughes, J.P., 0154, 0155
Hugo, E., 0502
Huxtable, K.A., 0541

I

India, Department of Health Services, Kerala., 0080
India, Ministry of Health and Family Planning., 0593
India, National Institute of Community Development, Hyderabad., 0694
India, State Health Education Bureau, Trivandrum, Kerala., 0081
Infante, A.D., 0204
Institute for Development Research, Copenhagen., 0637
Institute of Child Health of the University of Lagos, Lagos., 0594
Institute of Rural Health and Family Planning, Gandhigram., 0082, 0284, 0453, 0454, 0477, 0542, 0595, 0596, 0597, 0598
Intermediate Technology Development Group, London., 0034, 0145

International Confederation of Midwives, London., 0246, 0524, 0525, 0526, 0527
International Federation of Obstetrics and Gynaecology, London., 0524, 0527
International Hospital Federation, Washington, D.C., 0633
International Union for Child Welfare, Geneva., 0685
Iran, Ministry of Health., 0312, 0609
Iwase, H., 0263

J

Jackson, P., 0313
Jain, A.M., 0247, 0248
Janer, J.L., 0156
Janssens, P.G., 0399
Jensen, R.T., 0455
Jimeno, C., 0406
John, R., 0083
Johnson, G.Z., 0157, 0249
Johnson, S., 0305
Jones, G., 0634
Jose-Williams, A., 0057
Josiah Macy, Jr. Foundation, New York., 0518
Joubert, C., 0285, 0501
Journal of the Indian Medical Association, Calcutta., 0035, 0205
Journal of Tropical Pediatrics and Environmental Child Health, Kampala., 0084
Judy, M., 0085
Junichi, Y., 0263

K

Kaempffer, A.M., 0165, 0217
Kafuko, G.W., 0086
Kapil, K.K., 0686
Karefa-Smart, J., 0036
Karunaratne, W.A., 0635
Kassel, M.B., 0363
Katsuta, K., 0636
Kaul, S.J., 0543
Kebbouche, M.L., 0675
Keitzman, B., 0575
Kenya, Ministry of Information and Broadcasting., 0093
Kerr, C.B., 0456
Kesic, B., 0158, 0457
Kettle, E.S., 0221
Kidane-Miriam, W., 0250
Killen, O.H., 0307
Kimmelman, D., 0083
King, M., 0159, 0160, 0216
Kirfi, M.B., 0057
Kiryat Hayovel Health Centre, Jerusalem., 0642
Kivlin, J., 0694
Kleinbach, G., 0037
Kohn, R., 0015
Korn, J., 0637
Korsah, K.K., 0528
Kpedekpo, G.M., 0161
Kretchmer, N., 0206, 0251
Kuzuo, N., 0263
Kwansa, E.V., 0576

L

Laha, N.M., 0347
Lange, W.G., 0400
Larsson, Y., 0616
Latham, M., 0577
Lathem, W., 0162
League of Red Cross Societies, Geneva., 0458
Lee, N., 0469
Letlhaku, L., 0357
Limcharoen, C., 0692
Litman, T.J., 0638
Lizana, J., 0670
Llinares, V.M., 0252
Loefler, I.J., 0459
Long, E.C., 0163, 0460
Lourie, I.M., 0407
Lucas, A.O., 0164, 0401, 0639
Lutwama, J.S., 0232, 0402
Lyman, K., 0038
Lythcott, G.I., 0253

M

Maar, S.A., 0314
Mabry, J.H., 0656, 0659
Mahmoud, A.H., 0540
Maichuk, Y.F., 0687
Maier, J., 0518
Majekodunmi, M.A., 0039
Malawi, Health Extension Service., 0016
Malawi, Ministry of Finance., 0040
Malik, S.M., 0548
Manisoff, M.T., 0599
Mann, K.J., 0041, 0087, 0088, 0403, 0404, 0642
Manning, O., 0649
Manson-Bahr, P.E., 0383
Manuwa, S., 0046, 0405
Margulies, H., 0640
Marsh, M.C., 0437, 0614
Marson, W., 0688
Martens, E.G., 0461, 0462, 0463
Martin, J.F., 0254
Martoy, J., 0255
Marwah, S.M., 0176, 0243, 0415
Masters, D., 0511
Mathews, M., 0089
Matovu, H.L., 0315
Matsushita, Y., 0263
McDermott, W., 0256
McGlashan, N.D., 0207
McKeown, T., 0641
McPhail, J.E., 0286
Mechanic, D., 0023
Medalie, J.H., 0642
Medical Research Centre, Nairobi., 0090
Medina, E., 0165, 0217
Mehta, S.A., 0166
Mellander, O., 0674
Mendia, L., 0554
Messinezy, D.A., 0464
Messing, S.D., 0167, 0222, 0650, 0673
Meyer-Lie, A., 0168
Mgobozi, P., 0364

Milbank Memorial Fund Quarterly, New York., 0231
Modi, J.A., 0660
Moghaddam, R., 0465
Moles, G., 0316
Molina, G., 0406
Mollaret, P., 0257
Montag, M.L., 0512
Moodie, A.D., 0258
Morley, D., 0365
Muangman, D., 0612
Mullins, C., 0601
Murphy, A.K., 0610
Musoke, L.K., 0259

N

Na Oruwariye, T.O., 0057
Nakao, A., 0636
Namboze, J.N., 0315
Narain, B., 0260
Nasr, K., 0099
Nath, B., 0223
National Convention of Medical Technologists, Santiago., 0551
National Library of Medicine, Bethesda, Md., 0017, 0018
Navarro, V., 0091, 0169, 0170, 0661
Nepal, Family Planning and Maternal Child Health Project., 0261
Nepal, Ministry of Health., 0171, 0208
Neumann, A.K., 0281, 0407, 0610
New York Academy of Medicine, New York., 0404
Newbery, A., 0162
Newkirk, D.D., 0209
Nicholson, T.F., 0028
Nigeria, Laboratory Assistants Training School., 0574
Nigeria, Ministry of Health., 0466, 0578
Niu, L.C., 0374
Nor Laily, A.B., 0611

O

O'Connor, M., 0198
O'Neill, J.V., 0467
Oakley, D., 0134
Odeku, E.L., 0408
Oduntan, S.A., 0408
Ogbeide, M.I., 0262
Ogunlana, A., 0126
Ogunlesi, T.O., 0122
Ohio Medlars Center, Columbus., 0019
Ojo, O.A., 0046
Okediji, F.O., 0122, 0172
Okojie, C.G., 0639
Olatunbosun, D., 0123
Omran, A.R., 0643
Ong, G.B., 0042
Onuaguluchi, G.O., 0046
Ordonez-Plaja, A., 0092
Organization for Economic Cooperation and Development, Paris., 0559
Orris, P., 0083
Ortega, R.B., 0579
Osuntokun, B.O., 0057

Otiende, J.D., 0093
Otitoju, E.O., 0408
Otolorin, M.P., 0173
Otoo, S.N., 0468, 0689
Owada, K., 0263
Owens, P.N., 0555

P

Pakistan Academy for Rural Development, Comilla., 0600
Pakistan Family Planning Board, Lahore., 0537
Pakistan Family Planning Council, Islamabad., 0521, 0533, 0601
Pakistan, Health Department of West Pakistan., 0644
Pakistan, Ministry of Health and Social Welfare., 0671
Pan American Health Organization, Washington, D.C., 0645
Pan American Sanitary Bureau, Washington, D.C., 0556
Panchal, R.M., 0366
Panyavanija, P., 0469
Participant Journal, New Delhi., 0264
Passos, C., 0174
Patel, B.P., 0175
Patel, T.B., 0366
Patino, J.F., 0094, 0095
Pearson, C.A., 0126
Pearson, R.J., 0023, 0656
Pene, P., 0470
Peng, J.Y., 0611
Pequignot, H., 0471
Perkin, G.W., 0601
Perlman, M., 0026
Peru, Department of Health., 0579
Philippines, Bureau of Health., 0580
Pike, M.C., 0619
Pillai, K.K., 0683
Pinkerton, J.H., 0383
Pisharoti, K.A., 0265
Planned Parenthood-World Population, New York., 0599
Population Reference Bureau, Bogota., 0679
Poulton, E.M., 0266
Prachuabmoh, V., 0612
Prasad, B.G., 0144, 0648
Prasada Rao, D.C., 0267
Pratt, K.A., 0046
Price, E.W., 0662
Prince, J.S., 0222, 0407, 0650, 0673
Prywes, M., 0096, 0409, 0410
Pugh, A.O., 0097

Q

Quartey-Papafio, E.K., 0413

R

Rabin, D.L., 0646
Radius, S., 0015
Radoli, O., 0224
Rahman, S., 0602
Ramalingaswami, V., 0043

Raman, M.V., 0647
Ramos, R., 0411
RAND Corporation, Santa Monica., 0014
Ranganna, M.G., 0648
Ransome-Kuti, A.O., 0639
Rao, G.K., 0367
Rao, N.M., 0368
Rao, N.S., 0176
Rao, P.S., 0317, 0318
Rapoport, M., 0037
Raska, K., 0268
Razaq, A.A., 0044
Rehabilitation Record, Washington, D.C., 0348
Reiff, R., 0045
Reinke, W.A., 0098, 0663
Reissman, F., 0045
Research Triangle Institute, North Carolina., 0690
Revista Saude Publica, Sao Paulo., 0664
Revzin, M.E., 0544
Reyes, W.L., 0177
Reyna-Barrios, J.M., 0631
Reynolds, J., 0691
Rhodesia, Government of Rhodesia., 0472, 0473
Richard, J., 0317, 0318
Roberts, J.M., 0319
Robins, L., 0638
Rochac, A., 0178
Roemer, M.I., 0210, 0218, 0320, 0649, 0665
Roemer, R., 0613
Rojas, F.A., 0395
Romulo, C.P., 0503
Ronaghy, H.A., 0099
Rosa, F.W., 0269, 0474
Rosenfield, A.G., 0612, 0692, 0693
Rosinski, E.F., 0475
Ross, A., 0656
Rothert, F.C., 0270
Roy, P., 0694
Ruderman, A.P., 0213
Rundle, F.F., 0412
Ryder, B., 0650

S

Sabas, L.E., 0504
Sagen, O.K., 0656
Sai, F.T., 0271, 0413, 0476
Salawu, F.A., 0617
Samarasinghe, C.E., 0369
Samarasinghe, J., 0529
Samater, H.N., 0505
Sandtner, P., 0483
Sansarricq, H., 0100
Santhanam, M.L., 0477
Saroukhanian, G., 0302
Sastry, K.R., 0477
Saxena, K.N., 0370
Saxena, M.N., 0370
Schamschula, R.G., 0545
Schulman, D.P., 0321
Schulman, S., 0321
Schultz, G.P., 0179
Schultz, T.P., 0695

Segall, M., 0322
Segersky, U.B., 0616
Seidman, D.R., 0136
Sein, M.M., 0478
Senecal, J., 0479
Sengupta, A., 0371
Seoul National University, School of Public Health, Seoul., 0323
Shah, K.K., 0696
Shah, M.H., 0366
Shah, N.K., 0101
Sharma, B.N., 0349
Sharpston, M.J., 0211
Shehu, U., 0617
Shelesnyak, M.C., 0272
Shepherd, P., 0324
Shibata, T., 0636
Shillman, J.B., 0530
Shivaswamy, M.K., 0604
Siddhu, C.M., 0381
Sidel, V.W., 0480
Sierra, C.A., 0395
Sims, P., 0481
Singh, K., 0102
Singh, S., 0697
Smith, H., 0352
Smith, O.I., 0352
Smith, R.A., 0046
Sofoluwe, G.O., 0047, 0273
Solon, F.S., 0482
Soriano, L.R., 0626
Sosanya, R.O., 0531
Soumah, A., 0325
South Pacific Commission, Noumea., 0497
Southgate, B.A., 0307
Speare, M.C., 0677
Spencer, F.J., 0475
Spoustova, V., 0483
Spruyt, D.J., 0650
Standard, K.L., 0299, 0414, 0437, 0484, 0569, 0614
Stanfield, J.P., 0698
Stanley, A., 0326
Stapleton, T., 0219
Stein, Z., 0103
Stewart, W.H., 0048
Stiernborg, M., 0532
Stoeckle, J.D., 0104
Stolten, J.H., 0581
Stone, B., 0105
Sugiono, M., 0372
Sundram, C.J., 0373
Susser, M., 0103
Swallows in India, Madras., 0274
Sweden Pakistan Family Welfare Project, Lahore., 0603
Swedish International Development Agency, Stockholm., 0651
Swiss Tropical Institute, Basel., 0485
Syme, S.L., 0275

T

Taba, A.H., 0212

Tait, H.P., 0106
Takada, S., 0263
Takeshita, K., 0636
Tanzania, Ministry of Health., 0486, 0618
Taylor, C.E., 0180, 0276
Taylor, D., 0107
Tekirli, N., 0652
Ten Have, R., 0277
Thach, P.N., 0108
Thailand, Ministry of Public Health., 0278
Thapa, R., 0107
Theberge, J.D., 0220
Thomas, W.C., 0150
Tiglao, T.V., 0653
Tiwari, I.C., 0415
Torrey, E.F., 0109
Transactions of the Royal Society of Tropical Medicine and Hygiene, London., 0181
Tribhuvan University, Kathmandu., 0615
Truswell, A.S., 0258
Tsai, J.F., 0374
Tseghe, Y., 0650
Turner, J., 0287
Twumasi, P.A., 0225
Tyrer, F.H., 0182

U

Ukeje, M.A., 0279
Unhanand, M., 0699
Universidad de San Carlos de Guatemala, Facultad de Odontologia San Carlos, Guatemala, Guatemala., 0547
Universidad de San Carlos de Guatemala, Guatemala., 0582
University of the West Indies, Mona, Jamaica., 0569
USA, Department of Health, Education and Welfare., 0487

V

Vahlquist, B., 0674
Valenzuela, V.C., 0375
Van Die Redaksie., 0183
Vaughan, J.P., 0488
Velasquez, G., 0416
Velazquez, G., 0184
Venezuela, Ministry of Health., 0185, 0583
Vidal, E.L., 0395
Viel, B., 0533
Villarreal, R., 0422
Vintinner, F.J., 0350
Vogel, L.C., 0110, 0327, 0328, 0329, 0489

W

Waddy, B.B., 0049
Wade, C.C., 0050
Wade, M.K., 0650
Wakatsuki, T., 0654
Walker, V., 0490
Wang, W., 0374
Ward, J.P., 0111
Weinerman, E.R., 0655
Wells, M., 0330
Wennen, E.C., 0186
West African Medical Journal, Ibadan., 0417
Westinghouse Learning Corporation, Health Services Division, Bladensbury, Md., 0467
Westwater, K., 0351
White, K.L., 0621, 0656
WHO, Alexandria., 0051, 0112, 0113, 0114, 0133, 0187, 0293, 0334, 0418, 0506
WHO, Brazzaville., 0052, 0188, 0331, 0491, 0492
WHO, Geneva., 0020, 0053, 0054, 0115, 0116, 0117, 0147, 0150, 0151, 0189, 0190, 0191, 0192, 0193, 0194, 0195, 0196, 0197, 0280, 0286, 0320, 0378, 0419, 0420, 0421, 0493, 0494, 0495, 0496, 0507, 0513, 0514, 0534, 0535, 0536, 0552, 0657, 0658, 0672
WHO, Manila., 0118, 0140, 0497, 0629
WHO, New Delhi., 0288
Wilkie, W., 0584
Wilkinson, J.L., 0352
Williams, E., 0490
Williams, G.A., 0408
Wilson, E.E., 0286
Wilson, J.M., 0197
Wittmann, W., 0258
Wolf, A.C., 0220
Wolfe, S., 0023
Wolstenholme, G., 0198
Wood, A.M., 0353, 0354
Wood, C.H., 0498
Woolman, A., 0332
Wurapa, F.K., 0281, 0413, 0620
Wyon, J.B., 0697

Y

Yankauer, A., 0422
Yen, Y.T., 0333
Yohannes, T., 0222

Z

Zachariah, S., 0700
Zaghloul, A.Z., 0119, 0334
Zaire, Department of Public Health., 0289
Ziai, L., 0282

Geographical Index

(figures refer to abstract numbers)

A

Afghanistan, 0418
Africa, *See also: regional name(s), e.g., East Africa and specific country name(s)*, 0052, 0054, 0062, 0100, 0105, 0127, 0129, 0138, 0145, 0152, 0154, 0157, 0161, 0188, 0210, 0224, 0225, 0254, 0257, 0262, 0298, 0303, 0311, 0313, 0316, 0324, 0325, 0327, 0328, 0329, 0331, 0332, 0335, 0343, 0355, 0358, 0391, 0417, 0431, 0475, 0481, 0486, 0488, 0491, 0492, 0493, 0511, 0515, 0517, 0525, 0528, 0529, 0530, 0531, 0538, 0546, 0570, 0573, 0575, 0577, 0589, 0590, 0594, 0662, 0673
Alaska, 0121, 0452
Algeria, 0084, 0493, 0675
Argentina, 0124, 0249, 0380, 0400, 0508, 0558
Asia, *See also: regional name(s), e.g., Middle East and specific country name(s)*, 0145, 0157, 0210, 0323, 0347
Australia, 0061, 0118, 0129, 0219, 0221, 0338, 0513, 0633

B

Bahrain, 0050, 0506
Bangladesh, 0187, 0588, 0600, 0602, 0671, 0685
Barbados, 0681
Belgium, 0513
Bengal, India, 0132, 0700
Biafra, 0235
Bolivia, 0409
Botswana, 0052, 0056, 0423
Brazil, 0130, 0153, 0163, 0361, 0411, 0513, 0632, 0633, 0664
Brunei, 0118
Burma, 0106, 0383, 0428, 0478
Burundi, 0573

C

Cambodia, 0412
Cameroon, 0052, 0325, 0377, 0458, 0470
Canada, 0098, 0129, 0163, 0338, 0432, 0461, 0462, 0463, 0513, 0560, 0561, 0562, 0563, 0564, 0633
Cape Town, 0258
Central Africa, 0234, 0573
Central African Republic, 0249, 0428, 0493
Central America, *See also: Latin America*, 0059, 0270, 0338, 0350
Chad, 0470
Chile, 0098, 0115, 0117, 0128, 0153, 0157, 0165, 0199, 0200, 0203, 0204, 0217, 0249, 0406, 0409, 0411, 0526, 0533, 0549, 0550, 0633, 0670, 0672
China PR, 0065, 0091, 0412, 0436, 0518, 0637, 0654
China R, 0025, 0026, 0067, 0098, 0117, 0118, 0129, 0147, 0150, 0238, 0239, 0333, 0374, 0518, 0591, 0592, 0663, 0695
Colombia, 0006, 0029, 0066, 0095, 0162, 0184, 0202, 0249, 0321, 0376, 0416, 0566, 0567, 0568, 0587, 0605, 0613, 0623, 0633, 0666, 0667, 0678
Congo, 0234, 0455
Costa Rica, 0249, 0338, 0518, 0556
Cuba, 0083, 0091, 0103, 0169, 0618
Cyprus, 0212, 0506
Czechoslovakia, 0098, 0195, 0483, 0518, 0672

D

Dahomey, 0458, 0470
Denmark, 0040, 0518, 0637, 0651

E

East Africa, 0105, 0181, 0201, 0224, 0259, 0303, 0311, 0319, 0327, 0328, 0329, 0335, 0343, 0353, 0358, 0444, 0449, 0459, 0486, 0573, 0662
Egypt, 0051, 0112, 0114, 0119, 0157, 0195, 0212, 0418, 0506, 0540, 0607, 0643
El Salvador, 0249, 0338
Ethiopia, 0031, 0034, 0055, 0065, 0068, 0109, 0133, 0167, 0168, 0222, 0250, 0324, 0397, 0418, 0428, 0433, 0455, 0464, 0474, 0489, 0506, 0622, 0650, 0662, 0673, 0674, 0682, 0684
Europe, 0013, 0527

F

Far East, 0070, 0323
Fiji, 0118, 0428, 0444, 0488, 0633
Finland, 0637, 0651
France, 0098, 0117, 0513, 0613
French Polynesia, 0118

G

Gabon, 0470
Gambia, 0052, 0157
Germany FR, 0613
Ghana, 0032, 0049, 0076, 0145, 0154, 0157, 0160, 0161, 0211, 0225, 0281, 0285, 0325, 0369, 0407, 0413, 0427, 0444, 0468, 0476, 0501, 0515, 0526, 0528, 0529, 0572, 0576, 0608, 0620, 0689

Gondar, 0433
Guatemala, 0085, 0290, 0362, 0428, 0460, 0546, 0547, 0582, 0631, 0645
Guinea, 0160, 0470

H

Haiti, 0145
Hong Kong, 0042, 0071, 0118, 0523
Hungary, 0215

I

India, 0033, 0034, 0035, 0043, 0058, 0060, 0064, 0078, 0079, 0080, 0081, 0082, 0089, 0098, 0106, 0117, 0129, 0132, 0144, 0145, 0147, 0150, 0157, 0160, 0162, 0166, 0175, 0176, 0181, 0195, 0205, 0223, 0226, 0229, 0230, 0237, 0242, 0243, 0244, 0247, 0248, 0249, 0260, 0264, 0267, 0269, 0274, 0284, 0286, 0287, 0288, 0291, 0292, 0317, 0318, 0341, 0344, 0347, 0348, 0349, 0356, 0366, 0367, 0368, 0370, 0371, 0377, 0379, 0381, 0388, 0390, 0415, 0424, 0453, 0454, 0455, 0477, 0518, 0519, 0526, 0539, 0542, 0593, 0595, 0596, 0597, 0598, 0604, 0610, 0647, 0648, 0658, 0680, 0683, 0686, 0688, 0690, 0694, 0696, 0697, 0700
Indonesia, 0065, 0372, 0412, 0518
Iran, 0051, 0073, 0084, 0099, 0112, 0114, 0145, 0187, 0212, 0228, 0282, 0300, 0302, 0312, 0378, 0418, 0465, 0506, 0609
Iraq, 0051, 0084, 0112, 0114, 0187, 0418
Israel, 0041, 0087, 0088, 0098, 0117, 0187, 0403, 0404, 0418, 0506, 0642, 0672
Ivory Coast, 0052, 0154, 0470

J

Jamaica, 0154, 0299, 0414, 0437, 0484, 0490, 0546, 0569
Japan, 0117, 0118, 0129, 0513, 0518, 0613, 0636
Jerusalem, 0088
Jordan, 0114, 0506, 0584

K

Kenya, 0008, 0052, 0055, 0062, 0090, 0093, 0110, 0138, 0139, 0224, 0259, 0303, 0306, 0307, 0308, 0311, 0319, 0327, 0328, 0329, 0335, 0337, 0338, 0339, 0340, 0342, 0343, 0354, 0382, 0428, 0441, 0443, 0445, 0455, 0518, 0637
Kerala, India, 0081
Khmer Republic, 0118
Korea R, 0118, 0140, 0323, 0585
Kuwait, 0187, 0506

L

Laos, 0118, 0412
Latin America, *See also: regional name(s), e.g., Central America and specific country name(s)*, 0025, 0059, 0063, 0115, 0128, 0145, 0153, 0156, 0157, 0174, 0185, 0199, 0210, 0220, 0231, 0252, 0295, 0361, 0400, 0411, 0422, 0457, 0551, 0555, 0556, 0587, 0679
Lebanon, 0418, 0506

Lesotho, 0332
Liberia, 0052, 0538
Libya, 0212, 0506

M

Madagascar, 0052
Malawi, 0016, 0040, 0052, 0207, 0216, 0234, 0365, 0428, 0441
Malaysia, 0098, 0102, 0118, 0157, 0249, 0296, 0373, 0412, 0426, 0509, 0611, 0649
Mali, 0157, 0458, 0470
Masasi, Tanzania, 0105
Mexico, 0115, 0409
Middle East, 0051, 0112, 0114, 0187, 0212, 0418, 0506
Mysore, India, 0604

N

Nepal, 0101, 0107, 0111, 0171, 0208, 0261, 0277, 0510, 0615
Netherlands, 0518, 0637, 0658
New Hebrides, 0118
New Zealand, 0118, 0129, 0513
Niger, 0052, 0458, 0470
Nigeria, 0021, 0025, 0028, 0034, 0039, 0044, 0046, 0047, 0057, 0122, 0123, 0126, 0137, 0145, 0154, 0164, 0172, 0173, 0181, 0182, 0186, 0206, 0235, 0241, 0245, 0273, 0298, 0313, 0316, 0325, 0338, 0377, 0394, 0401, 0408, 0428, 0442, 0455, 0466, 0499, 0518, 0522, 0531, 0574, 0575, 0578, 0594, 0617, 0639
North Africa, 0051, 0112, 0114, 0212, 0324, 0418, 0506
Norway, 0633
Nyasaland, 0098, 0157

O

Oceania, 0456

P

Pakistan, 0051, 0065, 0112, 0114, 0145, 0157, 0187, 0212, 0249, 0300, 0418, 0518, 0521, 0537, 0541, 0543, 0588, 0600, 0601, 0602, 0603, 0644, 0671
Panama, 0153, 0249, 0350
Papua New Guinea, 0118, 0412, 0488, 0545
Peru, 0025, 0115, 0150, 0387, 0513
Philippines, 0022, 0065, 0118, 0162, 0177, 0249, 0304, 0310, 0375, 0386, 0482, 0503, 0504, 0580, 0626, 0629, 0653
Poland, 0513, 0613
Puerto Rico, 0157, 0162, 0518, 0658, 0668
Punjab, India, 0064, 0697

Q

Qatar, 0187, 0506

R

Rhodesia, 0097, 0098, 0157, 0234, 0314, 0326, 0472, 0473
Rwanda, 0573
Ryukyu Islands, 0070, 0118

Geographical Index   153

S

Saudi Arabia, 0114, 0187, 0334
Senegal, 0052, 0428, 0458, 0470
Sierra Leone, 0030, 0352, 0513, 0517
Singapore, 0118, 0157, 0377, 0412
Somalia, 0114, 0212, 0505
South Africa R, 0183, 0258, 0305, 0332, 0346, 0360, 0364, 0434, 0513, 0658
South East Asia, 0347, 0456
South Pacific, 0475
Spain, 0034
Sri Lanka, 0065, 0135, 0157, 0195, 0249, 0263, 0532, 0672
Sudan, 0055, 0145, 0157, 0187, 0336, 0418, 0428, 0441, 0455, 0548, 0575, 0687
Sweden, 0098, 0150, 0613, 0616, 0625, 0672, 0674
Switzerland, 0513
Syria, 0051, 0114, 0187, 0195, 0293, 0418, 0506

T

Tanzania, 0008, 0052, 0098, 0105, 0160, 0259, 0325, 0343, 0409, 0428, 0441, 0448, 0450, 0455, 0485, 0486, 0498, 0557, 0616, 0618, 0637
Tasmania, 0061
Thailand, 0147, 0162, 0278, 0385, 0392, 0444, 0469, 0518, 0526, 0546, 0601, 0606, 0612, 0634, 0692, 0699
Togo, 0052, 0147, 0458, 0520
Tonga, 0118
Trinidad and Tobago, 0411
Tunisia, 0051, 0098, 0112, 0418, 0451, 0506, 0633
Turkey, 0025, 0073, 0074, 0084, 0098, 0141, 0150, 0212, 0300, 0309, 0586, 0652

U

Uganda, 0008, 0052, 0086, 0221, 0259, 0297, 0315, 0338, 0343, 0357, 0358, 0382, 0428, 0441, 0455, 0573, 0619, 0628, 0669, 0698
U.K., 0034, 0065, 0098, 0113, 0117, 0145, 0162, 0181, 0195, 0300, 0338, 0513, 0518, 0613, 0630, 0641, 0658
Upper Volta, 0325, 0458, 0470
Uruguay, 0255
USA, 0014, 0034, 0045, 0048, 0065, 0098, 0113, 0117, 0121, 0129, 0143, 0145, 0148, 0150, 0162, 0163, 0300, 0338, 0355, 0411, 0428, 0435, 0436, 0452, 0467, 0487, 0493, 0518, 0521, 0526, 0613, 0630, 0640, 0672, 0677, 0691, 0693
USSR, 0116, 0117, 0129, 0150, 0195, 0428, 0471, 0480, 0488, 0493, 0518, 0630, 0654

V

Venezuela, 0098, 0115, 0150, 0185, 0249, 0395, 0553, 0583
Vietnam DR, 0108, 0322, 0338, 0651
Vietnam R, 0077, 0118, 0143, 0412, 0544
Volta River, 0154

W

West Africa, 0030, 0164, 0225, 0298, 0313, 0316, 0338, 0431, 0458, 0499, 0501, 0515, 0517, 0524, 0525, 0528, 0529, 0531, 0538, 0590, 0594
West Indies, 0484, 0569, 0614
Western Samoa, 0118

Y

Yemen, 0114
Yugoslavia, 0098, 0518

Z

Zaire, 0052, 0209, 0283, 0289, 0359, 0430, 0470, 0570, 0624
Zambia, 0065, 0145, 0160, 0216, 0234, 0279, 0294, 0345, 0351, 0459, 0481, 0625, 0635

Subject Index

Note: *Sometimes by matching the numbers under two subject index terms, or sets of keywords, the reader can pinpoint specific information. For example, item 0569 under "community health worker" and "training manual" is actually a training manual for community health workers.*

(figures refer to abstract numbers)

A

Aborigine, 0061, 0296
Abortion, 0533, 0587, 0599, 0679
Abstracting Journal, *See also: bibliography,* 0009, 0010, 0011
Administrative Aspect, *See also: health services administration,* 0036, 0042, 0043, 0049, 0050, 0055, 0060, 0061, 0062, 0065, 0073, 0078, 0089, 0090, 0091, 0092, 0100, 0109, 0110, 0112, 0113, 0118, 0132, 0133, 0153, 0169, 0173, 0192, 0196, 0213, 0233, 0236, 0239, 0260, 0265, 0280, 0292, 0299, 0303, 0308, 0309, 0319, 0331, 0339, 0347, 0356, 0405, 0422, 0455, 0486, 0507, 0536, 0542, 0551, 0609, 0623, 0630, 0644, 0649, 0657, 0658, 0686
Admission Requirements, 0419, 0420, 0430, 0453, 0475, 0477, 0512
African Medical and Res. Foundation, 0297, 0335, 0337, 0343
Agricultural Sector, 0049, 0117, 0119, 0134, 0166, 0182, 0202, 0252, 0290, 0382
Air Pollution, 0192
Aircraft, *See also: flying doctor service, mobile health unit, transport,* 0055, 0335, 0342, 0353
All India Institute of Med. Sci., 0379
American Dental Association, 0544
Anaesthetist Job Description, 0408
Ante-Natal Clinic, 0327, 0332
APHA, 0227
Assistant Medical Officer, *See also: auxiliary health worker,* 0475, 0497
Assistant Medical Officer Training, 0475, 0497
Attitude, 0223, 0224, 0225, 0283, 0291, 0298, 0355, 0357, 0358, 0371, 0435, 0673
Audiovisual Aid, 0358, 0368, 0378, 0393, 0458, 0481, 0573, 0576, 0586, 0588, 0624
Auxiliary Curriculum, 0450, 0452, 0472, 0473, 0486, 0487, 0583, 0598
Auxiliary Health Worker, *See also: barefoot doctor, community health aide, dresser, family planning auxiliary, feldsher, medex, medic, medical assistant, midwife, nurse auxiliary,* 0003, 0008, 0009, 0012, 0019, 0020, 0022, 0028, 0029, 0030, 0031, 0034, 0035, 0036, 0037, 0039, 0040, 0043, 0044, 0045, 0046, 0049, 0050, 0054, 0055, 0056, 0058, 0062, 0063, 0065, 0066, 0067, 0072, 0075, 0077, 0078, 0080, 0081, 0085, 0091, 0098, 0099, 0106, 0113, 0115, 0121, 0124, 0138, 0140, 0141, 0142, 0144, 0145, 0146, 0155, 0162, 0167, 0169, 0185, 0186, 0189, 0196, 0198, 0204, 0209, 0211, 0222, 0225, 0227, 0228, 0230, 0233, 0234, 0236, 0244, 0246, 0248, 0269, 0278, 0282, 0284, 0286, 0289, 0290, 0296, 0303, 0306, 0308, 0309, 0310, 0316, 0319, 0323, 0330, 0333, 0335, 0336, 0339, 0342, 0356, 0361, 0363, 0366, 0368, 0374, 0375, 0376, 0377, 0379, 0380, 0390, 0397, 0407, 0412, 0414, 0417, 0423, 0424, 0425, 0426, 0427, 0428, 0429, 0430, 0431, 0432, 0433, 0434, 0435, 0436, 0437, 0438, 0439, 0440, 0441, 0442, 0444, 0445, 0446, 0447, 0448, 0449, 0450, 0451, 0452, 0453, 0454, 0455, 0456, 0457, 0458, 0459, 0460, 0461, 0462, 0463, 0464, 0465, 0466, 0467, 0468, 0469, 0470, 0471, 0472, 0473, 0474, 0475, 0477, 0478, 0479, 0480, 0481, 0483, 0484, 0485, 0486, 0487, 0488, 0489, 0490, 0491, 0492, 0493, 0494, 0495, 0496, 0497, 0498, 0501, 0508, 0509, 0513, 0515, 0517, 0519, 0522, 0525, 0529, 0531, 0535, 0537, 0541, 0543, 0545, 0555, 0558, 0560, 0562, 0565, 0567, 0568, 0569, 0572, 0575, 0578, 0579, 0580, 0581, 0583, 0587, 0598, 0603, 0605, 0606, 0608, 0609, 0613, 0614, 0616, 0631, 0637, 0645, 0650, 0668, 0693
Auxiliary Job Description, 0045, 0052, 0098, 0291, 0431, 0440, 0443, 0444, 0452, 0457, 0468, 0470, 0487, 0491, 0493, 0501, 0558, 0579, 0580, 0581
Auxiliary Selection, 0045, 0424, 0472, 0473, 0491, 0602
Auxiliary Supervision, 0022, 0034, 0049, 0050, 0054, 0068, 0089, 0100, 0113, 0189, 0246, 0303, 0337, 0377, 0424, 0428, 0439, 0444, 0463, 0487, 0491, 0529, 0539, 0614, 0629, 0631, 0650
Auxiliary Training, *See also: health manpower training, midwife training,* 0012, 0020, 0021, 0027, 0028, 0030, 0034, 0036, 0037, 0040, 0044, 0049, 0051, 0052, 0054, 0055, 0056, 0058, 0067, 0068, 0080, 0099, 0121, 0140, 0144, 0162, 0167, 0181, 0183, 0189, 0198, 0222, 0225, 0227, 0246, 0278, 0280, 0290, 0291, 0302, 0308, 0310, 0316, 0323, 0335, 0336, 0339, 0356, 0363, 0368, 0374, 0377, 0380, 0390, 0393, 0397, 0398, 0407, 0414, 0417, 0420, 0421, 0422, 0423, 0424, 0425, 0427, 0429, 0430, 0431, 0433, 0435, 0436, 0437, 0438, 0439, 0440, 0441, 0442, 0443, 0444, 0445, 0446, 0447, 0448, 0449, 0450, 0451, 0452, 0453, 0454, 0455, 0456, 0457, 0458, 0459, 0460, 0461, 0463, 0466, 0467, 0468, 0469, 0470, 0471, 0472, 0473, 0474, 0475, 0476, 0478, 0479, 0481, 0482, 0483, 0484, 0485, 0486, 0487, 0488, 0490, 0491, 0492, 0493, 0495, 0496, 0506, 0514, 0517, 0523, 0531, 0539, 0541, 0545, 0555, 0558, 0562, 0567, 0568, 0569, 0575, 0581, 0583, 0588, 0598, 0603, 0609, 0614, 0616, 0620, 0629, 0644, 0650, 0686
Auxiliary Training Centre, 0375

Auxiliary Training Course, 0448, 0457, 0466, 0508
Auxiliary Training Curriculum, 0609
Auxiliary Training Evaluation, 0463, 0483
Auxiliary Utilization, 0045, 0062, 0121, 0144, 0198, 0265, 0407, 0424, 0429, 0431, 0439, 0440, 0441, 0444, 0457, 0461, 0465, 0467, 0469, 0470, 0475, 0488, 0491, 0498, 0540
Ayurvedic Medicine, 0035

B

Ballabhgarh Project, India, 0379
Bantu, 0364
Bantu Health Educator, 0434
Barefoot Doctor, *See also: auxiliary health worker,* 0189, 0436
BCG Vaccination, 0683
Bibliography, *See also: abstracting journal,* 0001, 0002, 0003, 0004, 0005, 0007, 0009, 0010, 0011, 0012, 0013, 0014, 0015, 0017, 0018, 0019, 0020
Bilharzia, 0119
Birth Control, *See also: abortion, contraception, family planning, intrauterine device, oral contraceptive, vasectomy,* 0072, 0145, 0153, 0256, 0313, 0371, 0515, 0521, 0525, 0529, 0532, 0534, 0587, 0591, 0593, 0599, 0686, 0695
Blindness, 0345, 0348
Blindness Prevention, 0340
Brain Drain, 0022, 0046, 0050, 0065, 0072, 0181, 0503, 0634
Breast Feeding, 0587
Building Plan, 0325, 0327, 0328, 0329, 0330

C

Canadian Indian Health Service, *See also: US Indian health service,* 0432, 0463, 0560
Carolina Population Center, 0254
Cataract, 0062, 0340
CENTO, 0300
Central Government, 0090, 0110, 0114, 0123, 0189, 0205, 0358, 0629, 0644
Child, *See also: maternal child health, pediatrics,* 0105, 0145, 0206, 0209, 0248, 0249, 0251, 0256, 0280, 0295, 0332, 0518, 0535, 0569, 0645
Child Care, 0011, 0072, 0124, 0232, 0236, 0247, 0274, 0280, 0534, 0565, 0587, 0594, 0651, 0685
Child Health, 0219, 0241, 0245, 0247, 0262, 0267, 0365, 0429, 0674
Child Mortality, 0643
Cholera, 0080, 0089, 0263, 0694
Christian Medical College, Vellore, 0390
Clinic, 0006, 0302, 0325, 0481, 0636, 0670, 0691
CMC, 0292
Communicable Disease, 0005, 0009, 0051, 0081, 0097, 0118, 0130, 0135, 0296, 0439, 0568, 0587, 0671
Communication, *See also: mass communication, mass media, radio communication,* 0075, 0115, 0160, 0228, 0353, 0354, 0358, 0362, 0364, 0371, 0374, 0460, 0489, 0559, 0576, 0583, 0586, 0588, 0591, 0597, 0633, 0694
Community, *See also: social participation,* 0005, 0045, 0056, 0059, 0064, 0079, 0148, 0163, 0184, 0247, 0248, 0258, 0270, 0283, 0299, 0318, 0355, 0356, 0357, 0358, 0359, 0360, 0361, 0362, 0364, 0365, 0366, 0368, 0369, 0370, 0371, 0372, 0373, 0374, 0375, 0378, 0384, 0386, 0389, 0392, 0404, 0421, 0422, 0461, 0482, 0502, 0563, 0570, 0572, 0581, 0588, 0626, 0635, 0685
Community Development, 0041, 0083, 0115, 0124, 0178, 0196, 0248, 0260, 0290, 0350, 0356, 0363, 0366, 0367, 0368, 0375, 0379, 0385, 0402, 0446, 0463, 0476, 0484, 0508, 0562, 0568, 0618, 0645, 0653, 0658, 0666, 0667, 0694
Community Health Aide, *See also: auxiliary health worker,* 0437, 0490
Community Health Aide Training, 0437
Community Health Worker, *See also: auxiliary health worker,* 0432, 0461, 0462, 0463, 0560, 0561, 0563, 0569
Community Health Worker Training, 0432, 0461, 0462, 0560, 0561
Community Nurse, *See also: nurse,* 0509, 0522
Community Nurse Training, 0522
Community Organization, 0067, 0321, 0369
Conjunctivitis, 0687
Consumer Association, 0189, 0368
Contraception, *See also: intrauterine device, oral contraceptive,* 0237, 0242, 0278, 0357, 0371, 0540, 0599, 0678, 0681, 0693
Cost Benefit Analysis, *See also: economic aspect, financial aspect,* 0122, 0189, 0213, 0214, 0217, 0295, 0498, 0678
Cultural Aspect, 0119, 0160, 0215, 0221, 0223, 0224, 0225, 0240, 0279, 0324, 0361, 0424, 0435, 0487, 0679, 0694
Cultural Change, 0224, 0291, 0355, 0694
Curative Medicine, 0046, 0076, 0168, 0230, 0281, 0361, 0460, 0547, 0622, 0631
Curriculum, 0068, 0359, 0382, 0384, 0390, 0392, 0393, 0394, 0395, 0399, 0416, 0418, 0419, 0420, 0430, 0432, 0433, 0438, 0439, 0442, 0448, 0450, 0452, 0464, 0466, 0472, 0473, 0474, 0497, 0508, 0512, 0514, 0519, 0521, 0522, 0535, 0537, 0545, 0547, 0548, 0552, 0556, 0559, 0561, 0582, 0592, 0593, 0595, 0596, 0598, 0599, 0602

D

Dai, *See also: midwife,* 0265, 0269, 0366, 0368, 0539, 0600, 0700
Dai Curriculum, 0603
Dai Evaluation, 0539
Dai Job Description, 0539
Dai Training, 0539
Danfa Project, Ghana, 0161, 0281, 0407, 0413, 0476, 0620
DANIDA, 0040
Data Collecting, 0050, 0195, 0431, 0666, 0667
Decision Making, *See also: government policy, health services planning,* 0031, 0149, 0169, 0189, 0356, 0610
Demography, *See also: family planning, migration, population,* 0051, 0090, 0107, 0114, 0129, 0145, 0153, 0156, 0169, 0177, 0178, 0207, 0244, 0261, 0266, 0325, 0407, 0569, 0645, 0661, 0666, 0667, 0680

Dental Auxiliary, 0019, 0029, 0121, 0491, 0495, 0545, 0546, 0547, 0548, 0573, 0605
Dental Auxiliary Job Description, 0052, 0546
Dental Auxiliary Teaching Aid, 0573
Dental Auxiliary Training, 0121, 0545, 0546, 0547, 0548, 0573, 0605
Dental Auxiliary Training Manual, 0573
Dental Equipment, 0351
Dental Health, 0544
Dental Services Evaluation, 0121
Dentist, 0492, 0605
Dentist Distribution, 0605
Dentist Job Description, 0362
Dentist Teaching Aid, 0582
Dentist Training, 0544, 0582, 0605
Dentist Training Centre, 0544
Dentistry, 0351, 0572, 0573, 0605
Dermatology, 0370
Developing Country, 0012, 0014, 0023, 0027, 0031, 0036, 0037, 0038, 0043, 0048, 0053, 0055, 0056, 0060, 0065, 0072, 0075, 0091, 0096, 0120, 0125, 0129, 0131, 0132, 0134, 0138, 0141, 0142, 0145, 0146, 0149, 0150, 0157, 0159, 0160, 0163, 0167, 0173, 0180, 0181, 0182, 0193, 0194, 0196, 0198, 0201, 0210, 0219, 0227, 0233, 0239, 0240, 0246, 0249, 0251, 0264, 0266, 0272, 0308, 0319, 0320, 0339, 0366, 0377, 0378, 0382, 0392, 0396, 0399, 0405, 0410, 0429, 0433, 0438, 0439, 0443, 0446, 0455, 0472, 0473, 0475, 0479, 0484, 0488, 0489, 0491, 0513, 0516, 0521, 0526, 0527, 0533, 0554, 0591, 0592, 0632, 0640, 0658, 0693
Development Aid, *See also: food aid, health aid,* 0180, 0616, 0625, 0637, 0651
Development Planning, *See also: health services planning,* 0102, 0180, 0261, 0666, 0667
Diagnosis, 0113, 0297, 0345, 0570, 0572, 0698
Disease Control, *See also: endemic disease, infectious disease, mass campaign, parasitic disease,* 0004, 0005, 0021, 0022, 0051, 0080, 0100, 0113, 0114, 0124, 0147, 0152, 0157, 0177, 0188, 0193, 0223, 0230, 0233, 0243, 0245, 0248, 0252, 0255, 0268, 0273, 0292, 0310, 0319, 0361, 0558, 0565, 0572, 0584, 0587, 0654, 0662, 0675, 0687
Dispensary, 0006, 0035, 0077, 0105, 0145, 0223, 0298, 0324, 0431, 0486, 0578, 0616, 0619, 0688
Dispensary Attendant, 0575, 0578
Dispensary Attendant Training, 0575
Dresser, *See also: auxiliary health worker,* 0324, 0464, 0481, 0650
Dresser Training, 0397, 0464, 0481

E

Ecology, 0131, 0180
Economic Aspect, *See also: cost benefit analysis, financial aspect,* 0013, 0214, 0628, 0672
Economic Development, *See also: development planning,* 0025, 0122, 0129, 0145, 0150, 0153, 0164, 0166, 0177, 0178, 0181, 0194, 0195, 0220, 0226, 0446, 0618, 0640, 0664
Economic Development Index, 0664
Economic Planning, 0230
Elephantiasis, 0662

Endemic Disease, 0100, 0114, 0164, 0571, 0643
Environment, *See also: air pollution, sanitation, waste disposal, water pollution,* 0005, 0017, 0076, 0123, 0192, 0252, 0556, 0571, 0614, 0641
Environmental Health, 0193, 0554, 0555, 0657
Environmental Sanitation, 0009, 0080, 0124, 0508, 0558, 0567, 0572, 0666, 0667
Environmental Technology, 0553
Epidemiology, 0004, 0005, 0018, 0051, 0062, 0090, 0098, 0114, 0121, 0129, 0145, 0152, 0157, 0161, 0168, 0184, 0200, 0202, 0229, 0233, 0235, 0241, 0243, 0245, 0253, 0257, 0266, 0268, 0271, 0273, 0274, 0275, 0309, 0334, 0361, 0370, 0377, 0378, 0382, 0394, 0448, 0557, 0656, 0658, 0661, 0662, 0671, 0675, 0687, 0694, 0697
Equipment, *See also: health centre, hospital,* 0085, 0551, 0651
Eskimo, 0432, 0452, 0461, 0560
Evaluation, *See also: health centre evaluation, health services evaluation,* 0078, 0103, 0151, 0162, 0190, 0191, 0192, 0194, 0195, 0197, 0207, 0222, 0280, 0295, 0315, 0319, 0338, 0341, 0378, 0393, 0398, 0407, 0432, 0435, 0454, 0463, 0490, 0533, 0541, 0543, 0561, 0576, 0590, 0601, 0607, 0611, 0615, 0620, 0624, 0638, 0655, 0656, 0657, 0658, 0672, 0673, 0678, 0680, 0684, 0690, 0692, 0697, 0700
Eye Disease, *See also: blindness, conjunctivitis, onchocerciasis, trachoma,* 0062, 0297, 0340, 0348

F

Family, 0064, 0079, 0088, 0127, 0148
Family Health Educator, 0278
Family Health Manual, 0564
Family Planning, *See also: abortion, birth control, contraception, demography, intrauterine device, oral contraceptive, population,* 0020, 0227, 0272, 0569, 0599, 0603
Family Planning Auxiliary, *See also: auxiliary health worker,* 0026, 0265, 0269, 0454, 0456, 0518, 0521, 0525, 0532, 0539, 0541, 0585, 0586, 0587, 0588, 0590, 0592, 0596, 0597, 0598, 0600, 0602, 0603, 0611
Family Planning Auxiliary Training, 0026, 0521, 0525, 0530, 0532, 0533, 0537, 0564, 0585, 0590, 0591, 0592, 0593, 0595, 0597, 0598, 0600, 0601, 0602, 0603, 0686
Family Planning Curriculum, 0601
Family Planning Doctor, 0603
Family Planning Evaluation, 0681, 0691, 0693, 0694, 0695, 0696
Family Planning Manpower, 0542
Family Planning Manpower Training, 0519, 0542
Family Planning Officer, 0588, 0595
Family Planning Programme, 0060, 0067, 0069, 0073, 0080, 0081, 0082, 0090, 0102, 0105, 0107, 0112, 0114, 0134, 0153, 0166, 0177, 0214, 0226, 0228, 0237, 0238, 0239, 0242, 0244, 0246, 0254, 0261, 0264, 0265, 0269, 0274, 0276, 0277, 0278, 0280, 0281, 0282, 0284, 0292, 0304, 0312, 0327, 0341, 0366, 0371, 0456, 0460, 0467, 0515, 0518, 0519, 0524, 0525, 0526, 0527, 0530, 0532, 0533, 0537, 0539, 0540, 0541, 0542, 0543, 0585, 0586, 0587,

0588, 0591, 0592, 0593, 0594, 0595, 0596, 0597, 0601, 0602, 0604, 0609, 0611, 0637, 0652, 0671, 0677, 0679, 0680, 0681, 0682, 0686, 0688, 0690, 0691, 0692, 0693, 0694, 0695, 0696, 0699
Family Planning Supervisor, 0592, 0603
Family Planning Supervisor Training, 0603
Feldsher, 0034, 0116, 0436, 0471, 0480, 0495, 0583
Feldsher Job Description, 0471
Feldsher Training, 0480
Fertility, 0676, 0678, 0681, 0695
Field Study, 0333, 0610
Filariasis, 0243, 0431
Film, 0367
Financial Aspect, *See also: cost benefit analysis, economic aspect*, 0009, 0010, 0025, 0029, 0040, 0047, 0050, 0055, 0065, 0072, 0082, 0084, 0088, 0091, 0098, 0102, 0112, 0119, 0120, 0132, 0145, 0146, 0149, 0151, 0152, 0154, 0159, 0165, 0173, 0177, 0181, 0187, 0189, 0191, 0192, 0196, 0197, 0199, 0203, 0205, 0213, 0214, 0215, 0216, 0217, 0218, 0219, 0220, 0227, 0236, 0263, 0277, 0281, 0290, 0298, 0303, 0316, 0319, 0320, 0327, 0336, 0337, 0339, 0342, 0343, 0347, 0349, 0372, 0398, 0409, 0428, 0429, 0436, 0455, 0486, 0548, 0557, 0606, 0610, 0616, 0622, 0623, 0625, 0631, 0633, 0634, 0635, 0637, 0645, 0651, 0665, 0668, 0669, 0671, 0672, 0678, 0685, 0689
Flying Doctor Service, *See also: aircraft, mobile health unit, transport*, 0061, 0296, 0335, 0336, 0337, 0343, 0351, 0354, 0423, 0481, 0633
Folklore, *See also: history of medicine, tradition, traditional culture, traditional medicine*, 0223
Food, *See also: malnutrition, nutrition*, 0049, 0134, 0167, 0295, 0584
Food Aid, 0235, 0260, 0352

G

Government, 0173, 0273, 0409, 0422
Government Policy, *See also: health services planning, national planning*, 0021, 0033, 0035, 0040, 0057, 0065, 0074, 0090, 0114, 0115, 0118, 0119, 0134, 0149, 0162, 0186, 0204, 0213, 0250, 0254, 0255, 0282, 0312, 0358, 0376, 0518, 0580, 0606, 0609, 0610, 0617, 0629, 0632, 0639, 0640, 0650, 0666, 0667, 0671
Government Project, 0486
GPHCTC, 0650
Gynaecology, *See also: family planning, maternal child health, obstetrics*, 0527, 0587

H

Hadassah Medical Organization, 0088
Handbook, *See also: teaching aid, textbook, training manual*, 0580, 0594
Health Aid, *See also: development aid, food aid*, 0030, 0077, 0118, 0180, 0181, 0216, 0219, 0235, 0332, 0350, 0407, 0454, 0539, 0544, 0581, 0629, 0645
Health Centre, *See also: clinic, hospital, medical personnel, rural hospital, rural inpatient care, rural outpatient care*, 0006, 0029, 0032, 0033, 0035, 0041, 0043, 0044, 0047, 0049, 0055, 0059, 0060, 0061, 0065, 0068, 0071, 0072, 0074, 0075, 0077, 0078, 0079, 0080, 0081, 0083, 0084, 0088, 0089, 0093, 0097, 0098, 0099, 0101, 0104, 0105, 0106, 0107, 0110, 0111, 0112, 0114, 0117, 0119, 0124, 0127, 0128, 0133, 0138, 0139, 0140, 0142, 0144, 0145, 0146, 0148, 0153, 0157, 0158, 0160, 0168, 0169, 0175, 0179, 0189, 0196, 0198, 0199, 0202, 0208, 0211, 0216, 0223, 0229, 0233, 0237, 0244, 0248, 0250, 0255, 0258, 0260, 0264, 0266, 0269, 0281, 0282, 0284, 0285, 0286, 0288, 0290, 0291, 0292, 0293, 0294, 0295, 0296, 0297, 0298, 0299, 0301, 0302, 0303, 0304, 0305, 0306, 0307, 0308, 0309, 0310, 0311, 0313, 0314, 0315, 0316, 0317, 0318, 0319, 0320, 0321, 0322, 0323, 0324, 0325, 0326, 0327, 0328, 0329, 0330, 0331, 0332, 0333, 0334, 0340, 0344, 0350, 0356, 0357, 0360, 0364, 0365, 0366, 0371, 0374, 0376, 0381, 0386, 0388, 0392, 0401, 0404, 0407, 0413, 0415, 0422, 0423, 0424, 0428, 0433, 0438, 0441, 0443, 0445, 0448, 0449, 0450, 0455, 0460, 0466, 0474, 0475, 0476, 0478, 0481, 0485, 0486, 0487, 0489, 0490, 0509, 0522, 0523, 0528, 0537, 0540, 0551, 0566, 0572, 0579, 0580, 0583, 0594, 0595, 0607, 0609, 0610, 0616, 0618, 0619, 0620, 0623, 0625, 0629, 0635, 0637, 0642, 0643, 0648, 0650, 0651, 0653, 0658, 0668, 0671, 0677, 0681, 0682, 0686, 0690, 0696, 0698, 0699, 0700
Health Centre Administration, 0290, 0300, 0303, 0307, 0309, 0311, 0328, 0365, 0629, 0644, 0650
Health Centre Distribution, 0102, 0202, 0291, 0330, 0424, 0644, 0661, 0671
Health Centre Equipment, 0111, 0126, 0300, 0310, 0319, 0579, 0580, 0590, 0629, 0644
Health Centre Evaluation, *See also: evaluation, health services evaluation*, 0305, 0309, 0317, 0320, 0327, 0333, 0619, 0636, 0642, 0648, 0650
Health Centre Organization, 0090, 0303, 0311
Health Centre Planning, 0111, 0122, 0126, 0133, 0144, 0205, 0279, 0290, 0293, 0300, 0304, 0307, 0308, 0317, 0325, 0327, 0328, 0329, 0330, 0344, 0629, 0644, 0650
Health Centre Superintendent, 0427
Health Centre Utilization, 0057, 0279, 0293, 0300, 0330, 0374, 0579, 0639
Health Corps, Iran, 0228, 0302, 0312, 0609
Health Education, 0021, 0030, 0043, 0054, 0056, 0059, 0059, 0062, 0067, 0075, 0076, 0078, 0081, 0097, 0109, 0116, 0118, 0135, 0146, 0162, 0166, 0183, 0187, 0188, 0191, 0196, 0197, 0214, 0215, 0221, 0223, 0234, 0236, 0240, 0243, 0248, 0250, 0258, 0259, 0260, 0267, 0273, 0279, 0283, 0295, 0297, 0301, 0308, 0312, 0315, 0325, 0341, 0343, 0355, 0356, 0357, 0358, 0359, 0360, 0361, 0362, 0364, 0365, 0366, 0367, 0368, 0369, 0370, 0371, 0372, 0373, 0374, 0375, 0379, 0380, 0382, 0390, 0401, 0402, 0432, 0434, 0436, 0453, 0454, 0462, 0474, 0481, 0482, 0489, 0504, 0505, 0532, 0545, 0557, 0558, 0562, 0564, 0565, 0571, 0572, 0576, 0577, 0581, 0584, 0585, 0586, 0588, 0591, 0599, 0600, 0609, 0618, 0619, 0620, 0624, 0625, 0629, 0633, 0635, 0639, 0653, 0658, 0684, 0686, 0687, 0688, 0694
Health Education Evaluation, 0357, 0371, 0373, 0390, 0686

Low-Cost Rural Health Care and Health Manpower Training

Health Educator, 0453, 0477
Health Educator Training, 0453, 0477
Health Insurance, 0010, 0168, 0199, 0203, 0210, 0213, 0218, 0654
Health Manpower, 0008, 0010, 0013, 0016, 0019, 0021, 0022, 0025, 0026, 0030, 0042, 0044, 0045, 0046, 0050, 0051, 0052, 0054, 0068, 0079, 0085, 0103, 0106, 0108, 0111, 0112, 0130, 0132, 0160, 0177, 0184, 0212, 0233, 0244, 0250, 0262, 0263, 0301, 0302, 0354, 0375, 0377, 0379, 0380, 0390, 0397, 0402, 0411, 0417, 0418, 0427, 0452, 0462, 0477, 0487, 0491, 0492, 0506, 0511, 0517, 0528, 0531, 0540, 0543, 0566, 0599, 0615, 0622, 0625, 0633, 0650, 0654, 0658
Health Manpower Distribution, 0032, 0046, 0072, 0130, 0182, 0302, 0436, 0439, 0460, 0491
Health Manpower Evaluation, 0047, 0050, 0074, 0605, 0606, 0607, 0608, 0610, 0611, 0612, 0613
Health Manpower Planning, 0012, 0021, 0022, 0023, 0024, 0025, 0026, 0027, 0028, 0030, 0031, 0033, 0034, 0035, 0036, 0037, 0038, 0039, 0040, 0041, 0042, 0043, 0044, 0045, 0046, 0047, 0048, 0049, 0050, 0051, 0052, 0053, 0054, 0074, 0080, 0094, 0098, 0111, 0112, 0121, 0122, 0123, 0124, 0137, 0141, 0144, 0145, 0149, 0152, 0163, 0177, 0196, 0205, 0227, 0264, 0312, 0363, 0375, 0385, 0391, 0400, 0408, 0410, 0411, 0418, 0425, 0426, 0434, 0438, 0446, 0447, 0452, 0455, 0459, 0462, 0479, 0487, 0491, 0492, 0496, 0497, 0506, 0508, 0509, 0513, 0515, 0516, 0517, 0521, 0528, 0529, 0536, 0539, 0545, 0554, 0556, 0613, 0637, 0644, 0650, 0671
Health Manpower Training, 0008, 0009, 0013, 0016, 0023, 0026, 0028, 0029, 0031, 0059, 0074, 0086, 0118, 0123, 0160, 0168, 0188, 0236, 0244, 0257, 0302, 0307, 0344, 0380, 0393, 0397, 0398, 0411, 0414, 0417, 0423, 0425, 0426, 0433, 0439, 0447, 0455, 0459, 0460, 0465, 0476, 0478, 0479, 0482, 0489, 0494, 0498, 0500, 0501, 0530, 0536, 0550, 0552, 0554, 0555, 0577, 0613, 0615, 0616, 0622, 0635, 0637, 0645, 0649
Health Manpower Utilization, 0084, 0540
Health Manpower Wage Structure, 0122
Health Planning Course, 0411
Health Service, 0001, 0002, 0006, 0009, 0013, 0014, 0015, 0016, 0017, 0018, 0021, 0024, 0027, 0031, 0036, 0039, 0041, 0042, 0043, 0044, 0048, 0060, 0066, 0070, 0073, 0079, 0084, 0089, 0095, 0099, 0101, 0107, 0110, 0112, 0115, 0117, 0119, 0120, 0125, 0129, 0135, 0136, 0142, 0155, 0157, 0159, 0160, 0162, 0163, 0167, 0169, 0176, 0181, 0182, 0184, 0187, 0199, 0200, 0202, 0203, 0210, 0212, 0213, 0215, 0219, 0220, 0223, 0228, 0231, 0236, 0239, 0242, 0245, 0246, 0248, 0249, 0253, 0259, 0271, 0276, 0277, 0285, 0288, 0290, 0291, 0292, 0297, 0299, 0304, 0306, 0308, 0310, 0315, 0319, 0320, 0322, 0325, 0328, 0331, 0334, 0342, 0348, 0351, 0354, 0356, 0366, 0372, 0376, 0377, 0382, 0384, 0386, 0392, 0403, 0404, 0409, 0412, 0415, 0422, 0429, 0446, 0449, 0452, 0455, 0463, 0465, 0467, 0482, 0487, 0488, 0489, 0491, 0493, 0498, 0502, 0505, 0514, 0518, 0520, 0545, 0590, 0591, 0604, 0608, 0610, 0611, 0616, 0621, 0629, 0633, 0638, 0641, 0645, 0648, 0655, 0657, 0658, 0668, 0672, 0678, 0680, 0686, 0689, 0690, 0696
Health Services Administration, *See also: economic aspect, financial aspect*, 0026, 0033, 0042, 0055, 0057, 0064, 0069, 0071, 0074, 0075, 0076, 0077, 0080, 0082, 0083, 0086, 0089, 0092, 0094, 0096, 0097, 0098, 0101, 0102, 0103, 0104, 0105, 0110, 0112, 0114, 0115, 0118, 0119, 0146, 0158, 0174, 0180, 0189, 0192, 0213, 0214, 0217, 0228, 0230, 0239, 0259, 0261, 0263, 0265, 0266, 0298, 0329, 0356, 0375, 0468, 0489, 0567, 0617, 0619, 0627, 0628, 0629, 0630, 0632, 0640, 0644, 0649, 0650, 0651, 0652, 0664, 0675, 0687
Health Services Distribution, 0032, 0044, 0056, 0057, 0061, 0083, 0098, 0105, 0107, 0121, 0126, 0129, 0130, 0137, 0143, 0145, 0146, 0168, 0178, 0181, 0188, 0189, 0199, 0200, 0201, 0202, 0203, 0204, 0205, 0206, 0207, 0208, 0209, 0210, 0211, 0225, 0227, 0250, 0312, 0325, 0330, 0337, 0347, 0349, 0609, 0617, 0622, 0630, 0639, 0644, 0654, 0661, 0666, 0667, 0668, 0669, 0670
Health Services Evaluation, *See also: evaluation, health centre evaluation*, 0013, 0050, 0068, 0087, 0090, 0098, 0105, 0121, 0168, 0189, 0227, 0250, 0262, 0305, 0309, 0318, 0327, 0337, 0360, 0604, 0616, 0617, 0618, 0620, 0621, 0622, 0623, 0625, 0626, 0627, 0628, 0630, 0631, 0632, 0633, 0634, 0635, 0636, 0637, 0639, 0640, 0641, 0642, 0643, 0644, 0645, 0646, 0647, 0648, 0649, 0651, 0652, 0653, 0654, 0659, 0660, 0661, 0662, 0663, 0664, 0665, 0666, 0667, 0668, 0669, 0671, 0674, 0675, 0676, 0677, 0679, 0682, 0683, 0685, 0687, 0688, 0689, 0694, 0697, 0698, 0699
Health Services Implementation, 0314
Health Services Integration, 0112, 0114, 0153, 0189, 0239, 0279, 0291
Health Services Organization, *See also: economic aspect, financial aspect*, 0009, 0010, 0029, 0033, 0042, 0047, 0056, 0057, 0059, 0061, 0063, 0065, 0068, 0069, 0070, 0071, 0074, 0075, 0079, 0080, 0081, 0083, 0084, 0085, 0087, 0088, 0089, 0090, 0091, 0092, 0093, 0094, 0095, 0096, 0097, 0098, 0099, 0100, 0101, 0102, 0103, 0104, 0106, 0107, 0108, 0109, 0111, 0112, 0113, 0114, 0115, 0116, 0117, 0119, 0124, 0128, 0152, 0168, 0171, 0174, 0180, 0189, 0195, 0200, 0202, 0205, 0208, 0215, 0223, 0224, 0229, 0232, 0233, 0234, 0236, 0237, 0239, 0247, 0253, 0254, 0255, 0259, 0261, 0265, 0268, 0269, 0270, 0272, 0277, 0279, 0282, 0291, 0292, 0297, 0298, 0322, 0336, 0356, 0357, 0363, 0369, 0385, 0436, 0458, 0460, 0471, 0486, 0528, 0549, 0567, 0579, 0616, 0617, 0618, 0619, 0621, 0624, 0626, 0628, 0629, 0630, 0631, 0633, 0634, 0635, 0636, 0637, 0640, 0641, 0643, 0644, 0650, 0653, 0654, 0655, 0666, 0667, 0669, 0670, 0686, 0687
Health Services Planning, *See also: decision making, economic aspect, financial aspect*, 0012, 0013, 0021, 0025, 0030, 0034, 0045, 0047, 0049, 0057, 0059, 0060, 0066, 0068, 0072, 0082, 0086, 0087, 0095, 0097, 0098, 0102, 0106, 0109, 0112, 0118, 0120, 0121, 0122, 0123, 0124, 0125, 0126, 0127, 0129, 0130, 0131, 0132, 0133, 0134, 0135, 0137, 0138, 0139, 0140, 0141, 0142, 0143, 0144, 0145, 0146,

0147, 0148, 0149, 0150, 0151, 0152, 0153, 0154, 0155, 0156, 0157, 0158, 0159, 0160, 0161, 0162, 0163, 0164, 0165, 0166, 0167, 0168, 0169, 0170, 0171, 0172, 0173, 0174, 0175, 0176, 0177, 0178, 0179, 0180, 0181, 0182, 0183, 0184, 0185, 0186, 0187, 0188, 0189, 0190, 0191, 0192, 0193, 0194, 0195, 0196, 0197, 0198, 0200, 0202, 0204, 0205, 0213, 0216, 0217, 0218, 0220, 0221, 0225, 0226, 0227, 0229, 0233, 0235, 0237, 0238, 0239, 0240, 0241, 0242, 0243, 0245, 0246, 0247, 0248, 0250, 0253, 0254, 0257, 0258, 0262, 0265, 0268, 0271, 0272, 0275, 0276, 0278, 0279, 0280, 0282, 0292, 0293, 0301, 0304, 0325, 0328, 0336, 0342, 0347, 0348, 0356, 0357, 0359, 0360, 0368, 0373, 0380, 0384, 0411, 0423, 0433, 0445, 0447, 0454, 0458, 0463, 0494, 0507, 0509, 0550, 0565, 0566, 0568, 0583, 0587, 0588, 0610, 0616, 0623, 0624, 0625, 0634, 0635, 0640, 0659, 0660, 0661, 0662, 0663, 0664, 0665, 0666, 0667, 0671, 0676, 0679, 0686
Health Services Utilization, 0148, 0203, 0211, 0318, 0656, 0661, 0670, 0677, 0694
History of Medicine, *See also: folklore, medicinal plant, traditional medicine,* 0058, 0081, 0294, 0329, 0343, 0358, 0390, 0517, 0538
Hospital, *See also: clinic, health centre, health manpower training, medical personnel, mobile health unit, rural hospital, rural outpatient care,* 0006, 0010, 0032, 0033, 0039, 0041, 0049, 0050, 0051, 0055, 0065, 0071, 0080, 0085, 0090, 0098, 0101, 0104, 0105, 0113, 0115, 0117, 0119, 0127, 0135, 0142, 0146, 0159, 0165, 0174, 0179, 0184, 0186, 0196, 0207, 0209, 0211, 0283, 0284, 0289, 0294, 0298, 0299, 0303, 0313, 0314, 0316, 0319, 0324, 0325, 0330, 0339, 0341, 0343, 0357, 0364, 0376, 0390, 0394, 0406, 0422, 0428, 0448, 0450, 0472, 0473, 0475, 0485, 0486, 0499, 0572, 0573, 0616, 0618, 0623, 0625, 0628, 0634, 0635, 0636, 0641, 0644, 0651, 0656, 0671, 0686, 0688, 0689, 0691, 0700
Hospital Administrator, 0408
Hospital Administrator Training, 0408
Hospital Construction, 0168
Hospital Dispensary, 0623
Hospital Laboratory, 0549
Housing, 0134, 0632, 0685
Hygiene, 0009, 0010, 0067, 0258, 0357, 0358, 0370, 0375, 0394, 0563, 0587, 0673

I

Ibarapa Project, Nigeria, 0401
IBRD, 0637
Illiteracy, 0072, 0458
ILO, 0052
Immunization, *See also: vaccination,* 0076, 0124, 0259, 0292, 0356, 0365, 0558, 0572, 0587, 0594
Indian Medical Association, 0205
Industrial Worker, 0210, 0559
Infant Feeding, 0011, 0587, 0589
Infant Mortality, 0011, 0124, 0157, 0200, 0350, 0678, 0679
Infectious Disease, *See also: disease control,* 0049, 0062, 0065, 0097, 0167, 0175, 0202, 0241, 0258, 0352, 0360, 0370, 0439, 0449, 0489, 0697, 0698

Information Dissemination, 0116
Information Retrieval, 0136
Information Service, 0136
Information System, 0136, 0190, 0228
Internal Migration, 0063
International Cooperation, 0030, 0040, 0068, 0090, 0118, 0181, 0227, 0254, 0281, 0401, 0450, 0539, 0629, 0637, 0644, 0650, 0671, 0685
Intrauterine Device, 0543, 0585, 0591, 0593, 0599, 0600, 0601, 0686, 0694, 0696
IPPF, 0281
Iranian Army, 0609
IRHFP, 0082, 0284, 0453, 0454, 0477, 0542, 0595, 0596, 0597, 0598

J

Jamkhed Project, India, 0060, 0291, 0292, 0356, 0424
Job Description, 0021, 0026, 0050, 0052, 0303, 0333, 0408, 0427, 0432, 0462, 0467, 0475, 0497, 0504, 0532, 0559, 0560, 0570, 0580, 0585, 0587, 0588, 0590, 0592

K

Kitchen Equipment, 0174
Kniporos Project, Kenya, 0327, 0328, 0329
Kwashiorkor, 0105, 0235, 0262, 0549, 0571

L

Laboratory, 0085, 0485
Laboratory Auxiliary, *See also: medical technologist,* 0040, 0050, 0052, 0185, 0301, 0316, 0392, 0492, 0549, 0552, 0574
Laboratory Auxiliary Distribution, 0491
Laboratory Auxiliary Training, 0316, 0552, 0574
Lady Family Planning Visitor, 0537, 0602
Lady Health Visitor, 0541, 0596, 0686
Land Reform, 0115, 0167
League of Red Cross Societies, 0458
Legal Aspect, 0021, 0022, 0044, 0114, 0191, 0192, 0197, 0203, 0223, 0280, 0467, 0472, 0473, 0475, 0487, 0495, 0499, 0511, 0513, 0515, 0525, 0528, 0531, 0535, 0536, 0580, 0599, 0606, 0609, 0613
Leprosy, 0060, 0063, 0090, 0124, 0143, 0186, 0223, 0291, 0345, 0431
Leprosy Clinic, 0223
Life Expectancy, 0153
Living Conditions, *See also: social change,* 0178, 0230, 0263, 0358, 0361, 0374, 0618, 0632, 0639, 0673
Local Government, 0092, 0110, 0138, 0189, 0330, 0356, 0358, 0562, 0609, 0629
Local Level, 0083, 0180, 0187, 0189, 0196, 0291, 0357, 0368, 0561, 0563, 0580, 0592, 0598, 0658
London School of Tropical Med., 0401

M

Makerere University, 0358
Malaria, 0063, 0080, 0102, 0105, 0114, 0115, 0119, 0124, 0140, 0142, 0233, 0277, 0431, 0489, 0694
Malnutrition, *See also: kwashiorkor, nutrition,* 0048, 0049, 0063, 0097, 0105, 0106, 0115, 0135, 0167,

0178, 0202, 0234, 0235, 0241, 0256, 0258, 0259, 0332, 0350, 0352, 0360, 0361, 0489, 0571, 0590, 0674, 0698

Management, 0090, 0189, 0265, 0303, 0356, 0375, 0623, 0660

Mass Campaign, *See also: disease control, preventive medicine, sanitation,* 0100, 0147, 0255, 0675, 0687

Mass Communication, *See also: communication, mass media, radio communication,* 0193, 0214

Mass Media, *See also: communication, mass communication, radio communication,* 0116, 0358, 0367, 0368, 0586, 0588, 0633, 0694

Maternal Child Health, *See also: child, pediatrics, pregnancy, prenatal care,* 0016, 0020, 0032, 0056, 0060, 0076, 0080, 0097, 0105, 0106, 0112, 0119, 0124, 0135, 0145, 0153, 0157, 0164, 0206, 0214, 0227, 0232, 0234, 0237, 0238, 0239, 0244, 0250, 0251, 0253, 0258, 0259, 0260, 0261, 0264, 0266, 0269, 0274, 0277, 0279, 0280, 0282, 0292, 0304, 0313, 0315, 0325, 0332, 0352, 0356, 0357, 0370, 0388, 0489, 0508, 0515, 0517, 0518, 0520, 0523, 0524, 0525, 0527, 0528, 0529, 0532, 0534, 0535, 0539, 0558, 0565, 0567, 0569, 0570, 0572, 0585, 0587, 0589, 0592, 0594, 0599, 0607, 0618, 0620, 0625, 0629, 0635, 0645, 0651, 0652, 0677, 0678, 0679, 0682, 0686, 0689, 0690, 0698, 0700

Medex, *See also: auxiliary health worker,* 0034, 0436

Medic, *See also: auxiliary health worker,* 0487

Medical Assistant, *See also: auxiliary health worker,* 0039, 0040, 0225, 0330, 0428, 0450, 0459, 0464, 0486, 0495

Medical Assistant Job Description, 0428

Medical Assistant Supervision, 0428

Medical Assistant Training, 0039, 0428, 0450, 0459, 0464, 0486

Medical Assistant Utilization, 0428

Medical Institutions, Directory, 0006

Medical Personnel, *See also: auxiliary health worker, barefoot doctor, dentist, health manpower, nurse, physician, traditional practitioner,* 0014, 0024, 0031, 0078, 0093, 0101, 0102, 0116, 0119, 0132, 0142, 0148, 0150, 0173, 0175, 0182, 0184, 0191, 0197, 0211, 0236, 0242, 0261, 0280, 0282, 0286, 0299, 0308, 0309, 0312, 0320, 0333, 0342, 0376, 0377, 0382, 0386, 0409, 0417, 0433, 0439, 0445, 0456, 0467, 0485, 0489, 0496, 0518, 0519, 0543, 0589, 0606, 0610, 0612, 0623, 0634, 0656, 0671

Medical Personnel Training, 0024, 0078, 0142, 0260, 0382, 0392, 0409, 0422, 0496

Medical Records Maintenance, 0050, 0064, 0191, 0266, 0274, 0297, 0593

Medical Research Centre, Nairobi, 0090

Medical Technologist, *See also: laboratory auxiliary,* 0085, 0397, 0549, 0550, 0551

Medical Technologist Training, 0550

Medicinal Plant, *See also: history of medicine, traditional medicine,* 0224

Mental Health, 0045, 0564

Methodology, 0666, 0667

Midwife, *See also: dai, lady health visitor, nurse auxiliary,* 0020, 0022, 0035, 0050, 0052, 0054, 0060, 0077, 0081, 0086, 0115, 0126, 0246, 0264, 0269, 0310, 0316, 0319, 0323, 0368, 0407, 0454, 0456, 0491, 0492, 0499, 0509, 0515, 0516, 0517, 0518, 0520, 0522, 0523, 0525, 0526, 0528, 0529, 0530, 0531, 0532, 0534, 0535, 0536, 0538, 0539, 0580, 0587, 0589, 0596, 0603, 0609, 0611, 0613, 0629, 0649, 0689, 0692, 0700

Midwife Curriculum, 0499, 0523, 0603

Midwife Job Description, 0052, 0517, 0523, 0524, 0529, 0532, 0539, 0590, 0601

Midwife Training, 0020, 0026, 0054, 0246, 0264, 0316, 0417, 0441, 0491, 0499, 0509, 0510, 0515, 0516, 0517, 0518, 0520, 0521, 0522, 0523, 0524, 0525, 0526, 0527, 0528, 0529, 0531, 0532, 0533, 0534, 0535, 0536, 0538, 0539, 0565, 0590, 0601, 0603, 0609, 0682, 0686

Midwife Training Evaluation, 0539

Migration, *See also: demography, internal migration, population, rural migration,* 0130, 0142, 0449, 0676

Military, 0143, 0228, 0282, 0312, 0609

Minority Group, 0045, 0435

Missionary, 0105, 0224, 0313, 0316, 0324

Missionary Hospital, 0332

Mobile Eye Unit, 0062

Mobile Health Unit, *See also: aircraft, flying doctor service, transport,* 0049, 0055, 0060, 0061, 0062, 0071, 0099, 0100, 0119, 0127, 0146, 0173, 0228, 0242, 0280, 0282, 0289, 0292, 0297, 0312, 0319, 0330, 0335, 0337, 0338, 0339, 0340, 0341, 0342, 0343, 0344, 0345, 0346, 0347, 0348, 0349, 0350, 0352, 0353, 0354, 0355, 0423, 0481, 0620, 0671

Mobile Health Unit Administration, 0349

Mobile Health Unit Equipment, 0297, 0338, 0349

Mobile Health Unit Organization, 0349

Morbidity, 0051, 0072, 0097, 0124, 0129, 0134, 0146, 0153, 0157, 0164, 0165, 0177, 0262, 0291, 0370, 0388, 0589, 0632, 0635, 0641, 0661, 0678

Mortality, 0060, 0124, 0129, 0134, 0135, 0146, 0153, 0157, 0165, 0177, 0231, 0249, 0261, 0262, 0310, 0583, 0589, 0632, 0641, 0645, 0647, 0661, 0678, 0697

Multipurpose Auxiliary, 0100

Myun-Eup Worker, Korea R, 0585

N

Narangwal Rural Health Centre, 0690

National Health Plan, 0664

National Plan, 0532, 0609

National Planning, *See also: government policy,* 0021, 0022, 0029, 0030, 0033, 0044, 0057, 0058, 0074, 0118, 0122, 0123, 0124, 0126, 0129, 0141, 0144, 0145, 0149, 0153, 0164, 0187, 0189, 0217, 0218, 0220, 0227, 0347, 0358, 0418, 0506, 0568, 0616, 0617, 0625, 0644, 0650, 0661, 0666, 0667, 0671

Nomad, 0505

Nurse, *See also: community nurse,* 0021, 0022, 0030, 0034, 0038, 0044, 0050, 0052, 0054, 0060, 0086, 0088, 0089, 0097, 0269, 0283, 0294, 0297, 0310, 0316, 0323, 0332, 0333, 0335, 0341, 0346, 0352, 0368, 0374, 0390, 0424, 0432, 0456, 0463, 0464, 0467, 0474, 0481, 0491, 0492, 0499, 0500, 0501, 0502, 0503, 0504, 0505, 0506, 0507, 0513, 0515, 0528, 0530, 0532, 0548, 0561, 0569, 0570, 0580, 0593, 0594, 0599, 0608, 0613, 0629, 0650

Subject Index 161

Nurse Anaesthetist, 0427
Nurse Anaesthetist Job Description, 0427
Nurse Auxiliary, *See also: auxiliary health worker, midwife,* 0029, 0035, 0115, 0284, 0321, 0323, 0332, 0335, 0464, 0492, 0508, 0509, 0511, 0512, 0513, 0514, 0561, 0563, 0565, 0566, 0596
Nurse Auxiliary Job Description, 0514, 0565
Nurse Auxiliary Training, 0508, 0509, 0565, 0566, 0596
Nurse Curriculum, 0499, 0571, 0593
Nurse Distribution, 0021, 0022, 0044, 0506
Nurse Job Description, 0021, 0022, 0052, 0368, 0408, 0432, 0507, 0532, 0570, 0601
Nurse Training, 0021, 0022, 0026, 0030, 0038, 0044, 0046, 0054, 0076, 0264, 0316, 0335, 0397, 0417, 0427, 0441, 0464, 0467, 0481, 0499, 0500, 0501, 0502, 0503, 0504, 0505, 0506, 0510, 0521, 0528, 0532, 0533, 0570, 0571, 0594, 0601, 0686
Nurse Training Evaluation, 0506
Nurse Training Manual, 0570, 0571
Nurse Utilization, 0022, 0061, 0368
Nutrition, *See also: kwashiorkor, malnutrition,* 0007, 0009, 0011, 0016, 0080, 0090, 0160, 0174, 0180, 0183, 0196, 0214, 0227, 0234, 0241, 0244, 0251, 0260, 0262, 0267, 0270, 0271, 0295, 0350, 0352, 0357, 0360, 0365, 0394, 0434, 0568, 0569, 0570, 0571, 0572, 0577, 0587, 0591, 0671, 0674, 0684
Nutrition Education, 0240, 0270

O

Obstetrics, *See also: gynaecology, maternal child health, pregnancy,* 0124, 0508, 0558, 0589, 0677
Occupational Health, 0155, 0164, 0182, 0202, 0285, 0364, 0371, 0382, 0608
OECD, 0559
Onchocerciasis, *See also: eye disease,* 0152, 0431, 0637
Oral Contraceptive, *See also: contraception, intrauterine device,* 0282, 0519, 0533, 0601, 0692, 0693
Outpatient Clinic, *See also: rural outpatient care,* 0298, 0313, 0327, 0328, 0329, 0332
Outpatient Clinic Evaluation, 0327, 0328

P

PAHO *See also: WHO,* 0115, 0153, 0661
Pakistan Academy for Rural Devt., 0600
Paraplegic, 0287
Parasitic Disease, 0048, 0182, 0202, 0263, 0568, 0571
Pediatrics, *See also: child, maternal child health,* 0011, 0124, 0251, 0422, 0558, 0589
Periodical, 0003, 0004, 0005, 0007, 0008, 0016
Pest Control, 0252, 0571, 0584
Pharmaceutical, 0186, 0236, 0297, 0319, 0572, 0575, 0580, 0594, 0606, 0610, 0619, 0651
Pharmacy Auxiliary, 0450, 0495
Physician, 0003, 0014, 0033, 0034, 0039, 0041, 0042, 0043, 0044, 0049, 0050, 0051, 0054, 0077, 0087, 0088, 0095, 0099, 0106, 0137, 0142, 0146, 0163, 0169, 0185, 0186, 0196, 0201, 0211, 0219, 0225, 0236, 0269, 0283, 0309, 0310, 0313, 0335, 0339, 0376, 0377, 0381, 0384, 0389, 0390, 0392, 0396, 0399, 0400, 0403, 0404, 0406, 0410, 0412, 0415, 0421, 0438, 0444, 0456, 0465, 0467, 0471, 0487, 0491, 0492, 0494, 0532, 0536, 0537, 0580, 0593, 0594, 0609, 0641, 0645, 0654
Physician Assistant, *See also: auxiliary health worker,* 0363
Physician Curriculum, 0046, 0385
Physician Distribution, 0044, 0060, 0061, 0065, 0072, 0202, 0205, 0225, 0313, 0330, 0378
Physician Education, *See also: admission requirements, curriculum, university,* 0003, 0022, 0026, 0027, 0028, 0031, 0033, 0034, 0036, 0039, 0041, 0044, 0046, 0054, 0090, 0094, 0095, 0137, 0141, 0162, 0181, 0202, 0225, 0300, 0309, 0310, 0330, 0335, 0349, 0376, 0377, 0378, 0379, 0380, 0381, 0383, 0384, 0385, 0386, 0387, 0388, 0390, 0391, 0393, 0394, 0395, 0396, 0397, 0398, 0399, 0400, 0401, 0402, 0403, 0404, 0405, 0406, 0407, 0409, 0410, 0412, 0413, 0414, 0415, 0416, 0417, 0418, 0419, 0420, 0421, 0455, 0467, 0482, 0485, 0492, 0496, 0530, 0532, 0533, 0541, 0607, 0618, 0620
Physician Evaluation, 0046, 0379, 0401, 0402
Physician Job Description, 0050, 0052, 0377, 0389, 0408, 0580
Physician Supervision, 0631
Physician Utilization, 0487, 0511, 0663
Pilot Project, 0041, 0082, 0088, 0205, 0227, 0277, 0290, 0309, 0323, 0327, 0328, 0329, 0361, 0371, 0379, 0401, 0486, 0487, 0500, 0519, 0594, 0658, 0685, 0686
Pilot Project Evaluation, 0309
Plague, 0263, 0637
Population, *See also: demography, family planning, migration, rural population,* 0129, 0146, 0530, 0616, 0676
Population Control, 0175, 0533, 0678
Population Increase, 0025, 0063, 0072, 0075, 0129, 0134, 0135, 0142, 0145, 0153, 0164, 0166, 0177, 0178, 0180, 0202, 0212, 0228, 0239, 0249, 0261, 0272, 0276, 0291, 0382, 0447, 0526, 0634, 0647, 0680
Poverty, 0105, 0119, 0148, 0167, 0178, 0202, 0223, 0258, 0262, 0449, 0489, 0626
Pregnancy, 0313, 0508, 0524, 0558, 0589
Prenatal Care, *See also: maternal child health,* 0589
Preventive Medicine, *See also: health education, health services administration, mass campaign, sanitation,* 0005, 0009, 0010, 0021, 0031, 0043, 0046, 0049, 0051, 0055, 0058, 0061, 0062, 0065, 0076, 0088, 0093, 0101, 0105, 0106, 0114, 0117, 0130, 0132, 0138, 0143, 0151, 0153, 0157, 0167, 0168, 0173, 0177, 0182, 0183, 0186, 0187, 0191, 0193, 0199, 0206, 0209, 0211, 0214, 0225, 0230, 0234, 0236, 0243, 0244, 0248, 0249, 0250, 0255, 0262, 0272, 0274, 0281, 0283, 0289, 0290, 0297, 0298, 0299, 0306, 0308, 0310, 0312, 0315, 0319, 0320, 0325, 0333, 0339, 0353, 0355, 0356, 0357, 0358, 0361, 0364, 0366, 0368, 0370, 0371, 0375, 0377, 0381, 0382, 0386, 0387, 0388, 0392, 0395, 0399, 0406, 0407, 0418, 0419, 0420, 0421, 0433, 0449, 0452, 0460, 0482, 0486, 0497, 0504, 0508, 0522, 0524, 0529, 0531, 0534, 0544, 0545, 0547, 0558, 0563,

0569, 0570, 0571, 0583, 0587, 0609, 0622, 0625, 0635, 0639, 0644, 0645, 0648, 0650, 0653, 0654, 0660, 0666, 0667, 0680, 0694, 0697

Q

Quality Standard, 0121, 0668
Questionnaire, 0492, 0541, 0611, 0612, 0673, 0699

R

Rabies, 0564
Radio Communication, 0055, 0335, 0337, 0343, 0367, 0368, 0481
Ramathibodi Hospital, 0385
Regional Planning, 0029, 0035, 0128, 0129, 0204, 0212, 0567, 0666, 0667, 0670
Rehabilitation, 0287, 0685
Reproduction, 0515, 0525
Research, 0023, 0024, 0050, 0058, 0074, 0082, 0088, 0090, 0095, 0104, 0132, 0138, 0149, 0151, 0181, 0184, 0190, 0191, 0196, 0206, 0214, 0222, 0231, 0245, 0256, 0257, 0258, 0267, 0271, 0273, 0281, 0287, 0309, 0314, 0317, 0327, 0328, 0329, 0333, 0376, 0377, 0379, 0382, 0390, 0407, 0454, 0492, 0541, 0542, 0597, 0604, 0607, 0610, 0613, 0620, 0626, 0628, 0629, 0634, 0638, 0649, 0655, 0656, 0658, 0659, 0662, 0671, 0673, 0676, 0680, 0683, 0690, 0691, 0694, 0697, 0700
Research Centre, 0257, 0386
Research Methodology, 0050, 0053, 0268, 0314, 0320, 0333, 0576, 0621, 0628, 0642, 0646, 0652, 0656, 0658, 0661, 0663, 0665, 0666, 0667, 0670, 0673, 0694
Research Project, 0666, 0667
Royal Society of Trop. Med., London, 0181
Royal Tropical Institute, Amsterdam, 0090
Rural Aid Centre, Ifakara, 0450
Rural Development, 0214, 0465
Rural Hospital, *See also: clinic, health centre, hospital, rural outpatient care*, 0128, 0285, 0287, 0549
Rural Inpatient Care, 0284, 0299, 0319
Rural Migration, 0063, 0178
Rural Outpatient Care, *See also: hospital, mobile health unit, outpatient clinic, rural hospital*, 0048, 0226, 0284, 0289, 0290, 0295, 0299, 0301, 0306, 0314, 0321, 0322, 0324, 0325, 0330, 0353, 0365
Rural Planning, 0129, 0558
Rural Population, *See also: population*, 0055, 0084, 0233, 0449, 0633, 0654, 0682

S

Sanitary Control, 0115, 0135, 0142, 0177, 0182, 0196, 0236, 0248, 0394, 0489, 0554, 0555, 0657, 0658
Sanitary Engineer, 0492
Sanitary Engineer Training, 0555
Sanitary Inspector, 0464, 0580
Sanitary Inspector Job Description, 0580
Sanitary Inspector Training, 0464
Sanitation, *See also: environment, mass campaign, pest control, waste disposal*, 0005, 0029, 0178, 0188, 0193, 0243, 0312, 0563, 0568, 0587

Sanitation Auxiliary, 0052, 0054, 0301, 0492, 0532, 0553, 0556, 0580, 0629, 0650
Sanitation Auxiliary Training, 0054, 0553, 0556, 0564, 0571, 0584
Sanitation Manpower, 0056, 0323, 0556
Sanitation Service, 0584, 0632, 0643, 0666, 0667
Schistosomiasis, 0152, 0361, 0431, 0643
School, 0232, 0247, 0248, 0280, 0504, 0535, 0662
School Health, 0090, 0357, 0364, 0368, 0674
SIDA, 0674
Skin Disease, 0370
Slum, 0258, 0321
Smallpox, 0114, 0263, 0671
Social and Cultural Anthropology, 0221, 0222, 0673
Social Change, *See also: living conditions*, 0562, 0588, 0643
Social Development, *See also: economic development*, 0026, 0150, 0194, 0195, 0372
Social Participation, *See also: community*, 0045, 0056, 0057, 0063, 0067, 0083, 0091, 0115, 0123, 0126, 0172, 0205, 0248, 0290, 0291, 0298, 0321, 0330, 0356, 0363, 0368, 0369, 0371, 0389, 0404, 0413, 0435, 0461, 0462, 0463, 0476, 0482, 0486, 0583, 0618, 0639
Social Planning, 0230, 0358
Social Problem, 0045, 0048, 0115, 0167, 0177, 0290, 0372
Social Security, 0203, 0210
Social Service, 0177, 0371
Social Stratification, 0694
Social Structure, 0569
Social Theory, 0225, 0358, 0368, 0371
Social Welfare, 0215, 0258, 0360, 0685
Social Worker, 0148
Socialism, 0618
Socioeconomic Aspect, 0001, 0002, 0065, 0130, 0134, 0149, 0223, 0225, 0279, 0364, 0371, 0377, 0632, 0653, 0666, 0667, 0694
Sociology, 0009, 0024, 0090, 0115, 0172, 0206, 0267, 0328, 0394, 0406, 0545, 0604, 0606, 0659
Statistical Analysis, 0046, 0068, 0122, 0177, 0217, 0628, 0673
Statistical Data, 0032, 0047, 0051, 0054, 0068, 0074, 0076, 0101, 0115, 0122, 0129, 0161, 0169, 0171, 0176, 0177, 0178, 0179, 0190, 0191, 0197, 0200, 0203, 0207, 0208, 0211, 0228, 0231, 0238, 0249, 0261, 0302, 0314, 0317, 0319, 0371, 0374, 0390, 0397, 0419, 0456, 0506, 0509, 0543, 0605, 0609, 0611, 0612, 0616, 0622, 0623, 0625, 0626, 0632, 0634, 0635, 0636, 0641, 0642, 0645, 0646, 0650, 0656, 0660, 0661, 0662, 0666, 0667, 0669, 0671, 0673, 0677, 0678, 0680, 0681, 0685, 0690, 0691, 0695, 0697
Surgery, 0077, 0085, 0111, 0137, 0348, 0349, 0400, 0418, 0573
Survey, 0161, 0193, 0195, 0314, 0381, 0612, 0647, 0653, 0669

T

Teacher, 0186, 0194, 0248, 0378, 0393, 0438
Teacher Training, 0393, 0420

Subject Index

163

Teaching, 0378, 0383, 0384, 0386, 0421
Teaching Aid, *See also: handbook, textbook, training manual,* 0367, 0368, 0458, 0557, 0570, 0573, 0574, 0575, 0576, 0578, 0580, 0585, 0586, 0588, 0591, 0595, 0596, 0599, 0600, 0603, 0686
Teaching Method, 0387, 0393, 0419, 0438, 0457, 0469, 0552, 0572
Tema Aluminum Smelter, Ghana, 0501
Textbook, *See also: handbook, teaching aid, training manual,* 0558, 0565, 0568
Trachoma, *See also: cataract, eye disease, onchocerciasis,* 0297, 0340, 0346, 0675, 0687
Tradition, 0115, 0167, 0223, 0224, 0225, 0291, 0375, 0426, 0583, 0673
Traditional Birth Attendant, 0246, 0515, 0516, 0525, 0528, 0531, 0534, 0535, 0538, 0689
Traditional Culture, 0224, 0225, 0673
Traditional Medicine, *See also: history of medicine, medicinal plant,* 0109, 0224, 0225, 0250, 0606, 0610, 0697
Traditional Practitioner, *See also: auxiliary health worker, traditional birth attendant, traditional medicine,* 0035, 0127, 0224, 0292, 0356, 0375, 0456, 0539, 0604, 0610
Training Centre, 0030, 0034, 0052, 0089, 0093, 0101, 0194, 0284, 0316, 0323, 0335, 0417, 0450, 0472, 0473, 0486, 0487, 0489, 0491, 0499, 0512, 0514, 0517, 0523, 0531, 0532, 0537, 0538, 0550, 0596, 0629, 0685
Training Course, 0160, 0393, 0453, 0469, 0477, 0481, 0494, 0512, 0519, 0535, 0552
Training Evaluation, 0021, 0022, 0026, 0052, 0227, 0427, 0458, 0462, 0481, 0506, 0551, 0559, 0571, 0614, 0629
Training Manual, *See also: handbook, teaching aid, textbook,* 0020, 0160, 0557, 0558, 0560, 0562, 0563, 0564, 0565, 0566, 0567, 0568, 0569, 0571, 0572, 0573, 0575, 0577, 0579, 0580, 0581, 0583, 0584, 0587, 0588, 0590, 0594, 0599, 0600, 0601
Training Method, 0160, 0494, 0508
Transport, *See also: aircraft, flying doctor service, mobile health unit,* 0055, 0061, 0105, 0288, 0339, 0347
Trichinosis, 0564
Tropical Disease, 0004, 0005, 0263, 0571, 0590
Tropical Zone, 0399, 0584
Trypanosomiasis, 0152, 0431
Tuberculosis, 0022, 0060, 0063, 0080, 0102, 0114, 0143, 0202, 0229, 0230, 0255, 0345, 0364, 0431, 0557, 0564, 0643, 0683
Typhoid, 0089, 0263

U

Uchawi, 0224
UCLA, 0281
UN, 0129
Under-Fives' Clinic, 0060, 0126, 0279, 0292, 0311, 0327
UNICEF, 0030, 0084, 0281, 0288, 0539, 0671
Universidad Austral de Chile, 0550
University, *See also: curriculum, education, physician education, research,* 0034, 0039, 0095, 0142, 0153, 0162, 0169, 0176, 0181, 0185, 0206, 0281, 0290, 0309, 0333, 0376, 0377, 0378, 0383, 0384, 0386, 0392, 0394, 0395, 0396, 0399, 0406, 0415, 0417, 0418, 0421, 0485, 0530, 0544, 0550, 0650
University of Chile, 0204
University of Ibadan, 0401
University of Lagos, 0401
University of Saigon, 0544
University of Sao Paulo, 0664
Urban Area, 0072, 0079, 0098, 0102, 0114, 0127, 0199, 0201, 0202, 0203, 0211, 0249, 0325, 0330, 0330, 0377, 0384, 0471, 0592, 0654, 0671, 0687
Urban Population, 0210, 0211
Urbanization, 0129
US Indian Health Service, 0121, 0435, 0452, 0487
USAID, 0030, 0227, 0254, 0281, 0539

V

Vaccination, *See also: immunization,* 0236, 0248, 0256, 0292, 0568, 0571, 0606, 0694
Vasectomy, 0521, 0694
Venereal Disease, 0332, 0564
Village, 0035, 0055, 0067, 0097, 0105, 0119, 0187, 0202, 0260, 0289, 0290, 0298, 0310, 0318, 0330, 0333, 0349, 0350, 0355, 0366, 0372, 0386, 0392, 0413, 0424, 0485, 0517, 0606, 0612, 0652, 0654, 0680, 0697
Village Leader, 0598
Village Leader Training, 0598
Voluntary Organization, 0030, 0056, 0205, 0304, 0358

W

Waganga Healers, 0224
Wage, 0538
Waste Disposal, *See also: environment, sanitation,* 0084, 0115, 0193, 0243, 0298, 0563, 0569, 0571, 0584
Water, 0009, 0673
Water Pollution, 0193
Water Resources, 0193
Water Supply, 0084, 0157, 0187, 0298, 0312, 0486, 0632
Water Treatment, 0089, 0115, 0135, 0143, 0157, 0177, 0187, 0192, 0193, 0236, 0563, 0571, 0584, 0694
Wellcome Trust, London, 0181
WHO, *See also: PAHO,* 0038, 0051, 0052, 0054, 0061, 0078, 0084, 0112, 0113, 0114, 0118, 0153, 0163, 0176, 0187, 0189, 0190, 0192, 0193, 0194, 0195, 0212, 0280, 0281, 0325, 0398, 0411, 0417, 0418, 0420, 0446, 0464, 0491, 0492, 0494, 0506, 0510, 0527, 0534, 0637, 0649, 0655, 0657, 0658, 0671
Women, 0679

X

X-Ray Technician, 0050

Y

Yaws, 0431
Yellow Fever, 0431

Credits

Cover design: Opague Design, Ottawa
Editor: Marilyn Campbell
Photographs: Ministry of Health, Malawi, page 2
Barry Donath, pages 6, 142
Health and Welfare Canada, page 10
Graham Johnson, page 16

I have been unable to obtain a copy of the following work through my local library or bookshop. I request the help of the IDRC in procuring this material. Address coupon to: **Rural Health Care Bibliography, c/o Library, IDRC, Box 8500, Ottawa, Canada K1G 3H9.** *(Please type or print)*

VOLUME NUMBER _____

ITEM NUMBER _____ PAGE _____

AUTHOR/EDITOR _____

TITLE _____

NAME & TITLE: _____

ORGANIZATION: _____

ADDRESS: _____

_____

_____

I have been unable to obtain a copy of the following work through my local library or bookshop. I request the help of the IDRC in procuring this material. Address coupon to: **Rural Health Care Bibliography, c/o Library, IDRC, Box 8500, Ottawa, Canada K1G 3H9.** *(Please type or print)*

VOLUME NUMBER _____

ITEM NUMBER _____ PAGE _____

AUTHOR/EDITOR _____

TITLE _____

NAME & TITLE: _____

ORGANIZATION: _____

ADDRESS: _____

_____

_____

I have been unable to obtain a copy of the following work through my local library or bookshop. I request the help of the IDRC in procuring this material. Address coupon to: **Rural Health Care Bibliography, c/o Library, IDRC, Box 8500, Ottawa, Canada K1G 3H9.** *(Please type or print)*

VOLUME NUMBER _____

ITEM NUMBER _____ PAGE _____

AUTHOR/EDITOR _____

TITLE _____

NAME & TITLE: _____

ORGANIZATION: _____

ADDRESS: _____

_____

_____